THE
INDEPENDENT MEDICAL
TRANSCRIPTIONIST

Fourth Edition

Donna Avila-Weil
and
Mary Glaccum

Rayve Productions

Cover vistas: (top to bottom) Hawaii, South Carolina, Montana

Rayve Productions Inc.
Box 726 Windsor CA 95492

Senior Editor: Barbara F. Ray

First printing, 1991
Second printing, 1992
Third printing, revised, 1994
Fourth printing, 1996
Fifth printing, 1996
Sixth printing, revised, 1998
Seventh printing, 1998
Eighth printing, 1999
Ninth printing, revised, 2002

Printed in the United States of America

Library of Congress Cataloging-in-Publication Data
Avila-Weil, Donna
   The independent medical transcriptionist / Donna Avila-Weil and Mary Glaccum. -- 4th ed.
      p. cm.
   Includes bibliographical references and index.
   ISBN 1-877810-52-5 (alk. paper)

   1. Medical transcription. I. Glaccum, Mary. II. Title.
   R728.8.A98   2002
   653'.18--dc21   2002017802
                                                                              CIP

The authors and publisher have attempted to ensure accuracy and completeness of information in this book. Any errors, inaccuracies, omissions, inconsistencies or slights against people or organizations are unintentional.

To our blessed country, the United States of America,
for giving us her loving support in our yearning
for true independence.

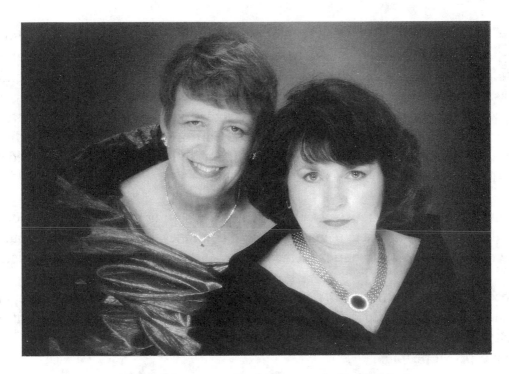

Mary Glaccum and Donna Avila-Weil

Donna Avila-Weil

Donna Avila Weil, RHIT, has been a transcriptionist since 1968. She received her ART credential in 1977, her CMT credential in the early 1980s, and has worked as an independent for 23 years. Donna was a founding member of the Central Valley Medical Transcribers Association, from which the American Association for Medical Transcription was born, and has served as a delegate of the California Association for Medical Transcription (CAMT) and as CAMT President. In 1991 Donna was honored as CAMT Member-of-the-Year.

Donna has worked extensively in the acute care setting and as an independent medical transcriptionist and consultant, and continues to do so. She is a popular keynote speaker, workshop presenter, and mentor to novice transcriptionists.

Recently, Donna fulfilled a lifelong dream to live in the tropics. With the support of her family and friends, she moved to the Big Island of Hawaii, a life transition that has given her opportunities to enjoy new professional networks and meet some special people.

Mary
Glaccum

Mary Glaccum has been a medical transcriptionist for 31 years. She received her CMT credential in 1981, and was an active member of the American Association for Medical Transcription (AAMT) from 1981-93, and the California Association for Medical Transcription (CAMT), serving as a delegate and chairing many committees. Mary founded the Central Coast Chapter of AAMT, serving as President from 1981-82, and as Newsletter Editor and Scholarship Committee Chair.

Mary taught medical terminology and transcription at Allan Hancock College in Santa Maria, California, for five years, and she worked in a variety of transcription settings before embarking on her career as a self-employed medical transcriptionist 15 years ago. Mary owns and operates The Dictation Station in the greater Los Angeles, California, area.

Mary has an 11-year-old adopted son, Robert, and enjoys being a PTA, roller hockey, Boy Scout, karate mom. Her spare-time passions are "countryfying" her home and transforming salvaged items into decorative art pieces such as the charming bird baths she creates from old clay pots.

Acknowledgments
Donna Avila-Weil

I want to thank all of the medical transcriptionists who have continued to support the profession over the years and who volunteer their time to mentor new professionals coming into the field. Positive influence and support is key to nurturing those who will follow in our footsteps.

Thanks to those who have taken the time to share their experiences through articles, books, and websites so that others can benefit from their knowledge and expertise.

I am especially indebted to two very special people and successful independent MTs here in Hawaii, Mary Whalen, a wonderful IMT in Kealakekua, Hawaii, who offered me sound advice regarding the local client base, shared equipment, and provided names of MTs and services I could contact for information about MT work; and Amy Geisser, an IMT on the island of Oahu, and newsletter editor for Hawaii Association for Medical Transcription (HAMT) for putting me to work!

I thank my family and friends for having faith in me, for supporting me, and tolerating my yearning to move on, and I thank God for watching over me and catching me when I stumble.

Last but not least, I thank Mary and Robert Glaccum, my lifelong friends, with whom I have shared so much joy . . . and some sadness. Our adventures just get better and better!

Acknowledgments
Mary Glaccum

To the old workhorses like me, who have been in business for themselves for many years, and to the new entrepreneurs in the field of medical transcription, thank you for sharing your successes as well as your missteps toward independence. Each and every one of you have shown great determination and ingenuity, and you continue to be a great inspiration to me.

To my family, thanks for reminding me to not take this thing called "life" too seriously and for believing in me these many years.

To my dear friend of 34 years and the lady who helped me believe I could be an MT, Grace Bach. Thank you for showing me the meaning of true grit and courage, Gradie Sue.

To my son, Robert, for your patience in giving up weekend trips to the skateboard park so I could sit in front of my computer working on this book, and for showing me the true meaning of love.

Last but not least, to Donna Avila-Weil, my coauthor. How many laptops do you think we can count on the beach?

"Trifles make perfection and perfection is no trifle."
—Michelangelo

Contents

Introduction

It has been just three years since the third edition of the *Independent Medical Transcriptionist* was published, but in that short time technology in our industry has advanced more than in the entire past decade. As a result of these remarkable advances, and increased opportunities in the global marketplace, there is a great deal of new information to share with those considering careers in medical transcription, and, more specifically, for those pursuing careers as independent medical transcriptionists.

Even though an abundance of generalized material about working independently has been published, it has left many specific questions unanswered and not satisfied the needs of those seeking more comprehensive information. These astute individuals, who see the rapid changes that continue to transpire in the medical transcription industry and the increasing emphasis on the home office as an alternative workplace, require an even more comprehensive book addressing these issues.

We are happy to report that independent medical transcription is alive and well! Your authors, Mary and Donna, have continued to promote working independently, and in our travels throughout the country have had the pleasure of networking with many people. These experiences have aided our research and work on this edition and reinforced our commitment to helping meet the need for this comprehensive and up-to-date resource for working independently as a medical transcriptionist.

Although our personal lives have evolved, we both continue to work as independent medical transcriptionists. As it was when we wrote the first edition of this book, our experiences are based on two perspectives: "Country Mouse" (Donna Avila-Weil) and "City Mouse" (Mary Glaccum). Donna has recently followed her dream and relocated to Hawaii, where she is experiencing firsthand the trials and tribulations of re-establishing herself as an independent medical transcriptionist in a new environment and market. These experiences have become very helpful in updating this latest IMT book. Mary still lives and works in the Greater Los Angeles area.

During our many years as medical transcriptionists — sometimes employed by others, sometimes independently employed — we have experienced diverse and exciting careers. Professionally, we have also taught, lectured, conducted seminars, served as mentors, written articles, developed our own IMT newsletter, and advised hundreds regarding details of self-employment and the how-to's of establishing a medical transcription business.

Through years of trial and error, we planned, studied, and endured numerous frustrations as we traveled the circuitous road to independent transcription success. No straighter road was available at the time. Few resource materials existed. Until this book there were few, if any, comprehensive sources to educate or refer to if questions or difficulties arose.

On the following pages we share with you our knowledge of the medical transcription field and the requirements, benefits, pitfalls, and methods of becoming an independent transcriptionist. The facts, figures, and vignettes are provided as guidelines for those interested in pursuing careers as medical transcriptionists and independent medical transcriptionists.

We have enjoyed assisting intelligent and talented transcriptionists as they pursued successful careers. We wish you the greatest success, too.

What Is Medical Transcription?

"The future belongs to those who believe
in the beauty of their dreams. "

— Eleanor Roosevelt

Medical Transcription

The translation of sound into organized,
well-expressed written statements that
communicate medical meaning.

Medical transcription has existed since the dawn of civilization and the beginning of experimentation. Rudimentary medical record keeping in the form of drawings was scratched onto prehistoric cave walls, evolving to clay tablet records, hieroglyphics, papyrus, parchment, and finally paper.

In mid-fifth century B.C. Greece, during the time of Hippocrates, who is often referred to as "The Father of Medicine," physicians' notes established new heights in rational, empirical medical reporting. They served not only as a written record of current medical actions, but also provided reference information for future patient care. Comparisons, conclusions and research were developed from medical record reviews, and medical information was shared to nurture medical education.

Over the centuries, medical records have become increasingly important. With expanding medical specialization, new developments in technology, and government and health care regulations, accurate documentation is critical. The medical record has expanded voluminously to meet these demands.

Until the twentieth century, physicians were both providers of medical service and scribes for medical communities. In the 1900s, medical stenographers began to take dictation in shorthand directly from physicians. Soon, a succession of voice recording machines evolved. The invention of magnetic tape storage in the form of cassette tapes launched medical stenographers into medical transcription careers.

Today, medical transcription is a vital link in the health care industry, a highly respected profession, and one of the most fascinating and rewarding of allied health careers. We have moved from handwriting to dictation, from shorthand to typewriting and transcription, and now, in the 21st century, we are moving into interactive data capture and template-based systems, speech recognition dictation, and interactive direct input.

From the shorthand and steno pad to interactive technology, medical transcription has grown into an international multi-billion dollar industry. The technology industry continues to create products and services to increase the profitability of medical transcription, provide easy access to documentation of patient encounters, and allow immediate access to medical documents which improves patient care. Speech recognition technology continues to improve as it is integrated into language processing systems and Internet technologies.

THE HEALTH CARE INDUSTRY

Health care is one of the most technologically diversified industries of this decade. The expanding scope and specialization of health care has created a growing demand for processing, coordinating, and communicating accurate documentation of clinical information. Now more than ever, timely, reliable, accessible, accurate health care information is needed to facilitate quality patient care, and this need has increased the demand for experienced, well-qualified medical transcriptionists.

The upkeep of the medical record has been called the "invisible profession." As the upcoming decade advances toward the "paperless record," the increasing challenge will be how to maintain quality, accuracy, and information integrity in the patient record.

In yesteryear's health care setting, when medical procedures were less sophisticated, state and federal regulations minimal, and malpractice lawsuits practically unheard of, physicians routinely documented patient progress in longhand. Today, however, our health care system is complex and handwritten reports are no longer appropriate.

INFORMATION MANAGEMENT (IM)

In the current environment, health care is focused on caring for "populations," not individual patients. To meet the information requirements needed for this paradigm shift, the effective and efficient delivery of patient care requires organized information management (IM). Health care organizations require organized systems information management to avoid scattered data bases (e.g. duplication of data gathering, inconsistent reports and inefficiencies in the use of economic resources).

The following are generally accepted objectives of health care information management.

1. Identify the information needs of the organization in providing patient care services.

2. Evaluate the existing data for accuracy, availability, accessibility, security, necessity, and performance.

3. Develop action plans to enhance and improve organizational performance in patient care, governance, management and support processes to meet the goals of the organization.

4. Improve turnaround time of results.

5. Reduce unnecessary duplication of data entries.

6. Provide timely access to information throughout the organization.

7. Provide patient-centered information systems and technology.

8. Provide for the collection, generation and analysis of data.

All of the above apply to the transcribed medical documentation provided through services inside or outside of the organization.

THE IMPORTANCE OF TRANSCRIBED REPORTS IN HEALTH CARE TODAY

Documentation is an integral and necessary part of health care with content and format influenced by legislation, compensation mechanisms, and liability exposure. As a result, today's health care records must be accurate, detailed, legible, and easily duplicated.

All health care providers face increasing demands to provide quality patient care as quickly as possible, documented by ever-more-thorough records. To meet these demands, reliance is placed on skilled physicians and other medical team members, state-of-the-art technology, and well-trained transcriptionists for accurate recording of patient care and treatment.

Transcriptionists are medical language specialists. The reports they produce are indispensable to modern health care because handwritten reports — especially quickly written reports that may contain illegible phrases or errors — not only waste time, but also present serious potential problems in quality assurance, risk management, professional recertification and licensing, and third party reimbursement.

Dictated reports are generally more thorough than handwritten reports. When dictating reports to be transcribed, physicians tend to record more detail about exams, conversations with the patient, medical decisions, advice dispensed, and laboratory and pharmacy information. In addition, it is easy for doctors to send copies of transcribed reports to associates, which improves patient care and reduces physician correspondence.

Transcribed reports are less likely to be misinterpreted by clinicians, referring physicians, attorneys, and others who make decisions based on information in the medical record. As a result, the health care provider experiences fewer interruptions of his or her work, spends less time in review and response, and faces fewer requests to appear in court to interpret handwritten reports.

The litigation crisis that has developed in recent years compels doctors and health care administrators to focus on accurate, comprehensive patient records. These superior medical records — in conjunction with other quality control measures — improve patient care, reduce risk exposure, lower insurance costs, and bring greater peace of mind to patients and health care providers.

THE MEDICAL RECORD AND QUALITY ASSURANCE

The quality of patient care is directly related to the quality of the medical record. Whether in an acute-care facility, convalescent hospital, physician group practice, or other medical setting, the many caregivers who attend the individual patient refer to, and depend on, accurate medical records to provide quality continuity in patient care.

Although doctors, nurses, and other members of the hands-on-health care team bear the primary responsibility for immediate, handwritten patient-care documentation, the medical transcriptionist also plays an important role as transcribed reports become a legal part of the medical record.

Medical records provide the means by which standards of care are evaluated. The quality and accuracy of the information in the health care record is continuously examined, and physicians are legally required to attest to the accuracy of the recorded diagnoses and procedures in patients' records.

At the administrative level, health care facilities depend on accurate medical records to meet ethical and legal standards of patient care and to provide accurate documentation of patient-care history for future reference during accreditation or medical/legal situations.

The medical record documents the facts of a patient's illness, symptoms, diagnosis, and treatment. This includes the daily care and treatment of that patient. Health care facilities, in accordance with accepted professional standards and practices, are required to maintain a medical record for each patient These records must be complete, accurate, current, readily accessible and systematically organized. Where patient care is concerned, the medical record is the principal means of communication between health care professionals. The medical record is an important patient-care planning tool which accomplishes the following:

1. Records the course of the patient's treatment and changes in the patient's condition.

2. Documents communications between the practitioner responsible for the patient and any other health professional who contributes to the patient's care.

3. Assists in protecting the legal interests of the patient, the organization and the practitioner.

4. Provides a data base for use in statistical reporting, continuing education and research.

5. Provides information necessary for third-party billing and regulatory agencies.

ILLEGIBLE ENTRIES — WHY TRANSCRIBED DOCUMENTATION IS IMPORTANT

Handwriting has long been a major problem in interpreting the events surrounding the care of patients, but illegible handwriting can no longer be tolerated in the modern health care environment. The American Medical Association (AMA) urges physicians to print, type or computerize prescriptions. A Harvard study found that " . . . penmanship was among the causes of 220 prescription errors out of 30,000 cases."

Today it is essential that medical record entries be legible, clear, and meaningful to each patient's course of treatment. Illegible medical records may have adverse effects on the performance of other health professionals who read the record and act on what they read. Illegible records may also make it difficult or impossible for caregivers or facilities to defend themselves.

Licensure rules and regulations contained in state statutes generally describe requirements and standards for the maintenance, handling, signing, filing and retention of medical records.

The failure of a medical facility or physician to maintain a complete and accurate medical record may affect the ability of that facility or physician to obtain third-party reimbursement (e.g., from Medicare, Medicaid, or Blue Cross). Under federal and state laws, the medical record must accurately reflect the treatment for which the facility or physician seeks payment. Third-party payers rely on timely and accurately dictated and transcribed documents in the record for determining reimbursement. Thus, the medical record is important to health care facilities and physicians for medical, legal and financial reasons.

It is important to remember that just as though it were set in stone, the medical record is a document that cannot be erased once a recording has been made.

LEGAL PROCEEDINGS AND THE MEDICAL RECORD

The importance of complete, accurate, and timely medical records as an evidentiary tool in legal proceedings cannot be overemphasized. The integrity and completeness of the medical record is extremely important in reconstructing the events surrounding any alleged negligence in the care of the patient.

Medical records aid police investigations in providing information for determining the cause of injury or death, and the extent of injury in workers' compensation or personal injury proceedings.

When health professionals are called as witnesses in legal proceedings, they are permitted to refresh their recollections of the facts and circumstances of particular cases by referring to the medical records. Under such circumstances, a complete, accurate and timely medical record is vitally important for accurate testimony. Furthermore, if medical records are proved to be inaccurate or incomplete or made long after the event they purport to record, they may be used as damaging evidence against health care facilities and medical caregivers.

CONFIDENTIALITY OF THE PATIENT RECORD

All health care professionals who have access to medical records have a clear legal, ethical, and moral obligation to protect the confidentiality of the information in the records. The communications between a physician and his or her patient and the information generated during the course of the patient's illness are generally accorded the protection of confidentiality. Thus, the information in the medical record must be dealt with in a confidential manner; otherwise, a medical facility or organization could incur liability.

WHAT IS HIPAA?

Although the Health Insurance Portability and Accountability Act (HIPAA) was introduced in 1996, we are just beginning to understand the impact it will have on the health care profession. Everyone agrees that privacy of health information

(PHI) is an important issue in our society. Many people feel they have lost control over their personal information and the way it is used, including their medical records, which contain sensitive information about their physical and mental health, behaviors and relationships. Intrusions into privacy can result in loss of trust, with an unwillingness to confide in health care professionals. Unauthorized disclosures of intimate information can cause embarrassment, stigma and discrimination.

HIPAA is a multifaceted piece of legislation covering three areas, including the following:

- Insurance portability — implemented
- Fraud enforcement (accountability) — implemented
- Administrative simplification — implementation pending

Our focus here is on the third component of this legislation, administrative simplification, which focuses primarily on three areas: 1) standardization of electronic formats for certain transactions, 2) ensuring the privacy of certain patient information, and 3) ensuring the security of electronic health information and electronic signatures. The final rules were implemented in 2001 and the health care industry will have two years to implement the requirements set forth by the regulations. Because much of our work is done via telecommuting, access to electronic information systems must be governed by protocols to ensure secure and confidential transactions. Policies and procedures that ensure privacy and security during operations will govern all access to patient information.

As MTs, we must comply with HIPAA rules so our internal procedures ensure that only authorized personnel will be able to gain access to private health information. In other words, your policy should address workstation access and log-in procedures. If you have hospitals as clients, you can request a copy of their information security policy and/or related policies to utilize as a guide to establish a policy for your own MT business.

Computerization facilitates acquiring, manipulating and disseminating vast amounts of information. This data is used for numerous health-related purposes, including clinical care, quality assurance, utilization review, reimbursement, research and public health. The HIPAA act of 1996 recently issued a final rule providing systematic nationwide health information privacy protection. The rule is extensive in its scope. It applies to personally identifiable information in any form, whether communicated electronically, on paper or orally. The rule affords patients rights to education about privacy safeguards, access to their medical records, and a process for correction of records. It also requires the patient's permission for disclosure of personal information. April 14, 2001 was set as the "effective date" for the rule, beginning a phase-in period requiring full compliance by April 14, 2004. The rule provides the first systematic nationwide privacy protection for health information. Violations to the rule can result in civil and criminal penalties up to a $250,000 fine and 10 years in prison.

The rule reaches virtually all those who use medical and financial information in the health care system, creating a national standard of privacy protection. The rule applies to health plans as well as health care clearinghouses which process information (e.g. transcription, coding and billing services), also known as business associates. HIPAA does not directly authorize the Department of Health and Human Services to regulate the use and redisclosure of health information by the business associates of health care providers, such as contractors mentioned above; however, the rule imposes a duty on entities to obtain assurances that business associates will comply with the privacy standards. In other words, to ensure that you protect patient privacy, your clients can request proof of your policies showing your compliance with the privacy standards.

THE FUTURE OF HEALTH INFORMATION PRIVACY

The intense political debate sparked by health information privacy continues in the U.S. Congress and involves two strong perspectives: 1) Privacy advocates seek patient autonomy over personal information, including access to medical information and control over use and disclosure; 2) The health care industry seeks less burdensome and costly procedures and freedom to use information for treatment, payment, research and other health-related purposes.

It is very likely that there will be modifications to the HIPAA rule to permit compliance but its significance is historical, because it is the first adopted national health information privacy standard in the United States.

NEW TECHNOLOGY DEMANDED

The importance and value of the medical record will be even greater in the future. With increasing numbers of individuals receiving medical care, and as patient information systems continue to merge with patient financial systems, the information demands of users of medical record information will increase. As a result, increasingly sophisticated technology must be continually developed to meet these demands.

According to the U.S. Department of Labor, by the year 2008, the need for technicians skilled in database and information technology may increase by as much as 102%. In this rapidly emerging and ever changing industry, medical transcriptionists will continue to play a vital role.

THE COMPUTERIZED PATIENT RECORD (CPR)

Although the health care industry lagged behind most other fields in becoming initially computerized, today's health professionals depend on computers. They are found in the admitting office, business office, operating room, nursing unit, pharmacy, laboratory, medical imaging, satellite unit and medical records departments.

Computers are efficient, offer great flexibility and have unlimited capacity to store data. They are definitely here to stay! The medical record is no longer a conglomeration of handwritten entries but includes fetal monitoring strips, electrocardiogram strips, electroencephalogram strips, electronic output from the laboratory, pharmacy and radiology services, nursing documentation, medication administration, etc.

The computerized patient record has been introduced in an effort to improve productivity and quality of patient information, and to provide the economic benefit of reducing costs. In addition, the CPR can support clinical research, be interactive, and facilitate computer-assisted diagnosis.

The CPR is used in telecommunications around the world on a real-time basis to transport picture graphics between nations. For instance, radiographic images that may have been taken in a hospital in Saudi Arabia at 3 a.m. can be reviewed on a real-time basis in the United States.

Critical lab values can immediately be communicated electronically. Via software, a physician can be notified when he or she has ordered medications; about risks, benefits, complications; and when to renew orders. Transcribed medical documents are an integral part of the CPR.

There are some disadvantages to the CPR. Although computers are a necessity in modern health care, they are not infallible. Several problems have been identified including lack of technical knowledge and support to integrate systems; loss of confidentiality and unauthorized disclosure of information, which have necessitated the development of sophisticated security systems; equipment unreliability; and concerns regarding the accuracy and reliability of data input by computer operators.

Another major problem slowing down health care's leap forward into the CPR age is the lack of system responsiveness. For peak efficiency, a system must respond quickly to any request for information. Some do not.

Often, computer communication and response time is negatively impacted by the operator's lack of ability to use the hardware effectively. Many health care organizations attempting to undergo computerization have underestimated the size and design of the system required to integrate effectively. Not only is the selection of adequate hardware and software needs essential, but the technical training required to operate these systems and keep them up and running has been a huge problem. It is wonderful to have technology at your fingertips, but if you don't know how to use it, what good is it?

HIPAA COMPLIANCE — THE BUSINESS ASSOCIATE AGREEMENT

As health care providers, including hospitals, clinics and physician practices, prepare to come into compliance with new HIPAA privacy and security laws, medical transcriptionists who provide transcription services working from home or in an office setting may be required to sign a *business associate agreement*, which is a contractual arrangement designed to safeguard protected health information against potential privacy and security risks. This agreement may address 1) who has access to protected health information, 2) e-mail communication, 3) computer access codes, 4) training and competency on privacy and security standards (annually or more often), 5) availability of contractor by phone and/or e-mail during working hours, and 6) availability for on-site inspection. An example of this business associate agreement is included in the appendix of this book.

Is Independent Medical Transcription the Profession for You?

"I do not know anyone who has got to the top
without hard work. That is the recipe.
It will not always get you to the top
but should get you pretty near."

—Margaret Thatcher

You are intrigued with the idea of self-employment and have decided to investigate freelancing. We look forward to helping you reach your goal.

In this book we focus on the medical transcription profession, but the general information we provide, and the methods we recommend, may also be utilized as research and marketing tools for other personal service specialties.

THE ENTREPRENEURIAL PERSONALITY

According to the Small Business Administration, research indicates that successful small business entrepreneurs have a number of characteristics in common. The following questions will help you evaluate your personality and entrepreneurial potential. How do you measure up?

_____ I have a strong desire to be my own boss.

_____ Win, lose, or draw, I want to be master of my own financial destiny.

_____ I have significant specialized business ability based on both my education and my experience.

_____ I have an ability to conceptualize the whole of a business; not just its individual parts, but how they relate to each other.

_____ I develop an inherent sense of what is "right" for a business and have the courage to pursue it.

_____ One or both of my parents were entrepreneurs; calculated risk-taking runs in my family.

_____ My life is characterized by a willingness and capacity to persevere.

_____ I possess a high level of energy, sustainable over long periods, to make my business successful.

While not every successful home-based business owner starts with a "yes" answer to all of these questions, three or four "nos" and "undecideds" should be sufficient reason for you to stop and think twice before going it alone.

EXPERIENCE

Do you have the necessary tools to be a successful independent transcriptionist? Independents are generally paid by production — by the line, page or character count. If you are highly productive, capable of transcribing accurately and quickly, your earnings might be excellent. On the other hand, if you are a low volume producer, you should carefully consider whether self-employment is the right career move for you.

How much medical transcription work experience do you have? If you have been employed specifically for medical offices, clinics, or other specialties and feel you are well qualified, it is probably best to concentrate your independent transcription work within your field of expertise.

RURAL VERSUS CITY TRANSCRIPTION

Some transcriptionists are more comfortable in a rural setting; others prefer the city. In more rural locales, your clients will probably be close to your home. You will become familiar with physicians in your area, their styles of dictating, and their idiosyncrasies, especially if you work for small clinics or one doctor's office. On the other hand, if you work in a large metropolitan area, the chances that you will be transcribing for doctors located near your home are slim, and you will probably experience a greater variety of dictation.

In either setting, you also have the option to market your services to clients outside your geographical area through telecommuting.

DIALECT DIFFICULTIES

Dialects present great difficulty for many transcriptionists. Some find dialects totally impossible, and even transcriptionists with an ear for languages generally find dialects challenging. This writer still shudders from the vivid memory of hearing her first "ezofeygous" for "esophagus" and wondering if she was ever going to make it through the day.

Hospitals and medical offices frequently send dictation they do not wish to deal with to outside services (e.g., self-employed transcriptionists). This dictation usually includes a variety of different dialects. On average, if your account is a large facility, many dictating doctors will be foreign-born. If you do not have an ear and an aptitude for dialects, you may find it difficult or impossible to service these accounts.

HOSPITAL VERSUS MEDICAL OFFICE TRANSCRIPTION

There is a great difference between hospital transcription and doctors' office transcription. In general, doctors' office transcription is more focused on patient histories and physical examinations, chart notes, and referral letters to other health care professionals. In contrast, hospital transcription covers many specialties, extensive procedures, operative reports, radiology, pathology, and numerous other subspecialties.

Hospital work can be an exciting and rewarding market, but do not assume you will succeed with hospital transcription if you have had no hospital transcription experience. Only an experienced hospital transcriptionist, or certified medical transcriptionist, should attempt hospital accounts.

If you have not been trained and do not have experience in hospital specialties, it would be a disastrous mistake for you to accept hospital accounts under the assumption you could transcribe the dictation adequately. Gain hospital transcription experience first, gradually increasing your knowledge of each specialty. We have seen many people attempt self-employment only to fail because they did not have adequate training and experience. Wise transcriptionists learn as much as possible and allow additional time for the seasoning of experience.

OPPORTUNITIES FOR THE
VISUALLY IMPAIRED TRANSCRIPTIONIST

Many MTs remember what office practices were like before the personal computer. The messy carbon paper, chunky typewriters clogged with eraser debris, and that awful "white out." People who are blind probably do not remember all that, because it was difficult, if not impossible, for anyone but a sighted person to use that equipment! Technology has opened many doors for people who are blind or visually impaired the last ten years or so. With personal computers and assistive technologies such as voice synthesizers, large screen displays, refreshable Braille, and scanners, office occupations are accessible in a practical manner.

There are visually impaired transcriptionists working in the health care field. There are courses available that provide them the skills to transcribe medical reports from tape to print in a hospital or health facility. Also, these skills can be used in a self-employment situation. A course can include training in the use of Microsoft Word in the word processing sequence. The length of the medical transcription course can vary from institution to institution but a good curriculum involves the study of medical terminology, anatomy and physiology, drug terms, and preparation of various medical reports. Textbooks and dictionaries are used, plus tapes, which are dictated by actual physicians. The individual is provided with an extensive word and phrase base in 15 medical specialties. One such program is available through Littlerock World Services for the Blind. For more information on their program and how to enroll at LWSB contact them at the numbers listed below.

- **Littlerock World Services for the Blind**
  P. O. Box 4055
  Little Rock, AR 72214
  501-664-7100
  www.lwsb.org

SPEECH SYNTHESIS TECHNOLOGY

For the visually impaired medical transcriptionist's home transcription system, a speech synthesizer is utilized, dedicated text-to-speech and software to make the synthesizer operate. This enables the MT to hear what she is typing. For example, a program called Jaws for Windows reads everything on the screen from text in a document to drop-down menus and key choices using a process that is exactly the opposite of speech recognition. Instead of converting speech to text, "Jaws" converts text to speech and plays it back to the listener. Adapting to this type of transcription equipment can require a great deal of patience. The technology does allow access to the Internet, which will give the visually impaired transcriptionist an excellent opportunity to network with peers, learn more about the profession and broaden horizons.

There are a number of technologies on the market by vendors that manufacture speech synthesizer programs and large print programs. The more popular ones now are JAWS for voice and ZoomText for large print. You can learn more about this technology and other information regarding resources for blind and visually impaired individuals by contacting resources beginning on page 420 of this book.

OPPORTUNITIES FOR COURT REPORTERS IN MEDICAL TRANSCRIPTION

Medical transcription has become a growing and challenging career in the labor market and has become an attractive career alternative for court reporters and "scopists." Combining course work in medical transcription with stenographic machine theory and speed building, a transcriptionist can prepare for a rewarding and flexible career.

The average court reporter spends three or more years in training. They learn keystroke, response to the spoken word, and grammar; and they work hard to develop the dramatically high speeds required to be successful court reporters. For many, even though they may have studied intensely and practiced rigorously, the incredibly rapid speed is not attained and, therefore, the court reporting goal is not reached. Generally, however, the speed they have attained is adequate for medical transcription.

Speed is not enough, however, to be a successful medical transcriptionist. In fact, court reporters who move into medical transcription have to accept and implement different transcription parameters that are not based on speed if they are to be successful.

While SPEED of production is paramount in court reporting, QUALITY of the finished product is the focus of medical transcription.

Court reporters are trained to respond to the spoken word, to keystroke the spoken word instantaneously, verbatim, without stopping. At the time they are transcribing, they pay little attention to details like punctuation and spelling. This is done at a later time (away from the actual recording setting) by the reporter or by a "scopist."

The scopist, who is knowledgeable in legal terminology and proceedings, proofs and corrects the court reporter's computer generated transcription, often relying on dictation to aid in the proofing. The scopist will scan the document and correct punctuation, but the *verbatim* dictation remains the same. Working as a scopist is an excellent background for someone wanting to become a legal or medical transcriptionist.

Medical transcriptionists must pay close attention to detail as they are transcribing, and they do not necessarily transcribe verbatim. They edit as they progress through their reports, which must be grammatically correct, with format and content completely accurate. Medical transcriptionists use a tape and transcribing machine to do their transcription, allowing them to stop, back up and listen again to what the dictator is saying. They may reformat material, spending additional time on details of sentence composition, adding or deleting unnecessary punctuation.

Court reporters who do not already have a medical transcription background will face considerable training if they are to make a successful transition into medical transcription. They will need solid skills in grammar, medical terminology, and anatomy/physiology, and they may need training or retraining on medical transcription technology and transcription practice using tapes of actual physician dictation.

COURT REPORTING TECHNOLOGY FOR MEDICAL TRANSCRIPTION

Some court reporting programs offering stenographic computer-aided medical transcription courses support the theory that a computerized machine shorthand writer, writing accurately at 140 words per minute, will perform medical transcription of medical reports much faster than standard keyboarding by a medical transcriptionist. Computer-assisted transcription "CAT" has turned the stenotype machine into a microcomputer. When a given key press or set of key presses is in the reporter's computerized database (dictionary) a match results and the key presses are transcribed with minimal effort in the transcription process (similar to the macro or shorthand programs that MTs are familiar with). However, the transcript produced by CAT should only be thought of as a first draft. Words that are not included in the dictionary won't automatically transcribe. This is where the "scoping" or editing of the document will take place.

The equipment court reporters utilize costs approximately three times as much (sometimes $10,000 and up) as the equipment required for medical transcription (approximately $3000). Can court reporters use their technology to do medical transcription? Yes. There are court reporters who successfully generate court documents and medical transcription using their court reporting technology.

Some court reporting equipment, such as the *RAPIDTEXT®* steno captioner, has been successfully adapted for use in medical transcription. This stenographic equipment is very effective. RAPIDTEXT entry uses a steno machine to input data or information into a computer at speeds of 120-200 or more words per minute. Although the concept of using this technology for general industry use is fairly new, the court reporting industry has successfully applied a similar technology to produce "legal documents" for the past decade. RAPIDTEXT utilizes the same theory of writing steno, but has the added instant display of translated English and word processing functions and capabilities available with the steno keyboard. For more information, contact RAPIDTEXT.

- **RAPIDTEXT**
  949-399-9200

Other educational products are available, as well as an entire home study program. For information, contact the following company:

- **Health Professions Institute (HPI)** — Training
  P.O. Box 801
  Modesto, CA 95353
  209-551-2112

Establishing an Independent Medical Transcription Business

"Whatever your goal in life, be proud of every day
that you are able to work in that direction."

— Chris Evert

The key word here is "business." You need to plan for, and take action regarding, all aspects of organizing and running a business. That means developing your marketing strategy, your business operations strategy, and your financial strategy. You need to set goals and put systems in place to achieve those goals. And you must make a personal commitment to work hard to make it all happen.

According to the Robert Half firm, 47% of those who voluntarily leave their jobs (some of which become self-employed) do so because they believe their jobs offer limited opportunity for advancement; 26% leave because they feel they suffered a lack of recognition; and the remainder leave for other causes, including dissatisfaction with their salaries and benefit packages.

Our motivation for working at home is the pleasure of independence and flexibility. Your motivation may be something different — a desire for greater income, career growth, prestige, recognition in the business world. Whatever, you must be motivated to succeed in order to withstand the monumental challenges that occur in business management.

THE INDEPENDENT TRANSCRIPTIONIST'S WORKSITE

We live in a highly mobile, competitive, ambitious society in which enterprising entrepreneurs often seek rewarding self-employment when it is a feasible alternative to traditional workplace jobs. In the medical transcription profession, there are various worksite alternatives, and working at home has been a viable option for many years.

The number of home-based workers is on the rise. In the past five years, fewer than 50% of the 5.6 million displaced workers have found full-time replacement jobs. But more than 440,000 of those 5.6 million have gone into business for themselves. Over the last decade in some areas of the country, the number of home-based independents grew by 122%, in contrast to the number of all other workers which increased by only about 22%. In 2001 there were more than 30 million people telecommuting from home, and forecasters predict that this number will increase by 28% by 2004.

ADVANTAGES OF SELF-EMPLOYMENT

The home-based career has definite advantages. It offers freedom, flexibility, and best of all, professional respect and unlimited opportunity for success and fulfillment. The independent medical transcriptionist establishes personal goals, sets a schedule that meets lifestyle needs, and manages daily activities. In short, she or he is in control.

As an independent, duties are performed with little or no supervision, and decisions are made without a great deal of red tape or waiting indefinitely for someone higher on the management chain-of-command to approve a task that could have been accomplished immediately.

The independent transcriptionist determines the work schedule, work pace, and work hours — day or night.

Office colors and styles are personal favorites. Business equipment and furniture are rearranged whenever and however desired.

The program of work is designed to allow time for other interests — creative projects, professional and community organizations, classes, sports, friends, and family.

Each day's schedule determines work attire — casual, classic, sporty — and bare feet are acceptable on the home-front. The independent is free to wear bold perfume, bright jewelry, listen to classical, country or rock music, snuggle a pet, laugh out loud, whistle, sing, talk to friends or family on the phone, and generally enjoy life with no fear of disturbing co-workers or being scolded for wasting company time.

The independent medical transcriptionist does not have to pay for expensive day care for children, arise before dawn and arrive home after dark, fight daily commute traffic, scramble for parking spaces, tolerate an uncomfortable office setting, endure office politics, withstand autocratic supervision, avoid low-producing co-workers or suffer through intolerable working hours!

If "home-based" sounds good to you, as it does to so many, consider the following important factors.

THE MULTI-TALENTED TRANSCRIPTIONIST

Becoming self-employed requires many talents beyond those that propelled you into business in the first place. First and foremost, you must be seriously committed to your career as an independent. In addition, advanced planning and preparation will be essential if you are to succeed.

Evaluate your professional knowledge and skills proficiency. Rate yourself as objectively and as honestly as possible, and don't be tempted to rationalize about areas where knowledge is lacking or skills are weak. If you are not certain you are completely prepared to accomplish the goals you have outlined, take additional classes to improve your skills and increase your confidence.

DOING YOUR HOMEWORK BEFORE
GOING INTO BUSINESS

Don't reinvent the wheel . . . or medical transcription. Learning basic information, ways to be more efficient, and how to avoid professional pitfalls from someone who has already been there will save you time, money, and prevent headaches.

Do your homework before attempting to establish a business. Gather as much information as you can from a variety of sources, including your competition.

However, be cautious when opinions are offered. Good advice can be invaluable, but beware of naysayers with negative attitudes, who may never have taken a risk or were stymied by adverse experiences. Learn to differentiate fact from fantasy. Sit down and make a list of the benefits and drawbacks of being self-employed. Then make your own educated decisions.

JOINING PROFESSIONAL ORGANIZATIONS

Join local medical transcription organizations and participate in professional activities that will inform and inspire you. Networking with transcriptionists offers you important professional exposure, visibility, and encouragement. In addition, you will maintain a competitive edge as current professional information is shared, and you will enjoy opportunities for state and national networking as your career progresses.

Consider joining other professional organizations, too. Your local chamber of commerce, word processing and secretarial groups, home-based workers groups, and other business-oriented groups offer excellent opportunities for personal and career development, interaction with a variety of professionals, and community involvement. You will discover that extra hours invested in organizational meetings and community participation can yield exciting rewards.

There is an association for most every group, cause, idea or occupation now in existence. They all have membership lists and a good many of them publish newsletters. Investigate the various associations in your area and consider joining some of them. This is where you'll meet your community's "movers and shakers," learn valuable business tips from individuals and newsletters, and you may even pick up some referrals.

Professional organizations also hold conventions, and if you think conventions are designed just to meet annual organizational requirements and take care of board of directors' business, think again. The main reason conventions are held is to provide optimum opportunity for the dissemination of information and for interaction with other professionals. In one or two hours at a convention, you can make more GOOD CONTACTS than in two weeks of cold-calling.

Every major city has a convention bureau because convention business represents a sizable share of a city's revenue. Find out who's holding what and where, or get convention resource information from the convention bureau. To attend a convention, you will generally only have to pay a registration fee. For this, you will receive a program, sometimes a list of attendees, and you will have access to numerous vendors, products, workshop presentations, and professionals in your field.

BUSINESS ALLIANCES

National Association for the Self-Employed (NASE) — If you are in business for yourself, there are many associations and organization that would be of benefit to you in your day-to-day working environment. One of the most well-known is the National Association for the Self-Employed (NASE).

Not only is this organization very active in promoting legislation that will help and empower the self-employed, it also offers many benefits such as health insurance, discounts on business services, products and travel, and business legal advice. NASE also publishes a bimonthly newsletter that reports details of recent legislation affecting our businesses, new products and available services as well as asking for reader feedback. The thing we like most about this organization is that its leaders welcome feedback from members — suggestions and new ideas — and encourage members to be proactive in their personal and professional lives. Having a strong membership base, NASE is able to greatly influence positive changes for the self-employed. For more information, contact NASE.

- **National Association for the Self-Employed (NASE)**
  800-232-NASE
  www.nase.org

Women Incorporated (WIC) — Women Incorporated is located in Sacramento, California. WIC welcomes all self-employed entrepreneurs, including men. During the past few years, Women Incorporated has been instrumental in forming alliances with the Money Store Investment Company and the Small Business Administration to procure start-up financing for new businesses as well as financing to expand member businesses. Before WIC was organized, it was difficult for women business owners to get financial backing, but with WIC's help, that has changed throughout the country. WIC also offers group rates for health insurance, discounts, and a quarterly magazine. In addition, Women

Incorporated sponsors the annual National Conference for Women in Business. For more data, contact WIC.

- **Women Incorporated (WIC)**
  800-930-3993
  www.womeninc.com

BUSINESS PUBLICATIONS FOR INDEPENDENTS

Numerous publications, far too many to list here, are helpful to the self-employed. We recommend that you do an Internet search, where you'll quickly find abundant printed resources, many of which are published specifically for the medical transcription industry.

Being home-based and disconnected from the outside world for the most part, it is very important that we become involved with business groups that will not only enhance the way we run our businesses, but also will fight for the changes necessary to compete successfully.

WHEN IN DOUBT, CONFER WITH AN EXPERT

Don't hesitate to consult experts for help in areas where your knowledge and experience are limited. Smart entrepreneurs seek guidance and support, and build a stronger business by including accountants, bankers, attorneys and other skilled professionals in their management team. Access to the Internet has also opened up many opportunities to network with these professionals through e-mail, chat rooms, newsgroups, webpages, etc.

TELEPHONE QUERIES FROM NOVICES

There is great misunderstanding about the medical transcription field and what is required to be a competent transcriptionist. Many believe that anyone who can type and knows a few medical terms can transcribe medical reports. However, medical transcription is a language skill and not a typing/keyboarding skill.

Individuals interested in becoming home-based transcriptionists often contact us. Unfortunately, many of these people do not have the education and skills necessary to succeed. Some have had experience as medical office receptionists, insurance billers, or hospital admission clerks. One physician's wife explained that although she lacked some technical training, she did know how to type and her husband was willing to help her decipher the medical terms.

During our years as transcriptionists, we have encountered people who dreamed of rewarding medical transcription careers but entered the field ill-equipped for the job. It was a painful experience for them and their employers or clients. Many of these transcriptionist hopefuls had never seen a transcribing machine and didn't know how to use a headset. Others couldn't use a foot pedal, preferring instead to stop and start the tape by hand.

Some had poor grammar skills and were unable to spell correctly or punctuate sentences. Many did not understand the necessity of, and were not interested in, taking courses in medical terminology, anatomy, and physiology to develop transcription competence.

To be a skilled medical transcriptionist, one should know something about the basic elements of language because medical terminology is a mix of Latin and Greek word parts, roots, prefixes, suffixes, English, and a smattering of miscellaneous other foreign terms. A working knowledge of biology, human anatomy and physiology is also necessary to understand dictation. And excellent grammar, spelling, and punctuation are essential for creating a document that is correct, professional looking and interpretable to others.

Word processing skills are important, too. Gone are the days when transcriptionists used manual typewriters and got by typing 60 wpm. Today, the minimum acceptable typing speed for medical transcription work is over 80 wpm, and well-trained MTs efficiently use computers, a variety of software programs, and other technological devices that give them a competitive edge. For the new medical transcriptionist, technical training is a necessity, usually in the form of vocational or technical college, medical transcription programs, or an accredited medical transcription home-study program.

Most of us "old-timers" learned transcribing via "OJT" (on-the-job training). Unfortunately, that option is rarely open to new transcriptionists today. Hospitals, clinics, and physicians, faced with budget cutbacks, limited staff, and pressures to produce transcribed records as quickly as possible, seldom hire trainees. However, a few still take on inexperienced transcriptionists so consider contacting prospective employers in your area.

BREAKING INTO THE FIELD THE RIGHT WAY

There are several paths to medical transcription success. Many colleges offer courses in medical transcription and terminology, and there are also home study programs available, which are discussed in this book. Find the path that's right for you, make a commitment to excellence, and a bright future awaits. Network with other transcriptionists, develop your communication skills, and become more confident and assertive in the workplace, and you will soon reap professional benefits.

Increasingly, formally educated individuals are coming into the medical transcription field as crossovers from other career fields like finance, education, marketing, communication and other health care professions, to name a few. For financial and economic reasons, or even just to change careers, they are seeking self-employment as medical transcriptionists, bringing with them skills from their former professions, which puts them well ahead of the game in many respects.

THE COMPETENT HOME-BASED MEDICAL TRANSCRIPTIONIST

As an independent home-based MT, you will face daily challenges. You will be responsible for transcribing many different types of medical reports, dictated by a variety of practitioners, with an assortment of accents that will require a good ear for deciphering dialects. You will have to be a stickler for detail and learn new medical terms on a daily basis. You will have to remain focused, concentrating on individual projects over long periods of time. You will be "plugged into a machine," typing for eight or more hours a day.

A quick mind, solid basic skills, and fingers that fly across the keyboard are independent transcription essentials, for you will be paid by production. Correctly transcribed production. Quantity combined with quality.

While building your business, you may need to forego vacations, sick days, and weekend leisure. Health insurance and retirement benefits may be unaffordable luxuries for an indefinite period of time.

As an independent business person you will be responsible for marketing, public relations, quality control, troubleshooting equipment problems, delivering and picking up work, and general bookkeeping and billing. Simply stated, YOU will be the business!

Until the advent of the computer, very few medical transcriptionists enjoyed the option of working independently. Technology, however, has opened new doors for medical transcription entrepreneurs.

Businesses are outsourcing everything these days. Contract employment has never seen such a boom as companies look to outside expertise to get the job done. After a decade of seeing the rise and fall of many large medical transcription services, the health care industry is discovering what independent transcriptionists have always known — that small is better. Small is more flexible, small is closer to the customer, small means quality, small means speed and SMALL IS SMART.

Independent medical transcription services are establishing their own niche in the medical transcription industry, each focusing on a microslice of the market, which enables them to provide maximum service to their clients. These dynamic small companies are creating significant pressure in a once large-service-dominated industry and the competitive battles are shifting. As information technology gets better, independent services are finding it easier to provide excellent service and compete with large services.

Global telecommunication has reached the medical transcription industry and is redefining the meaning of "BIG." According to the United States Department of Labor there are between 20 and 30 million telecommuters using technology at home. It just keeps getting "smaller" out there. With a PC, fax, desktop publishing, and data base management software one person can do the job it took several people to do fifteen years ago. If you add telecommunication to this, an independent entrepreneur can do things that used to require a huge organization.

The key words here are *responsiveness*, *flexibility* and *independence*. Independent services are enormously successful in today's competitive marketplace because 1) they thoroughly understand every aspect of their business and its position in the marketplace, and 2) they understand the need for, and are willing to make, immediate business transitions to provide continuing excellent service and to remain competitive. Indeed, independent services eagerly anticipate opportunities for positive change, and because of their small size, often have a distinct advantage over large, monolithic businesses.

Successful independents know there is always room for improvement and take personal responsibility for bringing about that improvement. They don't depend on or wait for directives from industry "experts," who are often out of touch with independent career variables, are content with the status quo or are slow to react to market issues. Independents waste no time. They read, study, and evaluate facts and alternatives and, based on their unique business situation and location, make sound decisions that move their business forward. They control their destiny. They take the risks and they get the rewards.

Before walking across the threshold of entrepreneurial independence, commit yourself to excellence and develop your potential. Obtain an appropriate education and practice your skills. After that, evaluate your skill level, and if you feel you are ready for the challenging world of self-employment, by all means, proceed.

This book was designed to be an informative and helpful guide, taking you step-by-step through the complicated maze of establishing yourself as an independent medical transcriptionist. Success and respect await those with excellent skills, diligence, integrity, and a passion for their profession. May success be yours!

TESTING THE WATERS

Evaluate your lifestyle and your goals for the future. How far do you want to go, and how big do you want to become? Will it be feasible for you to be self-employed? Are you doing it for the income, because you want to be your own boss, to be independent, have flexible working time, work at home, or other reasons?

If you are not completely sure of the answers, you may want to "test the waters" before plunging completely into self-employment.

CONSIDER MOONLIGHTING

Moonlighting has launched many businesses and may be the ideal way for you to try out a new career path. Assuming that you are employed, we advise you to **hang onto that job while determining whether you want to be independent**. Regular salary checks can alleviate that sink-or-swim feeling while you experience the real world of independence, allowing your business to develop while you continue to feed the family.

It is possible, of course, to earn a fine wage if you are an industrious individual and a high-volume producer, but few entrepreneurs start out at such a comfort level. And if you discover that you are a low volume producer — which may occur for a variety of personal and professional reasons — you may decide that self-employment will not be suitable for you.

WORKING FOR A SERVICE

Another alternative to consider is working for a transcription service that uses the talents of home-based medical transcriptionists. A transcription service will give you greater flexibility, allowing you to decide how much work you wish to take each day.

Medical transcription work can be mailed, picked up and delivered by hand or transmitted via modem. Larger services often provide pickup and delivery to home-based transcriptionists unless they are using a digital dictation system. In that case, the finished product is modemed to either the service or the health care institution where the work originated. If you work for a smaller medical transcription service, however, you will probably have to personally pick up and deliver the work to the service. Services generally provide necessary formats, physician lists and stationery. The independent medical transcriptionist provides the labor.

Working for a service of any size is a great learning experience. You will see how a service functions, giving you an edge over less experienced persons just entering the field of medical transcription. Some services utilize their own dictation equipment and have 800 numbers that make it convenient for medical transcriptionists to call in and download dictation. Most services use state-of-the-art technology so you may be required to have a high-tech computer setup to interact with their systems.

PRODUCTIVITY PAYS

Independents are generally paid by production, and a low-volume producer may not be as successful as an independent. For instance, if a transcriptionist earns more working at an hourly rate for an employer than she earns by the line, character count, etc., as an independent, she is probably a low-volume producer and may not succeed self-employed.

33

In addition to covering living expenses, the self-employed independent must also cover business expenses such as office equipment, supplies, insurance, twice the amount of FICA an employer would withhold, and allow for health, accident and other benefits normally provided by an employer. Self-employment may not be practical unless there is another stable income to fall back on.

HOURS IN YOUR WORK WEEK

Successful self-employed transcriptionists are those who are aware of and prepare for the more difficult side of independence. The profession is not all fun and games, and not everyone is suited to the challenge. Individuals must examine their goals, skills, schedule, and lifestyle carefully to determine whether or not they are likely candidates for an independent transcriptionist career.

Will your working commitment be a part-time venture, two, four, or six hours a day, a few days a week, or are you planning to do this full-time, perhaps at least 40 hours per week? This may be difficult to judge at first, if you are completely new at freelancing.

Much depends on knowing your own transcription production limits by hour, line, character, minute, tape, etc. There are many variables. To plan ahead and make accurate projections, it is important to know your professional capabilities. As your service grows and your management responsibilities increase, these will be very important revenue production factors.

DETERMINING YOUR PRODUCTION CAPABILITIES

If you are not sure of your production capabilities, begin slowly with a few hours and gradually increase as you become comfortable with your output. This may take a few weeks or months depending on the type of accounts you assume. Generally, production can be determined on minutes of dictation and lines transcribed. With new equipment technology on the market today, it is quick and easy to monitor production rates accurately and you should do this on a regular basis.

> *"Before walking across the threshold of entrepreneurial independence, commit yourself to excellence and develop your potential."*

> *"The demand for more detailed and accurate medical records will increase in direct proportion to the growing complexity of our health care system."*

RATE OF PRODUCTION FORMULAS

There are several simple formulas for determining the rate of production: Minutes of dictation, lines transcribed, hours worked. Minutes of dictation divided by hours worked = minutes transcribed per hour, divided by total hours = lines transcribed per hour. In monetary terms, charging by the line, lines transcribed x $ per line = $ earned, by hour, and by job (total lines). This is a simple formula for determining production by minutes, lines and, of course, dollars earned.

If you are choosing physician office dictation, it may take more than one account to reach a volume that is comfortable for you. If, on the other hand, there are three physicians in the practice, the volume from that single office may be sufficient. To be on the safe side, work with new accounts, determining average time commitment and volume (which generally increases in a positive working relationship) before soliciting more transcription clients.

Since the first edition of this book was released, we have answered many questions about medical transcription. One question frequently asked has been: "How can I net $40,000 per year in my business?"

The good news is that it is possible to net that amount; the bad news for new people entering the field is that in order to do so you will probably have to work anywhere from 17-31 hours per day!

If you intend to **net** $40,000 per year, you must first **gross** approximately $80,000 per year. In other words, your revenue received from billing your services should be $80,000 if you want to end up with $40,000 net income from your business. You determine taxable income by subtracting your business expenses ("tax deductions") from your revenue. (See example on pages 381-382.)

The table at the top of the following page demonstrates what it takes to achieve about $80,000 per year in billings according to lines transcribed per day, line rate charged, and working five days a week.

LINE RATE BILLED	LINES BILLED PER DAY	GROSS YEARLY BILLINGS
10 cents	3100	$80,600
12 cents	2550	$79,560
13 cents	2350	$79,430
14 cents	2200	$80,080
15 cents	2050	$79,950
16 cents	1900	$79,040
17 cents	1800	$79,560
18 cents	1700	$79,560

The following three tables show you how many billable hours you need to work per day at various billing rates in order to achieve your $80,000 annual billings goal if your typing speed is 200, 300, or 400 lines per hour.

200 LINES/HOUR	LINE RATE
15.5 hrs/day	10 cents
12.75 hrs/day	12 cents
11.75 hrs/day	13 cents
11 hrs/day	14 cents
10.25 hrs/day	15 cents
9.5 hrs/day	16 cents
9 hrs/day	17 cents
8.5 hrs/day	18 cents

300 LINES/HOUR	LINE RATE
10.3 hrs/day	10 cents
8.5 hrs/day	12 cents
7.8 hrs/day	13 cents
7.3 hrs/day	14 cents
6.8 hrs/day	15 cents
6.3 hrs/day	16 cents
6 hrs/day	17 cents
5.6 hrs/day	18 cents

400 LINES/HOUR	LINE RATE
7.75 hrs/day	10 cents
6.3 hrs/day	12 cents
5.8 hrs/day	13 cents
5.5 hrs/day	14 cents
5.1 hrs/day	15 cents
4.7 hrs/day	16 cents
4.5 hrs/day	17 cents
4.2 hrs/day	18 cents

NOTE

If your billing is based on character count instead of gross line count, you should reduce the above tables by 15% to 20%.

Most experienced medical transcriptionists using the latest computer technology including macro abbreviation programs can average between 300-400 lines per hour or higher, depending on the type of dictation. As stated earlier, if you are new to the field and only typing 100 lines per hour, your expectations must be scaled down realistically.

Also take into account that the above formula is just for hours transcribed, not for the one to two additional hours per day (unless your work is modemed) you will spend printing, logging and delivering the work. Those extra hours must also be factored into your work day, billable hours available, and billing line rate chosen.

Medical Transcription Education

*"Education is a private matter between the person
and the world of knowledge and experience,
and has little to do with school or college."*

—Lillian Smith

Do you know what skills and training are necessary to be a competent and successful medical transcriptionist? Are your education and skills sufficient for professional success? Affirmative answers to these questions are essential. Solid educational preparation is the basic foundation underlying every successful transcriptionist's career.

I know several medical transcriptionists who have learned transcription through extensive training in independent study or community college classes and a couple of years hospital internship. After only four or five years, they are making almost as much as I do after thirty-one years as a medical transcriptionist. I should point out, however, that I learned on the job and took college courses in my spare time over the years, boot-strapping my way up.

A bright, industrious student can make it big in medical transcription work — with hospital training, after extensive book learning and transcription of **authentic** physician dictated reports. However, this takes a tremendous amount of effort and does not happen with a six-week-crash-course.

Generally speaking, you will not find training programs within the work setting today. In our modern health care era, hospitals, clinics, and most doctors' offices do not have the time nor the personnel necessary to educate inexperienced trainees in the complexities of medical transcription. Transcriptionists must seek basic training elsewhere.

AAMT'S COMPRO

To better evaluate your medical transcription qualifications, the American Association for Medical Transcription (AAMT) offers a competency profile, COMPRO, which lists competencies necessary for medical transcription professionals.

BEYOND THE BASICS

To build a more solid foundation for working in the medical transcription field, we recommend including a college level anatomy and/or physiology course.

An extensive medical terminology class (more than eight weeks) is essential. There is an excellent study guide for medical terminology published by W.B. Saunders, *The Language of Medicine*, by Davi-Ellen Chabner, B.A., M.A.T. This guide is particularly helpful when used in conjunction with a medical terminology class or simply as an independent study guide. Audio tapes are also available, with Davi-Ellen pronouncing the medical terms. If the guide is used without the audio tapes, you will lose the advantage of learning the correct pronunciation of each medical term, which is crucial in transcribing medical reports.

JUNIOR COLLEGE COURSES

If your education consists of one eight-week medical transcription course at the local junior college, you probably need more education. Although junior college medical transcription courses can be helpful, usually offering general information about transcription equipment, as well as some medical terminology, they are often limited in scope and do not provide adequate medical transcription training. Frequently, such classes are designed for medical assisting students, not medical transcriptionists.

In one college we evaluated, the dictation courses employed dictators whose diction was perfect. They also used perfect sentence structure, indicated correct placement of all punctuation marks, and spelled all uncommon words. Let us assure you that this is not the real world of medical transcription!

FOR-PROFIT TRANSCRIPTION SCHOOLS

We are not opposed to for-profit schools that provide what they promise, but we have no patience with those that do not. Beware of these! In recent years, a number of ethically questionable medical transcription schools have sprung up. Like fast food restaurants, they promise to instantaneously satisfy the appetites of career-hungry people.

These schools extol the virtues of their training programs and ensure unsuspecting and eager students that in just eight to sixteen weeks they will be able to work as home-based transcriptionists, earning generous incomes. When that rosy scenario does not occur, few students are confident enough to protest.

The tuition for such schools is usually high, ranging from $2000-$7000. Some schools offer government sponsored student loans, which are paid directly to the school. Students must repay these loans.

> "I cna tpye 200 wrods per mniute! oHw fsat cna ouy tpy?e"

HOME STUDY COURSES

The end of the 1980s found us in a time of self-discovery and suffering from the I-want-it-now syndrome. Schools sprang up offering to teach medical transcription in a short three to six month home-study program. These schools marketed themselves aggressively, even advertising in *TV Guide* and *The Enquirer*. (You know the old saying, "If it's in *The Enquirer*, it has to be true.") The ads claimed that after completing their course, one could earn the grandiose salary of $35,000 a year. One school promised free job placement at the end of training, which consisted of nothing more than a two-year-old list of physicians.

Before selecting a transcription training program, make sure it is accredited. Ask other transcriptionists for their thoughts and advice when choosing a program. Remember, "If it looks too good to be true, it probably is."

SUM Program — Training like that provided by the SUM Program for Medical Transcription Training offered by Health Professions Institute is a very good educational reference that can be used in a course setting or as independent study material. The course utilizes actual physician dictation and was developed by certified medical transcriptionists.

As a medical transcriptionist, you will be required to produce quality work. However, this will be impossible if you have not had a solid medical transcription education.

When evaluating educational programs for quality, be sure to cover all the bases. Ask to see the course syllabus, which will give you the description, objectives and intended outcome of the course. Ask to see what subjects are taught and what textbooks are provided or are needed. Are textbooks well-written and thorough? How many are there? Is authentic physician dictation provided?

The course should include, but not be limited to, the following:

- anatomy and physiology
- computer training
- grammar, punctuation, editing and proofreading skills
- basic medical principles: laboratory values and procedures, drugs/pharmacology
- professionalism, ethics and medicolegal issues
- disease processes
- specialty courses
- transcription equipment
- reference books
- medical transcription practice
- externship/available networks

Ask about the teaching staff. What are their credentials, and what type of technical support can a student rely upon?

How long is the course? Is the course accredited? Is there college credit or a certificate-of-completion awarded?

Medical transcription is not easy, and to be a successful medical transcriptionist, your education must be thorough and well-rounded. You will also have to work hard to develop the many skills necessary in this highly skilled profession. All of this takes time, so don't expect to learn the basics and develop your skills overnight.

INTERNET RESOURCES FOR MT TRAINING

The Internet is a wonderful resource for accessing information on medical transcription education. Use a search engine such as "Google," which is a favorite of ours, and type in the words "medical transcription." You will find a multitude of MT resources to choose from. You will find student learning centers, virtual classrooms, home study courses reference books, technical school contacts and much more.

LESSONS AFTER SCHOOL

If you are ambitious and have recently completed a qualified course in medical transcription, you may have a burning desire to work as an independent transcriptionist.

With little or no experience as a transcriptionist, it will probably be difficult to break into the transcription field. However, there are several steps that may help you achieve your goal.

- Join the American Association for Medical Transcription (AAMT). Student membership category (available to nonemployed students enrolled in medical transcription courses at accredited schools) is a nominal fee. Fees for working transcriptionists are somewhat higher.

  AAMT membership provides you with excellent resource material, newsletters, meeting, seminar and convention information that you can use for networking with other transcriptionists and industry supporters. In addition, AAMT has local chapters that offer student membership.

- Find a mentor from the above sources. You will find this a valuable resource for information about techniques, skills, and trends in transcription practices.

- Review reference materials promoted in AAMT publications and other sources. Mentors are generally eager to share information and advise you regarding resource materials.

- Pursue continuing education through medical lectures, transcription practices seminars, and other related sources.

If you show a genuine eagerness to listen, learn, and work to improve yourself, you will find others willing to help you, providing the information, guidance and support you seek.

MEDICAL TRANSCRIPTION STUDENT NETWORK

Health Professions Institute (HPI) has formed the Medical Transcription Student Network (MTSN). This transcription network is open to all students actively participating in classroom study, home study, or in self-directed programs. Each student receives a free subscription to *Perspectives on the Medical Transcription Profession* magazine as well as discounts on all books from Health Professions Institute (HPI) and the Lippincott, Williams and Wilkins publishing company. For more information contact HPI or visit them on their student network website at www.hpisum.com. It has amazing things for students — self-assessments, study tips, articles of interest, etc.

- **Health Professions Institute (HPI)**
  209-551-2112

- **HPI Student Network**
  www.hpisum.com

CERTIFICATION OF HEALTH CARE PROFESSIONALS

The certification of health care professionals is the recognition by a governmental or professional association that an individual's expertise meets the standards of that group. The standards established by professional associations generally exceed those required by government agencies. Some professional groups establish their own minimum standards for certification in those professions that are not licensed by a particular state. Certification by an association or group is a self-regulation credentialing process.

The Medical Transcription Certification Commission (MTCC) is a nationally recognized, voluntary recertification program for medical transcriptionists, designed "to promote professional standards and improve the practice of medical transcription by giving special recognition to those professionals who demonstrate requisite knowledge, expertise, and performance through successful completion of the exam and who maintain certification through the fulfillment of stated requirements." According to the MTCC *Cert Alert*, there are more than 3000 medical transcriptionists certified.

Many dedicated and experienced medical transcriptionists seek this personal achievement. The certification examination consists of two parts, which are given separately.

Part I — The Written Exam — The written exam consists of 120 multiple-choice questions covering:

* medical terminology

* English language usage

* anatomy and physiology

* disease processes

* health care record

* professional development

Part II — The Practical Exam — Candidates must pass the written exam to be eligible for the practical exam. The practical exam requires transcription of original physician dictation in a wide variety of specialty areas and report types. Candidates who successfully pass the certification exam may then place the initials CMT (Certified Medical Transcriptionist) after their names.

To request information about the certification program contact MTCP.

* **MTCC** (Medical Transcription Certification Commission)
  800-578-9823; 209-527-9630
  Fax: 209-527-9636

MAINTAINING CERTIFICATION

After becoming certified, a transcriptionist must acquire continuing education credits to maintain certification, which is standard procedure in credentialed professions. Read the continuing education guidelines that accompany your certification information to learn about creditworthy activities that will allow you to receive continuing education credits (CECs). Keep track of your CECs on an ongoing basis and pay close attention to paperwork and any updates on information regarding recertification guidelines. Recertification fee is $60 per three-year cycle or $45 for early birds.

OTHER CERTIFICATION EXAMINATIONS

There are two other associations that offer certification examinations for medical transcriptionists:

- **American Association of Medical Assistants, Inc. (AAMA)** offers certification as a medical assistant (CMA), administrative (CMA-A), or clinical (CMA-C).

- **American Medical Technologists (AMT)** organization awards the Registered Medical Assistant (RMA).

For more information, contact AAMT, AAMA and AMT.

- **American Association for Medical Transcription (AAMT)**
  100 Sycamore Avenue
  Modesto, CA 95354
  800-982-2182
  Help Desk: 800-578-0308
  Fax: 209-527-9633
  www.aamt.org

- **American Association of Medical Assistants, Inc.**
  20 North Wacker Street, Suite 1575
  Chicago, IL 60606

- **Registered Medical Assistants of AMT**
  710 Higgins Road
  Park Ridge, IL 60068

NOTE

A medical transcriptionist does not have to belong to a professional organization to become certified or to maintain certification status. However, professional organizations can provide many opportunities and resources that will aid the transcriptionist in maintaining continuing education credits (CECs) for ongoing certification.

Building a Successful Home-based Business

"Confidence is an important part of any business venture.
If you don't think you can, you won't."

—Beatrice Gage

According to many resources, the number of home-based businesses continues to increase. This trend is occurring for a variety of reasons. Among them are four significant factors: 1) the accelerating global movement toward a service-based economy, 2) rapidly advancing technology that is continually creating new home-based career opportunities, 3) continuing mergers and downsizing of other businesses and professions, and 4) economic downturns within many industries that create massive work force layoffs.

In the medical transcription profession, working at home has been an option for many years. Today, industry consultants list home-based transcription as one of the top entrepreneurial career opportunities in the nation. This trend is now expanding globally into such countries as India, Mexico and the Philippines.

Statistics show that of all new businesses launched, 13% will fail within the first year. Why?

Businesses ultimately fail for many different reasons, but the basic element found in most failures is a significant lack of preparation prior to business start-up. The successful entrepreneur knows not only the skills of trade but the basics of business management, too.

Those who are not prepared establish businesses without a business plan and adequate analysis of their market. When they actually face the realities of a competitive marketplace, they are unable to resolve the multiplicity of unanticipated problems confronting them. Many fall by the wayside almost immediately, a few hang on for a time before giving up, and a minute number survive. But most poorly planned businesses fail sooner or later.

Business success cannot be guaranteed. Even with preparation, and under the best circumstances, business is a day-to-day challenge. The road to independence is full of sharp curves, detours and potholes, but if you prepare yourself realistically for the future, you increase your chances of succeeding.

BEFORE GOING SOLO

Before embarking on a freelance career, ask yourself the following questions:

- Can I earn an adequate income freelancing?

- Am I capable of managing my own business?

- Will I be working at what I like best?

- Am I willing to take on additional responsibilities, including other essential, but less glamorous, tasks such as sales, accounting and paperwork?

If the answer to all of the above is "yes," then ask yourself these questions:

1. Am I ready to make a COMMITMENT?

2. Am I SELF-DISCIPLINED?

3. Do I have enough EXPERIENCE?

FACING INDEPENDENT REALITY

In the early stages of your home-based career, be prepared to sacrifice much in order to give your business your all. Expect to do without a high quality personal life, free time, socializing with family and friends, and evenings out. This period of self-sacrifice won't last forever, it will be worth the effort, and it is actually not so bad if you are prepared for it.

Anticipate initial long days that do not end after eight hours. For a time, every day may seem like a Monday. You won't be able to call in sick and vacations will be out of the question.

You will discover that building your new business requires days and/or nights filled with mundane organizational tasks and responsibilities. And you will face daily distractions that interrupt your work schedule — nonbusiness telephone calls, salesmen, and friendly neighbors.

We know from experience that it takes drive and stamina to survive this period. Some transcriptionists find the pressure too great and decide that being independent is not their cup of tea. It takes a great deal of fortitude and self-discipline to follow through on commitments, especially when you are unsupervised. It may sound like fun to be your own boss, but without adequate self-discipline, it is very tempting to "kick back," put off the work, and miss deadlines.

You can do what you want! You will not punch a time-clock or have a time-conscious supervisor peering over your shoulder. You will decide your priorities and establish your work schedule. And it will be you, and you alone, who will determine your success or failure.

ESTABLISHING PRIORITIES

Do you have your priorities straight? Are you able to set up a work schedule for yourself and not deviate? You may find it tempting to put off working until the last minute, thereby jeopardizing your delivery and pickup times.

Take control! Schedule a specific set of hours in which you do nothing but work. Prioritize your time and have a set schedule or block of hours in which to transcribe.

THE EMPLOYER MENTALITY

It is imperative to step away from the employee mentality and get into the employer mentality. Remember that you are the owner of this business, therefore the boss, and that you must provide yourself with all the things that you have come to expect from an employer — health insurance, disability insurance, retirement benefits, sick days, vacation days, a five-day work week, setting up an accounting system, and paying estimated taxes.

MANAGING FAMILY LIFE

Being your own boss and working out of your home offers wonderful flexibility for home and community activities. Being home-based, you can spend more time with family and attend school and after-school functions with your children, participating more fully in their lives. It does take planning, however, to find the ideal balance between family and profession.

It is nearly impossible to maintain a set work schedule with children racing through the house, demanding attention, arguing over television programs, dancing to the boom box, answering doors or phones, and generally just being children! To eliminate this type of stress, it is imperative that you reduce noise, avoid interruptions, provide adequate child care, and maintain good communication with family members, particularly children.

It is essential to establish rules in the beginning. Ask your spouse to respect your work schedule by avoiding unnecessary telephone calls during your work hours, especially if the questions are, "What's for dinner?" or "Did you pick up my clothes at the dry cleaners?"

CHILDCARE

The most difficult issue to deal with is childcare. After all, if you choose to work at home in order to be near your children, what have you accomplished if you send them away to be taken care of?

If your children are preschoolers or young enough to require supervision after school, you may be faced with hiring at least part-time care for them. You may choose to have that childcare in your home or outside your home, depending on family members' personalities and your work setup. Either way, you will still be able to spend more time with your children.

Some home-based professionals find it convenient and satisfying to work in one part of the house while the children are cared for in another part of the house. This offers more parent/child contact during breaks and lunch and provides flexibility to answer your caregiver's questions and respond to emergencies.

If your children are at school full-time during the day, it isn't difficult to work around their schedule, hiring someone to come in for a few hours after school, if necessary.

Whether the children are in-house or out, the home-based professional can readily leave her office and adjust work hours to accommodate family and personal priorities.

FAMILY COMMUNICATION

Communication with your family is crucial, especially when the business is located in the home and is a new experience for everyone. Suddenly, household rules have changed. Certain rooms are off-limits. Mother (or Dad) is home but not home. The new regimen can be frustrating for all concerned.

Give your children as much information as possible about when and where you will be working, when you will and won't be available, who will be available when you can't be, and exactly what is expected of them. This will help to allay many fears and questions they may have.

Without the cooperation and support of the family, home-based self-employment is impossible. It takes family team work, and even then, it will be challenging in the beginning. By working together, your family members will soon wonder how you ever lived and worked any other way.

Marketing

"No one can arrive from being talented alone.
God gives talent, work transforms
talent into genius."

—Anna Pavlova

You have made the decision to freelance, and are moving ahead. You have studied hard, learned medical terminology, and honed your keyboarding skills. Now you must have a plan. Work is not likely to simply fall into your lap. You will have to go after it. You can work, you want work, but how do you go about getting it?

MARKET AND COMPETITION ANALYSIS

One of the first steps you should take is to do a market and competition analysis, which is not necessarily complex. In fact, it is essentially logical. It can be as simple as one, two, three.

1. Research adequate facts/information

2. Organize and study the facts

3. Develop a business plan

INNOVATIVE MARKETING — YOUR BLUEPRINT FOR SUCCESS

Resources state that 80% of new businesses that fail do so because they do not have enough clients. Determining the probability of success for your medical transcribing service, which will really determine the probability of success for the business, takes planning. Planning is the root for developing a successful business. Granted, many businesses succeed without planning; however, most businesses that do not plan do not succeed. Planning for business success is very much like planning for your vacation. In order to make sure that you can find your vacation destination, a map is secured and followed. The business plan is a tool to map your path towards success. There are various components of a business plan, however. Here we will focus on innovative and inexpensive ways of marketing your service. Within each business plan, there should be a marketing plan.

To develop this plan, do a feasibility study, which will consist of three basic components: the market, the competition and the opportunity for selling your service. Once you have done this, you will have a clear picture of what you are facing, and it will be a useful tool to support any needed requests for credit and financing your start-up.

Many states in the U.S. now have websites that can provide you with very useful information on new business start-ups. I found this out firsthand when I followed my dream to Hawaii.

THE MARKETING PLAN

The marketing plan should take care of many aspects within the business plan. It should concern itself with the following:

- Who are the potential clients in my market?

- How many potential clients are in my market?

- What are the needs of those potential clients?

- How well will my product or service meet clients' needs?

- What is the price of my product or service?

- How will my service be delivered to clients?

- Who are my competitors and what benefits do they offer?

- What promotional vehicles will I use to promote services to potential clients? By organizing the information listed above and committing to it on paper, a business can get a much clearer perspective regarding a service's potential for success.

Your market research should clearly answer the following questions:

- Who will buy my services?

- Why will they buy it?

- What do I need to charge to ensure a healthy profit?

- What services will mine be competing with?

- Am I positioning a service correctly? In other words, if there is much competition, you might want to look for a specialized market niche.

- What government regulations will my service be subject to?

Once your analysis shows that the service has a good probability for success, the promotional program is set into motion. Deciding where best to commit your advertising dollars will be determined in large part by who your clients will be.

BUSINESS PROMOTION AND ADVERTISING

By looking at the list of potential clients, you will discover logical groupings. Those groupings will determine how you will advertise and promote your services. For instance, if potential clients belong to associations and read professional journals, it might be beneficial to advertise your business there. Or if clients will be actively shopping for your services, perhaps a yellow-page ad will be best. Only by writing down who your clients might be, can you get a handle on what might work best for promotion.

PRICING

Pricing is an item that seems simple but can be the most complex issue of all. Small-business owners too often overlook factors that are essential in determining their total costs accurately. Most everything that you do to bring your services to market involve some cost. The cost for your equipment, utilities, insurance premiums, gas in your car, advertising and the time spent picking up tapes are all costs related to conducting business. Unless you enjoy giving money away in the form of those cost items, you should include those items in the price of your services.

Now that you have determined your target market, found the best promotional strategy to reach it and the distribution channels for getting to it, you need to make the sale.

SELLING YOUR SERVICES

Sales are rarely made without some type of human contact. Services do not sell themselves; people sell them. As a small business owner, be prepared to be your lead salesperson. To be a successful salesperson, it is necessary to be client-focused. To be client-focused, the clients' needs will become your needs. When clients can see that you have solutions that meet or exceed their needs, you have the opportunity for sales. By becoming a partner in satisfying your clients' requirements, you are well on the way to success.

Other factors in making the sale include price, delivery schedule, etc., but those details can usually be ironed out later. By assessing the needs of your client and being actively involved in satisfying those needs, you can develop the type of trust that is necessary to do business today.

Clients are becoming more concerned with value than with price. If your services are exactly like your competitor's services, then price, obviously, is extremely important. However, if you can distinguish your services from your competitor's, then it is up to you to sell the value of what you have to offer. Be creative in analyzing your services, and be prepared to offer what others do not. In short, develop a competitive advantage over your competitors. By having a competitive advantage, price will not be the central issue.

SIX SUGGESTIONS FOR SUCCESS

Here are some suggestions for doing business:

1. **Focus on a smaller market:** For every trend, there is at least one countertrend. It is sometimes better to focus on a smaller market — one nobody is serving because they are all catering to a bigger trend.

   If you are setting up a one-person medical transcription service, don't go after the large hospital accounts or even large clinic accounts. Let the bigger companies compete for those markets. Target local physicians and smaller clinics (four doctors or less).

   Ancillary departments in hospitals are an excellent resource for the smaller business. Most hospitals have emergency rooms, cardiac catheterization laboratories, gastroenterology labs, radiology and pathology departments, which are excellent sources of income for the smaller business since most of that work is now being outsourced.

2. **Beware of the negative:** Deal with all your clients in good faith and with integrity. Negative word of mouth, especially on computer bulletin boards and systems like the Internet, can cripple your business even more than positive public relations can help. Remember, physicians talk to one another. If a physician is pleased with your service, word-of-mouth referrals will follow.

3. **Be ready for change:** Medical transcription technology changes on a monthly basis, so be prepared to adapt accordingly. If your client wants a faster turnaround time than your competitors, consider installing a modem and sending all completed work back to the client's office to be printed. Or, to improve turnaround time even more, invest in a call-in-line system. Always think ahead and research business methods that will save you and your client time and money. What's more, your reputation as a heads-up professional will soar.

4. **Get on the ball:** Be ready to be *where* your client wants you, *when* your client wants you, with *what* your client wants. Just-in-time marketing is critical

as people become spoiled by 24-hour, seven-day-a-week customized products and services. Of course, you must set boundaries with accounts at the beginning of your relationship or some may treat you like a doormat. Under all circumstances, keep the lines of communication open at all times. Always listen carefully to what clients have to say, evaluate their comments and, if appropriate, do your best to meet their needs.

5. **Keep your clients:** Keeping clients is far more cost effective than finding new ones. Focus on relationships with existing clients and be creative in finding ways to keep them. Every client should be given a questionnaire to complete each year — something on the order of a report card — to measure your relationship with that client and his or her satisfaction with your service. Always ask for and encourage client input. If a client leaves, do as much research to find out why as you do to seek out new markets.

6. **Project a big image:** It doesn't cost anything to aim high. Think of yourself as owning a "macro" not a "micro" business. Remember, most home-based businesses are relatively small operations — but the smart ones don't advertise it.

Look around you, listen to other business people, analyze business advertising — newspapers, magazines, newsletters, television, signs — and become aware of all the marketing techniques you are subject to as you go about your day. Most of this advertising has been produced by top professionals. Try to build on these ideas and apply them to your business in ways that fit what you are selling. There are no new ideas under the sun, just different ways to use them.

You may find creative marketing a challenge at first. Although being innovative isn't difficult, trying new ideas isn't easy either. Don't be discouraged. With a little practice, you'll soon get a feel for it.

MONEY-SAVING MARKETING IDEAS

If you are on a budget, as most of us were when starting our businesses, here are some very inexpensive ways to market your service.

1. **Develop a 30-second commercial:** It is very important to market yourself at every opportunity. The best tool for this is a rehearsed 30-second commercial

about yourself and your business. State your name, the name of your business, where it is located, what type of business it is, how long you have been in business and your specialties. End your commercial by handing that person your business card. If you catch someone's interest, you will have time to expand their understanding and may even gain a new client or a referral.

2. **Become an expert:** Television and radio programs, especially local shows, are always looking for programming. Many business organizations are looking for speakers for meetings. Become an expert who is available and agree to appear without charge. Become such an interesting, informative guest that word begins to spread about your speaking abilities and the great information you have to share. Schedule at least one appearance monthly. The medical transcription home-business industry is growing by leaps and bounds. Who better to be an expert than you?

3. **Get your business mentioned in the media:** Develop both a press kit containing interesting and pertinent information about you and your business and a media list (a list of all newspapers, radio and TV stations, and publications in your community) of those sources that communicate with and reflect the demographics of the group you believe will buy your services. Using a newsworthy "hook" (an interesting and attractive idea), write your own one page press release. Distribute the release to the media list you have developed. Within one week, contact every source on your list and sell them on running your story. The best part, it won't cost you a dime.

4. **Utilize the Internet:** The Internet is an innovative advertising tool to get your name into cyberspace. Some sites offer free advertising, and you can also develop your own webpage or site to promote your business. In addition, you may be happily surprised at the many benefits you derive from online networking with other MTs. Using the Internet, you can reach more potential clients than through any other resource.

5. **Advertise in newsletters:** Many associations publish newsletters which are mailed directly to members at their cost. These newsletters may target individuals or groups that you really want to reach. Often they sell ads at minimal rates. Identify the newsletters you want to reach and send a press release, flier or advertisement to the membership. Also, think about advertising in your local medical association newsletter. Every county has a medical association and most will take advertising. These newsletters are sent to every doctor in your county who is a member.

6. Network, network, network: Networking is more than just going to special business events to specifically market your business. Networking is a way of life.

Every day, everywhere, every person you meet socially, professionally or athletically is a part of your network. You should always sell yourself and your business. Remain open to going to new places and meeting new people. You never know where that next contact will lead.

Contact the medical staff secretary at your local hospitals to see about possible referrals. These people are the first contacts that new doctors make when moving to a new community and setting up practice.

7. Have a positive, professional attitude: Treat people with respect. Be honest. Be consistent. Be credible. Be nice. Great service is never forgotten.

ESTABLISHING A BUSINESS PLAN

As stated earlier, numerous businesses fail within the first year because of poor planning. Ask any successful business owner, and he or she will tell you that the first step for assuring success is developing a business plan.

There are three main reasons for having a business plan.

1. It helps you to visualize your business before it actually gets off the ground.

2. It is required if you seek financial help from lenders or investors. They want to see that your business idea has been well researched and well thought out.

3. You will be able to determine from the business plan if the business has a reasonable chance of succeeding.

Here are steps toward developing a business plan:

• Define your business mission and your business goals. What do you hope to accomplish? List your personal as well as your professional goals.

• Describe your anticipated market and client base. Indicate your fee structure and develop a marketing plan.

- Prepare revenue and expense projections on a monthly basis for two years. Determine how much profit you want from your business. Be realistic. Carefully evaluate whether your projected net income will satisfy your personal financial needs.

- Define your market and your competition. Demonstrate that you can generate enough work to produce your projected revenue.

- Indicate the legal form of your business. Is it going to be a sole proprietorship, a partnership or a corporation?

- Indicate how your home business will physically operate. Is your home or apartment large enough to accommodate living quarters and the business you are considering?

- List the assets required to operate your business and estimate their costs. Determine how much money will be needed to meet all start-up expenses, including your living expenses during the hungry start-up phase. Refer to Budget Assumptions on the next page.

- Identify actual and potential funding sources for your business.

- Indicate if you will need additional personnel to get your business underway and as it grows. If so, identify potential personnel sources.

- Evaluate risks involved with the business and decide what measures you need to take to cope with these risks.

Using these steps, you should have a highly detailed statement as to why your business is being formed, what personal and monetary goals can be realistically achieved, and where and how it will operate.

If the plan looks good, then GET INTO ACTION. If it looks dismal, keep your full-time position and postpone your plans for a home-based medical transcription business for a year or two — or until the prospects for success can be improved.

It is very important to have a business plan. You should closely evaluate what type income you are expecting to generate from your business and if you are being realistic in your income and expense expectations. In order to help you assess this, we have included a budget assumptions list for your use.

Estimate your monthly expenses by reviewing your actual expenses for the prior six months. After you have completed this form, you will have an excellent idea how much money you will need to make every month in order to meet your obligations.

Since some of you are just starting your businesses and have not yet paid quarterly taxes, use the formula found in the finances section of this book to guesstimate what your taxes would be for the amount of income you expect to earn based on your plan.

BUDGET ASSUMPTIONS
FOR HOME-BASED BUSINESSES

CATEGORY	ASSUMPTION
Gross Income	_____
Advertising	_____
Automobile	_____
Bad Debts	_____
Business Gifts	_____
Business License	_____
Continuing Education	_____
Depreciation	
• Office Space	_____
• Office Equipment	_____
• Car	_____
Insurance	
• Health	_____
• Disability*	_____

- Life*
- Liability
- Equipment

(*for corporations only)

Interest (business loans)   _____

Office Equipment   _____

Office Supplies   _____

Lease Payments   _____

Marketing Promotions
- Brochures   _____
- Mailing Lists, etc.   _____

Rent   _____

Repairs & Maintenance   _____

Payroll (employees)   _____

Subcontractors (outsourcers)   _____

Subscription/Dues   _____

Taxes
- FICA   _____
- Federal Income   _____
- State Income   _____
- State Disability   _____
- Payroll Taxes   _____

Telephone   _____

Utilities   _____

In the appendix is an example of an effective budget worksheet from the book *Easy Financials for Your Home-based Business*, which you can photocopy.

GETTING FACTS/ADEQUATE INFORMATION

- Total market and demand

- Competition

- Industry trends

- Your target market

Familiarize yourself with the resources in your area. If you have been established in an area for some time, this can be an advantage as you may already be familiar with the available market. On the other hand, if you are new to an area, there are various resources for obtaining market information.

YOUR TARGET MARKET

The medical transcription marketplace is broad. Determining **your** target market, zeroing in on the specific area for **you**, is important, and it isn't difficult to do.

Evaluating your background experience will help determine your target market. Are you a student of medical transcription who is considering self-employment upon completion of your education? An experienced, currently employed transcriptionist? Are you crossing over from a related profession or an unrelated profession? If so, you will discover that each of the above will have a different target market.

If you are new to the field of medical transcription, your target market will probably be limited. We recommend starting with one medical specialty, focusing on that specialty until you have developed a high level of skill and confidence. At that point, consider expanding your business.

WARNING

Don't take on too much too soon.

Medical transcription is a challenge even for experienced professionals. If you are a novice transcriptionist, you will be wise to allow yourself time to develop additional skills, insights into your work style, professional contacts, and confidence. Spreading yourself too thin at the beginning of your career may result in unnecessary failure.

With adequate experience, your career future offers exciting opportunities and your business will grow. The more experience you have in medical transcription, the more diversified your service will become. Your service will be in demand by hospitals, medical clinics, physicians, and others within your market area.

Evaluate the overall transcription service need of the medical community in your area and then target a specific segment of that need. This is your target market.

You may decide to transcribe for hospitals and medical clinics, or limit your accounts to physicians' office records.

You may prefer to work as an independent, on-site/off-site, for a transcription service, home-based, or develop another option. There are various directions you can take, depending on your qualifications and experience.

Identifying the total market is the basic step. Make a list of what is available in your area.

DIRECTORIES

If you live in a large metropolitan area and decide to target hospital accounts, the best source for getting names and addresses of hospitals is *The Thomas Guide*, available in major book stores. In the back is a list of all hospitals within the county.

Another excellent tool is the yellow pages section of your telephone directory. Not only are hospitals listed, but also physicians within the area you are targeting. Directory information includes addresses, phone numbers, and in larger institutions and clinics, departments. Physicians are listed alphabetically and by specialty. If you are marketing your service outside the area in which you live, review the telephone directories for every county and city on file at your local library.

Local medical societies also have directories. Call or write for a physician reference directory. Classified "help wanted" ads provide additional information.

The Little Blue Book is a comprehensive directory that includes physicians, pharmacies and related health professionals in 157 metropolitan areas. It lists physicians in alphabetical order, and includes their specialty, address and phone number. This publication, which costs $15.00 plus $1.50 for shipping, is a great marketing tool. To see if *The Little Blue Book* is available for your area, contact National Physician's Data Source. You can also access DocFinderPlus through their website.

- **National Physician's Data Source**
  800-345-6865
  www.thelittlebluebook.com

As you network and become familiar with your area, you will discover other directories that will be helpful in your marketing. Be on the lookout for them.

ADVERTISING IN THE YELLOW PAGES

The Yellow Pages Publishers Association (YPPA) in Troy, Michigan, reports that almost 60% of all adults use the yellow pages weekly. Eighty four percent read two or more ads, suggesting that users are not just looking up telephone numbers but are shoppers who can be influenced by the quality of the ad. For those of us on a budget, this is an excellent advertising alternative.

There are about 6000 yellow pages directories nationwide. Some areas are served only by one, but others have many. Los Angeles County has 28. Telephone companies publish the most widely used directories, but many are now published by independent companies. The cost of an ad in an independently published yellow pages directory is usually less expensive (often one-tenth as much!) as an ad in a phone company directory. However, an independent directory may not give you the exposure you are seeking.

A yellow pages sales rep will pressure you to place ads under several headings (e.g., Medical Secretarial Services, Medical Transcription Services, Secretarial Services, Word Processing). That may be a good investment, but be careful; investing in many headings is usually a waste of money. The best way to find the most productive heading is to look where the competition places its ads. If you see competitors under the same headings year after year, you should be there, too. Remember, however, that sales reps work on commission and may also pressure you to use color, have large ads or use other expensive options.

Consider using an outside agency or graphic artist. Yellow pages advertising is different from conventional print, so if you decide to use someone other than a sales rep, use only a person with experience in this medium. You may even discover that you are the expert in designing your own ad.

Always track your ad responses or you will never know what works and what doesn't. Make sure you ask every caller how they learned about your service — from a friend, physician or hospital referral, one of your speaking engagements, an ad, etc. — and write down their responses. If they saw your ad, and if it is appearing in more than one directory, ask callers for the ad's page number, which will tell you what directory they are using. This way you will know exactly how many sales each directory or listing produces.

EVALUATE THE COMPETITION

It is important to research service demand in your area. Is there a need for additional transcription services or is the local market pretty well saturated?

For information regarding the industry, contact local employment agencies, employment development departments, personnel departments and other medical personnel service agencies, trade schools, and community colleges that offer courses in medical transcription. Do not hesitate to make phone inquiries and check out the trends in your area. Review the yellow pages of the phone book for transcription services and talk to managers in clinic and hospital personnel departments to see if there is a need for medical transcriptionists.

When you have completed your investigation, carefully analyze the facts you have gathered and determine the potential market for your transcription services.

TRANSCRIPTIONIST NETWORKING

Communication and networking with other medical transcriptionists is beneficial in fact-gathering. Make a list of local transcription services and file information you obtain about self-employed transcriptionists in your area. If you are not already online, consider accessing the Internet. There are approximately 750-1000 MTs online networking via chat rooms or through newsgroups.

INTERNET INFORMATION RESOURCES

Today, the Internet is the world's most valuable resource for general information and, more specifically, for medical transcription information. In the past four years the availability of information at our fingertips has increased in phenomenal proportions until our online resources are now limitless. Here are a few examples of topics, websites and e-mail addresses you will find useful for medical transcription research:

- National medical transcription companies
- Job listings
- Company profiles, home-based jobs
- Dictation and transcription equipment
- Web-based transcription/dictation service providers
- Medical transcription books
- MT chat rooms and public forums
- MT websites and e-mail addresses
- Websites for new medical terms
- Websites for business information
- Resource sites for physician names and addresses
- Long distance telephone rates
- Paper resources for transcription
- Transcription software programs
- MT consultants and investors
- Work-at-home websites
- Health information websites
- Top speech technology sources

It is not possible to list every website or e-mail address for MT resources. However, you can easily conduct your own search via a number of sites such as Yahoo, Netscape, GoTo, HotBot, Infoseek, Excite, Dogpile, Google, and others. One of my favorites is Google. Simply type in the keywords "Medical Transcription" and you will have a world of resources before your eyes. Use any combination of words — MT jobs, MT education, MT equipment, MT services — to get a reference, cross-reference, resource, or pages of information. Be careful, it can become addictive, so allot only an hour or two for browsing each week. Don't allow your net surfing to consume all of your "productive" time.

COMPUTER ONLINE INTERACTIVE INFORMATION AND COMMUNICATION SERVICES

Networking is a key element in any successful business because the more people you connect with, the more business you will obtain through referrals. If you don't have access to a local networking group, consider joining one of the computer online services. To get started, all you need is a computer, a telephone line, a modem and a basic online service package. Many personal computers and modems are now being marketed with online services preinstalled. You can get a membership kit, which includes software for connecting to the service and often a usage credit, from the online service you have subscribed to. Kits cost about $30. Most of them have bulletin boards for every facet of business including medical transcription.

It's great fun talking with MTs all over the country. Heard a new word that you can't document or need a business question answered? No problem. Your question can be answered twenty-four hours a day on a bulletin board.

HIGH-SPEED INTERNET ACCESS WITH DSL

The digital subscriber line (DSL) is exciting new technology that offers computer users high-speed Internet access which was previously reserved for only a few. With this technology, you will be able to transmit vast quantities of data very quickly. Technically, DSL technology uses standard copper wiring that already exists in almost every home and office in the United States, and it is becoming increasingly popular for professional and personal use. DSL's high-speed transmission is made possible by special hardware that is installed at the switch end and the user's end (i.e. your office or home) of telephone lines. Contact your local Internet service provider to learn how you can get a digital subscriber line. Most ISPs charge subscribers around $20 to $40 per month for DSL service. For more information, research DSLs online. Check out the following website to search for internet service providers that offer DSL in your area.

* **www.thelist.com**

GATHERING FACTS AT THE CHAMBER OF COMMERCE

The local chamber of commerce is generally helpful in providing and recommending resources for businesses. Visit your chamber office to find out what is available.

Consider joining your local chamber of commerce, which offers many benefits to members: informative speakers; educational presentations; business tours; fact-filled seminars; fun-filled business open houses and parties; well-researched booklets, brochures, directories, and newsletters; information about state and national business trends; updates on relevant legal and tax issues; insurance programs; and other benefits specific to local chambers. Although some chamber programs and printed materials are available to the public, many are not, which gives chamber members an inside track in the race to business success.

Chamber of commerce membership dues vary from community to community so check with your local chamber office regarding its dues schedule. Most members find that business generated by referrals from the chamber office more than covers their annual chamber dues. In addition, dues are a tax-deductible business expense.

Chamber membership cannot substitute for your medical transcription association memberships, but it will build friendships beyond your medical transcription environment and broaden your knowledge of diverse businesses. To locate a chamber of commerce near you, contact your state's chamber of commerce office listed in the resources at the back of this book.

> *"Courage doesn't always roar. Sometimes courage*
> *is the quiet voice at the end of the day saying,*
> *'I will try again tomorrow.'"*
>
> —DeHerrmann Hill

STAYING ABREAST OF MT NEWS
AND INDUSTRY TRENDS

If you are beginning your independent medical transcription career with little or no background information, spend some time researching the history of medical transcription, current trends, and what is forecast for the future. You will benefit immediately, and developing good reading and research habits will help you remain professionally competitive in the future.

If you are an active member of AAMT, you will receive the bimonthly *Journal of the American Association for Medical Transcription (JAAMT)*. Health Professions Institute publishes *Perspectives. MT Monthly*, a monthly newsletter by Computer Systems Management contains word lists, new medications, and a variety of articles pertaining to the medical transcription industry.

ROMANCING THE $$$

In the past few years, in order to reduce overhead, there has been an industry trend toward contract services. This is good news for independents because contracting offers increased opportunities for skilled transcriptionists working outside a hospital or medical office setting.

A few years ago large medical transcription services dominated the medical transcription industry. They made huge investments to be on the cutting edge of technology because they realized that health care facilities were finding it increasingly more difficult and less cost effective to maintain in-house transcription departments. With increasing volumes of dictation and lack of physical space to expand, many facilities were contracting part or all of their transcription work to outside services. In many cases, it was not a positive experience. Some services failed to meet commitments for turnaround and transcription quality was poor. In addition, they had their own staffing problems, legal difficulties and so on.

Now the industry is fragmenting, with frequently breaking news of mergers, acquisitions and takeovers. The home-based business movement is definitely changing the marketplace and the future of the medical transcription industry. As information and technology become more affordable to one-person businesses, we are providing the same services as the industry giants, often at a lower cost and with better quality.

Everyone is romancing the client and there is a niche in the marketplace for all. Independent contractors are not capable of servicing 2500 bed facilities, but they are more efficacious for smaller hospitals, physicians, clinics, and hospitals in rural settings. Large services are romancing their clients for total contracts — extended contracts to guarantee their investment in equipment and technology. Some are even offering to place the technology on-site.

Many hospitals are now shifting direction and, with the help of their financial departments, discovering that they can decrease costs while bringing work back "inside." As a result, many hospitals are not renewing contracts with larger services. "If a service can utilize home-based medical transcriptionists, why can't we?" they ask. The answer is, of course, they can! So they are placing their own employees at home or are using independent transcriptionists with excellent results.

Competition is fierce, but there is more than enough work and funding for all skilled transcriptionists. Health care regulators now allow the use of contract services to be included in health care providers' operating expenses. This is good news for independent medical transcriptionists because it means more work is coming our way!

DEFINING YOUR MARKET

Define your market. Do you want to work for hospitals, offices, multispecialty clinics, or a combination of all three? Will you mail, modem or personally transport transcription work? How far are you willing to travel to pick up and deliver work? Remember, depending on the priority of work types, hospital work turnaround times will vary from two-, four-, or six- to twenty-four hours. Offices and clinics are generally more flexible. Turnaround time will also vary, of course, depending on clients' needs. With technology now available through telecommuting, the trend is toward shorter turnaround times, so make sure that you evaluate this factor when defining your market.

YOUR CLIENT BASE

Another key factor in success is determining the number of clients needed to support your business. A good rule of thumb is to follow the old adage: *Do not put all your eggs in one basket.*

A hospital overload account is wonderful, but it can be a fickle market. For instance, the hospital census may decline or a new medical records director may decide to keep all work in-house or switch to a larger service. If you are dependent on that one hospital account, you may suddenly find yourself with no income.

A market mix is much better, perhaps one hospital and two or more small accounts comprised of doctors' offices or clinic transcription. In this way, if one account disappears or declines, you may still have a solid business base and adequate revenues.

ANCILLARY DEPARTMENTS

Another excellent market is hospital ancillary departments, which include specialties such as cardiology, gastroenterology, radiology, pathology, physical therapy, occupational therapy, and emergency rooms. In the past, these ancillary departments relied heavily on the hospital's main medical records department for transcription service, but that is changing.

Recently, there has been a trend toward separating ancillary department work from that of the medical records department, mainly because the primary hospital transcription pool is finding it increasingly difficult to keep up with inpatient work, let alone outpatient services.

MAILING LABELS

Another great marketing tool is mailing labels, which may be ordered from a wide variety of marketing consultant firms. Search online to find multiple mailing-label resource sites.

When ordering, specify market type and target area by zip codes. You will receive lists, on preprinted mailing labels, of hospitals and/or physicians, by specialty if you wish, for a particular area.

NEWSPAPERS

Local newspapers are another good resource. Hospitals, clinics, and physicians often advertise their services in space ads. Review classified "help wanted" ads for transcription positions, and don't overlook any opportunity. Even if the advertisement is for an in-house position, consider interviewing for it. You may convince the interviewer to work with you instead. Stress the advantages of an outside service over a full-time or part-time employee, including dollars saved on benefits packages, vacations, sick leave, and holidays. Tell the prospective client that studies have been done that show it costs an employer between 45-75 cents a line to hire an in-house employee. Hospitals, clinics and physicians almost always respond to new ways to cut operating expenses.

PERSONAL ADVERTISING

There are many ways to reach your market, including business brochures, cold calling, fliers, and letters. You can network in elevators, parking lots, hospitals, office buildings, emergency rooms, and by word of mouth (doctor to doctor). You can advertise in the yellow pages, local newspapers, trade newsletters and journals, as well as local county medical society newsletters for a very nominal fee. The Internet offers great exposure. Many MTs are regularly tapping into resources by surfing the Net. Some are even publishing their own webpages.

THE BOTTOM LINE — OBTAINING CLIENTS

Medical transcription is a multibillion dollar industry and the competition, big or small, can be fierce. Read and learn EVERYTHING you can about marketing because if you are to succeed professionally, YOU MUST MARKET YOUR GOODS AND SERVICES. If you don't, your business will fail. Marketing should become second nature to you, and if it doesn't, seek help from someone skilled in marketing.

Be bold in promoting your transcription service. "Press the flesh" as often as you can. Tell everyone you ever knew or come into contact with that you are in business and would appreciate their business and/or referrals. Pass out your business cards and brochures as though your life depended on it . . . and when they're gone, order more. Business cards do you no good unless someone sees them. Plaster your fliers on every bulletin board you can find.

Consider giving clients a packet containing information on charges, turnaround, delivery, stat work, availability of services beyond basic transcription (e.g., DTP, fax, phone-in or modem capabilities, samples of reports and references).

The key word here is BENEFITS. Convince the client that the services you are providing are BENEFITS to them. The more BENEFITS you offer customers, the more work you're likely to get.

When approaching a potential client for the first time, present a personally addressed letter (not a form letter). Follow up with a phone call, and if there are no available openings, offer to fill in on an as-needed basis during employee vacations, holidays or other absences.

When soliciting new business, some transcriptionists offer to transcribe a tape of dictation or a few reports at no charge to demonstrate the quality of their work. This can be effective because the client feels no obligation to commit to using your service. HOWEVER, don't make the mistake one transcriptionist made. At the start of her independent career, she sent out a flier offering *one week of free transcription*. She got takers — absolutely! They bombarded her with tapes of transcription. Unfortunately, she could not complete the work, and had to return some tapes. It was not a good beginning for her business.

Don't be overly generous to clients even though you are anxious to get your business started. Clients may take advantage of your free offer and then bid you farewell. A large transcription service once offered a month's free transcription to a large hospital, hoping to impress the medical facility with quality transcription produced in a 24-hour turnaround time, which would result in a substantial transcription contract. The hospital bombarded the service with work. The transcription service hired numerous IMTs to service the account, and everyone was happy because they were working. Well, when the thirty days ended, the hospital said thanks and good-bye to the service, the service had no more work for the IMTs, and that was that.

This marketing tactic proved to be financially devastating for the service. It worked for 30 days free but still had to pay its IMTs and cover its overhead. The service could not pay its IMTs as agreed and everyone suffered from the trickle-down effect . . . except for the hospital, which came out smelling like a rose!

MARKETING YOUR SPECIALTY

If you have special knowledge in a certain area, that is the area you should promote. After all, that is where you "shine" and will "outshine" your competition.

BUSINESS CARDS

Do you have a business card? How effective is it? How do people react when they look at the business card you hand them? Do they simply put your card in their pocket or do they give it a second glance? If the latter is true, you have probably made a positive impression according to Paul and Sarah Edwards, authors of "Your Card: A Marketing Tool," which appeared in *Home Office Computing Magazine*.

The Edwardses, leading authorities on working from home, recommend reviewing business cards in your Rolodex and selecting those that stand out. What attracts you to them? How does yours compare? An effective business card is far more than a piece of paper containing your name, address, and phone number. It is a marketing tool that can serve several purposes. Think of your business card as a mini-billboard, a brochure, or an advertisement . . . even an order form.

There are a number of online desktop services that design and produce business cards. Business Cards, Etc. (BCE) produces full-color business cards and stationary personalized to meet your specific business needs.

- **Business Cards, Etc. (BCE)**
  www.bcardsetc.homestead.com.

- **Coordinate your business card, letterhead and stationery.**

  For continuity, use the same typeface and colors on all your print communications. The investment you make in designing a consistent visual image for your business will return to you in referrals.

  Select a readable typeface that is not complicated or ornate. A business card is small, so use no more than two typefaces. Create variety with sizing, boldface type, and spacing. Avoid printing with only capital letters, which makes your card less readable and detracts from a quality image. And don't crowd the card with type.

- **Make sure your card talks to your market.**

  What do potential clients expect from a business like yours? The creative and unusual? Quiet elegance and professionalism? Tried, true, and trusted? Design your card to meet the expectations of your target market.

Avoid cartoon characters, cute creatures, and hearts and flowers. They're unlikely to convey your professional image.

• **Cover the basics.**

Your business card should contain the name of your business, your name (if different from the business), title, and your phone number(s). Your business card will probably also display your address (optional) and logo. If you don't have a logo for your company, consider using the logo of your trade to enhance your credibility (e.g., a computer screen, dictating unit, or the medical caduceus).

NOTE

The logo for the American Association for Medical Transcription is the sole property of AAMT and therefore, cannot be used on stationery or business cards.

Make sure your phone number stands out prominently.

• **Be open to creative alternatives.**

Instead of simply using a standard business card, consider a card that fits a Rolodex. Or use a double-size card folded in half. Double-size cards become mini-brochures. Standard business information appears on the front; additional benefits and information appear inside. On the down side, bear in mind that such cards may be difficult to carry.

• **Add color.**

An additional color, which can make your card stand out, may add only $15 to $20 to your printing bill, depending on the color. If your budget simply won't allow two colors of ink, select a single color in addition to black, and use it creatively. Alternatively, choose a card stock other than white. Consider various textures to complement your image — high gloss, matte, and rag for example. Each creates a different impression.

- **Make the most of your business cards.**

   Don't let them sit in your office. Carry them with you at all times and give them to as many people as possible. Remember, as you distribute your business cards to new contacts, they will give you their business cards in return, resulting in excellent leads that you can follow up by phone or mail.

   If you want advice about your business card ideas or need help designing your business card, contact a professional. Local printers are generally more than happy to advise potential customers, and graphic artists are readily available for design work. To locate skilled professionals, check the yellow pages of your telephone directory or get a recommendation from an associate.

THE BUSINESS ADDRESS

A business address communicates respectability, substance, and permanence. If you are home-based, you may be hesitant to publicize your home address for safety and personal reasons. You are not required by law to show your address on your business cards; however, most states do require that you show a street address on your business stationery. If you are hesitant to advertise where you live, consider renting a post office box for business mail or better yet, use a mail-receiving service like MAIL BOXES ETC®, which in our opinion offers service that is superior to that of the U.S. postal system. And don't forget, rental of either a public or a private postal box is a tax-deductible business expense.

At the time of this writing under current California law, independent workers are required to list a physical address for their businesses. Noncompliance carries a $2500 fine and a maximum six-month jail sentence for those not disclosing their home address when using the word "suite" as their box return address. As with anything else, do your homework before taking any action, and find out what the laws are in your state.

THE COVER LETTER

Cover letters should accompany material you send or hand deliver to others. These letters should be brief and to the point, courteous, attractive, and accurate. The main purpose of a cover letter is to introduce yourself and provide basic information about you and your service. Include a description of any additional material you are enclosing or attaching. Request some action on the part of the letter's recipient — review of material provided, acceptance of your planned telephone call, scheduling an interview with you.

THE RESUME

Prepare and maintain an updated resume of your work experience. It will be helpful in promoting your service, especially if the content is professionally done. You can hire a professional resume writer to work with you or prepare the resume yourself, using resume-writing reference books that are available at bookstores and public libraries. Attach the resume to your flier, enclose it in packets of materials, or carry it with you to present on interviews.

FLIERS

Paul and Sarah Edwards point out that a flier is one of the easiest and least expensive advertising methods. Make it clever, to immediately capture the reader's attention, but don't make it too flowery or cute. Bunnies, kittens, or bridal bouquets may get immediate attention but will probably create a less-than-professional impression of your business!

Desktop publishing firms, and some printers who offer desktop design services, can be great help in creating a professional looking flier. Fees will be approximately $25-$35 an hour for the setup, a worthwhile expenditure if you are not able to design your own flier.

In your flier, state your objectives, the services you offer, and your background in medical transcription. At this point it is not necessary to quote a price and, in fact, we recommend against it. Pricing should be presented only after discussing the account with the client.

After you have created the flier, take it to a print shop (unless, of course, you are already working directly with a printer) and have it photocopied, preferably on colored paper. Colored paper costs a little more, but it generates more interest and creates a longer lasting impression. Select a color that coordinates with your business cards and, for a dynamic visual impact, add matching colored envelopes.

Be sure to paper clip or staple a business card to each flier before mailing. This will ensure that either one or the other is kept by the client for future reference. If your flier is really impressive, the client may keep one and pass the other on to a friend!

On the following page is a sample of a successful flier.

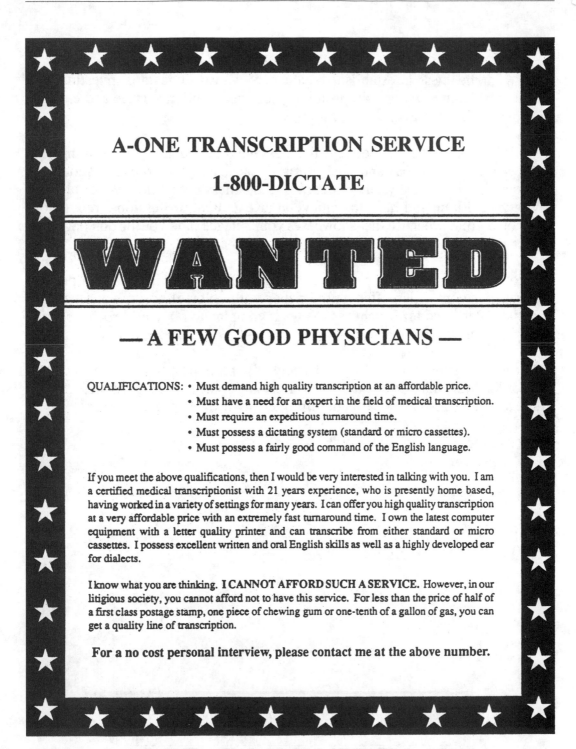

A-ONE TRANSCRIPTION SERVICE

1-800-DICTATE

WANTED

— A FEW GOOD PHYSICIANS —

QUALIFICATIONS: • Must demand high quality transcription at an affordable price.
- Must have a need for an expert in the field of medical transcription.
- Must require an expeditious turnaround time.
- Must possess a dictating system (standard or micro cassettes).
- Must possess a fairly good command of the English language.

If you meet the above qualifications, then I would be very interested in talking with you. I am a certified medical transcriptionist with 21 years experience, who is presently home based, having worked in a variety of settings for many years. I can offer you high quality transcription at a very affordable price with an extremely fast turnaround time. I own the latest computer equipment with a letter quality printer and can transcribe from either standard or micro cassettes. I possess excellent written and oral English skills as well as a highly developed ear for dialects.

I know what you are thinking. **I CANNOT AFFORD SUCH A SERVICE.** However, in our litigious society, you cannot afford not to have this service. For less than the price of half of a first class postage stamp, one piece of chewing gum or one-tenth of a gallon of gas, you can get a quality line of transcription.

For a no cost personal interview, please contact me at the above number.

BROCHURES

After your business is established, you may want to consider investing in a business brochure, which will promote your transcription service and enhance your professional image.

A well-designed brochure conveys the message that you and your transcription service are professional and successful — facts that are true and should be publicized. Don't be shy when it comes to business promotion. After all, you have worked long and hard to achieve your excellent professional reputation. Develop a great brochure that showcases your service, and you'll soon have new clients.

Use colored paper for extra panache, especially if you don't have a color printer. Many paper companies offer trifold paper with colorful borders and patterns especially designed for brochures. Note: If you plan to fax your brochure, stick with plain white paper.

Office and art supply stores stock a variety of paper types. In addition, specialty mail-order companies offer extensive variety and some real bargains. And, you'll find even more resources for paper products by browsing the Internet.

For a catalog call these suppliers:

- **Quill**
  800-789-5813

- **PaperDirect**
  800-272-7377

- **Queblo**
  800-523-9080

- **Idea Art**
  800-433-2278

> *"It is a good idea to send out fliers and brochures every four to six months."*

It is not necessary to design a complicated brochure. Your brochure can be as simple as an 8½" x 11" folded sheet of paper. By folding it twice, as you would a letter, then turning it upright so it opens like a book, you have the beginnings of a brochure.

On the outside, write a headline that stands out and gets the attention of the client. Immediately inside, elaborate on the headline's promise or claim. Then elaborate further about the benefits of your services in the remaining brochure space.

The overall look of your brochure is the key to making a good impression. Here are some ideas to help:

- Have the descriptive copy typeset in a fairly large size.

- Break up the copy with subheads.

- Add something unexpected visually. Avoid broad or slapstick humor, which may give the impression you are not serious or professional.

- The back of the brochure is a good place for a business biography or testimonials from satisfied clients. Briefly describe how your business began, how it has succeeded, and its current status. Include your professional affiliations (e.g., AAMT, state/regional association or local chapter of AAMT), any offices held past and present, any special schooling that you have received, etc.

- Add substance to your brochure by printing it on heavier paper stock than you would normally use for a flier.

Enclose your business card with the brochure. One or the other will generally be filed for future reference.

Don't be disappointed if after sending out a flier or brochure, your telephone doesn't ring off the hook. You may receive immediate responses, but prospective clients may not call for a few days or weeks. It isn't uncommon to receive calls even two years later.

It is a good idea to send out fliers and brochures every four to six months to ensure a steady work flow. As mentioned earlier, accounts will come and go for various reasons, and it is important to keep your name and business fresh in the minds of prospective clients.

MARKETING THROUGH NETWORKING

Networking with other transcriptionists offers excellent opportunities to share information and services and increase professional exposure.

As a member of your local AAMT chapter, you will be able to promote your business and word-of-mouth referrals will be readily passed on. At chapter meetings, announcements are made about who and where transcriptionists are needed. Don't be shy or hesitate to pass out your business cards at meetings, and do send thank-you notes for referrals. That personal touch showing your appreciation is important.

We recommend donating door prizes in your business name at appropriate professional functions. The door prizes will cost you very little, association members will remember you positively, and you'll discover that it's personally rewarding.

ADVERTISING IN TRADE PUBLICATIONS

Local chapters of AAMT offer business-card-size advertising space in their newsletters for as little as $15-$20 an issue. This is a cost-effective way to promote your business while contributing to your local professional newsletter. Consider advertising in other local publications and trade newsletters in your area. Look into the possibility of advertising in your local medical society bulletin, newsletter or physician directory. Don't forget the Internet!

Remember, marketing is an ongoing process. Successful entrepreneurs never stop promoting their business.

MARKETING THROUGH THE CHAMBER OF COMMERCE

Membership in your local chamber of commerce is another excellent way to market services. Through chamber activities, and with chamber support, your business will increase.

You will enjoy networking with men and women in a wide variety of businesses. These business people are dedicated to maintaining a strong economic base in their community, and they actively promote local businesses.

Medical doctors, chiropractors, podiatrists, and many other health care professionals are active in chambers of commerce, offering you added opportunities for one-on-one contact, professional recognition, and word-of-mouth promotion.

As a participant in chamber activities, you and your business will receive publicity in local media, and you will also receive coverage in the chamber newsletter.

WORD-OF-MOUTH REFERRALS

Word-of-mouth referrals are an excellent source of new business. Doctors talk to one another in elevators, operating rooms, and at business functions. If they have been provided with your business card, they can refer you to fellow physicians.

COLD CALLING FOR THE SELF-CONFIDENT

For those of you who are self-assured and assertive, cold calling may generate new clients. Spontaneous or semi-spontaneous introductions, when managed with a professional demeanor in a courteous manner, can be very effective. If you are energetic and have a spirit of adventure, give it a try.

Before setting out, verify that there are no local restrictions on cold calling, which is prohibited in some cities. And even if cold calling is legally permitted in an area, it may not be allowed in specific buildings.

When cold calling and meeting prospective clients, be positive about yourself and the transcription service you offer. Point out the exceptional qualities of your service and your skills, from which the client will, of course, benefit.

However, let us interject a word of warning at this point. Do not promise the moon to prospective clients! A foot in the door and enthusiastic self-promotion can be a heady experience. You may be tempted to offer more or better service than you can realistically provide. Don't do it! Know yourself and know your limits! Both you and your clients will be better served when you are able to follow through on professional commitments.

ARMED WITH BUSINESS CARD AND FLIER

Brief visits to medical offices and one-on-one contact with front-desk receptionists is an effective way to market your service. Select an appropriate medical building and go from office to office armed with your business flier and business card. Some transcriptionists also leave note pads and/or pens imprinted with their business name, logo, and telephone number. Introduce yourself to the receptionist and leave the material for later review. You may experience some rejection, but nine times out of ten the material will be accepted with a smile.

MANAGING "NO, THANK YOU"

Your service may be excellent and your promotion superb, but some professional contacts will say, "Thanks, but no thanks." Don't take it personally or let it get you down. Rejection happens. It's part of the keyboard of life! We can assure you that clients will come your way if you are persistent. In fact, the very next person you call on may be a new customer.

FIRST IMPRESSIONS LINGER LONGEST

"You don't get a second chance to make a first impression."
—Will Rogers

Long ago, humorist Will Rogers said, "You don't get a second chance to make a first impression." The statement is as true today as it was then. Your initial impact on business contacts will leave a lasting impression, so make your initial impact magnificent.

Before you open your mouth, the person standing before you will quickly review your appearance and demeanor, and make an instantaneous value judgment based on what he or she sees. You may be exceptionally competent, capable, intelligent, educated, and efficient, but if you don't look like a professional, your credibility will suffer.

When meeting a client for the first time, look as professional as possible. Basic squeaky-clean guidelines are a given, of course — face, hair, hands, nails, clothes, shoes. Leave the sweats and shorts at home. It isn't necessary to dress as though you are attending an afternoon tea at the Beverly Hills Hotel, but do dress for success. If you look professional and behave in a professional manner, you will generally be treated as a professional.

INFORMATIONAL PACKETS

Plan ahead. Well before a scheduled meeting, prepare and organize all appropriate materials in a neat packet . . . or several packets if you are scheduled for several interviews. The interviewer will be impressed with your organization and you won't be embarrassed by last minute fumbling . . . or missing information.

THE INTERVIEW

Be prepared for interviews. Have your resume up-to-date and readily available, as well as personal references attesting to your competence and skills. Some transcriptionists also provide a ready-to-sign contract, which demonstrates professional forethought and commitment.

Be ready to provide specific facts about your service to clients who ask for information regarding schedules, turnaround-time, and availability to clients who request this information. Give forethought to guarantees of service and confidentiality. Review your deadline procedures and backup systems for personal emergencies.

Be prepared to answer questions about your office and its location, type of equipment you use, your proposed method of operation, line counts, margin widths, type styles, quality assurance, and other facets of medical transcription.

When speaking, be as concise as possible, clearly explaining your service and how it will benefit the client. Point out areas of flexibility and offer to tailor your service whenever possible to meet the client's needs.

If the interview goes well and you negotiate a contract, state your terms succinctly and logically at the outset. Carefully explain your fees, billing dates, payment schedules, and other important business factors to avoid confusion later.

In an interview, **do not answer statements**. If a prospective client states that using an outside service is expensive, don't try to convince her otherwise. Smile pleasantly and allow her to express her opinion.

Do not criticize or belittle your competitors! If a prospect baits you by praising your competitor, do not respond with a laundry list of your competitor's flaws or snidely point out that if the competitor was actually so fantastic, the interviewer would already be using that service! Instead, respond with a relaxed smile and "Hmmm," "Very interesting," "Ah, yes," or another ambiguous comment.

If you are familiar with your competitor's service and are asked a specific question about it, respond as honestly and as directly as possible, but phrase your response so the final emphasis is on the excellence and benefits of **your** service. Emphasize **your** experience, training, background, continuing education, and awards you have received.

If a prospective client asks about your competitor's credentials or urges you to corroborate negative rumors, simply reply that you cannot speak for your competitor's credentials or personal life. And then get back to business.

Try to maintain control of the interview from opening formalities to final farewells, moving the meeting along with pleasant efficiency as you systematically explain your service program, answer questions, and conclude the meeting. Your professional position will be stronger if **you** bring the interview to an appropriate conclusion and avoid an unexpected or abrupt ending initiated by the interviewer.

When you have concluded your presentation, ask if there are any further questions. If not, thank the interviewer for meeting with you and indicate that you will look forward to hearing from her or him in the future, at which time you will be happy to answer any additional questions. That's it! End of interview!

DO NOT BEG FOR BUSINESS

Do not say, "Let's draw up a contract" or "Won't you please try my service on a short-term basis?" Do not beg for work or offer bargain prices. Hold your head high and exit.

You are a professional medical transcriptionist and professionals adhere to standards of excellence. Even if this is your first client prospect, it is important to maintain and communicate an aura of professionalism and independence. Although your service may not yet have reached the pinnacle of success, it will eventually. Believe it, work for it, and it will happen. Don't settle for anything less. Communicate your future success now!

ADVERTISING

There are different approaches to marketing, but the most efficient and economical are mailings and handouts. Utilizing the information you gathered from the yellow pages and various reference lists, mail your fliers, brochures or cover letter with your business card attached.

Focus on a few clinics each week, perhaps ten, and build a solid base from there. Don't be tempted to market more widely, to 50 or 100, even though you feel secure in your skills and are eager for accounts. Trying to manage too much too soon can result in overwhelming problems and possible business failure.

It's important to direct your mailings to medical record/transcription supervisors, office managers, or medical transcription supervisors in specific departments. Be sure you correctly identify the department and contact person on your dispatch or it may never reach the intended destination. It may end up in health care limbo!

After a week or so, follow up your mailing with a phone call. Introduce yourself, verify that you are not interrupting your contact's work (in which case you offer to call at a more convenient time), and ask if your announcement was received. If not, indicate that you will send another packet and call again soon. If the mailing was received, continue your conversation.

Request an appointment, at the supervisor's convenience, to discuss your services. If the facility currently has no need for your services, encourage the supervisor to keep your card on file for future reference.

Conveying a positive and professional demeanor on the telephone is not easy, especially when you are feeling rejected, but it's vitally important. Don't allow yourself to label the negative response as "a turndown," when in fact it is only "a turning aside." The supervisor didn't say, "No." She merely said, "Not now." Continue to radiate enthusiasm and energy, and you can be sure your business card will go in her file.

PUBLIC RELATIONS

Develop rapport with lead and other transcriptionists and office managers at medical facilities. Often, the in-house staff may initially feel intimidated by you or they may even feel jealous because of the income disparity between independents and in-house medical transcriptionists. Always maintain a positive and friendly attitude, even though at first it may seem that your friendliness is not being returned.

You may discover that because of their resentment toward you, in-house medical transcriptionists may be inclined to route sloppy work they don't want to do to you and other independent transcriptionists. Our recommendation is, do it! Once you do the "slop" you will become very valuable to those in-house people, and their attitudes will change because they know that they can depend on you. Yes, learn to do slop. Through it you'll "earn your stripes," increase and diversify your skills, and find all other transcription easier.

MAINTAINING A CLIENT BASE WITH CREATIVE FOLLOW-UP

In any service-oriented business, finding and keeping clients is an ongoing challenge. Having an established business doesn't mean that you can take a rest from pursuing and nurturing new accounts. Maintaining a solid client base requires follow-up and communication. There are various ways to do this including thank you notes, dependable service, prompt delivery of completed work, phone calls, personal visits, and other courtesies tailored to individual clients.

Call and make sure customers are satisfied with your services. Encourage comments and suggestions for transcription improvement, then respond positively and actively.

The cumulative effect of everything you say and do affects your clients' perceptions of you and your business, ultimately determining whether or not they continue with your service and refer others to you.

Whenever there is client contact, there should be regular, ongoing follow up. This demonstrates to clients that you are concerned about their business needs, not just the account income. Your excellent service and personalized care will make your clients happy; and happy clients are usually loyal clients.

FOLLOW-UP CHECK LIST

- Budget time for follow-up and make it a regular habit.

- Use 3 x 5 cards or a software program to maintain a client and prospective client database. Be sure to list business name, contact person, address, phone, fax, and e-mail address if available.

- Remember to send thank-you notes to clients after the first meeting. The simple courtesy will be long remembered.

- Contact new clients five days after beginning the service to ask if they have any questions or concerns. This establishes a strong communication link and helps resolve problems or potential problems.

- Always deliver your work as promised. If for some unforeseen reason the delivery schedule cannot be met, contact the client immediately, apologize, and explain the reasons for the delay. Specify the exact time the work will be delivered and make every effort to meet that goal.

- Always be honest. Clients respect a transcriptionist who has integrity. Don't give creative excuses for delays or other business problems. "Computer trouble," "stuck in traffic," "sick kids," and "brownout" work only so many times before the frustrated client stops calling for transcription and calls it quits instead.

- Communicate promptly. Some days will be disastrous to your work schedule, but don't keep your clients pacing back and forth waiting for work that should have been delivered hours earlier. Call your clients as soon as possible about any significant delay or change in schedule.

- Consider taking clients out to lunch or giving them gifts occasionally. These professional courtesies are tax deductible business expenses, so keep your receipts.

- Don't forget to follow up. Keep a tickler file, mark your calendar with colored pens, or use sticky notes to flag dates and people to contact.

  On the following page is a list of prospective clients to consider when marketing your medical transcription services.

A LIST OF PROSPECTIVE CLIENTS

Medical Doctors/Specialists
Cardiologists
Internists
Neurologists
Radiologists
Ear, Nose and Throat Doctors
Dental Clinics
Walk-In Clinics
Urgi-/Surgi-Centers
Word Processing Services
Hospitals Extended Care
Chemical Dependence Facilities
Urgent Care Clinics
Rehabilitation Centers
Military Installations
Imaging Facilities
Mental Health Facilities/State Hospitals
Cardiopulmonary Rehabilitation Centers
Clinical Psychologists/Counselors
Workers Compensation Clinic
Veterans Facilities
Pediatricians
Dentists
Osteopaths
Health Centers
Insurance Adjusters
Disability Offices
Podiatrists
Radiology/Medical Imaging Facilities
Workers Compensation Clinic
Ophthalmologists
Immunologists
Pathologists

Orthopedists
Court Reporters
Family Practitioners
Surgeons
OB/GYN
Correctional Facilities
Industrial Medicine
Ambulatory Care Clinics
Pathology Laboratories
Other Transcription Services
Hospitals Acute Care
Physical Therapy Clinics
Group Medical Clinics
Clinical Laboratories
Teaching Universities
Urologists
Oncologists
Neurosurgeons
Plastic Surgeons
Pulmonologists
Veterinary Clinics
Psychiatrists
Veterinarians
Oral Surgeons
Insurance Agencies
Legal Offices
Surgical Centers
Chiropractors
Private Investigators
Authors
Gastroenterologists

Business Ethics

"Character isn't inherited. One builds it daily
by the way one thinks and acts,
thought by thought, action by action."

—Helen Gahagan Douglas

An ethical person is one who lives by a set of principles of right conduct, that is, a system of moral values. These principles of right and wrong serve as guides and help the individual make decisions that will have positive impacts on his or her life and on the lives of others. In the same manner within professions, ethical rules or standards govern the conduct of each profession and its members.

MEDICAL RECORD CONFIDENTIALITY

Confidentiality of the medical record and protecting patient privacy has long been a major health care principle. In today's health care world, medical record confidentiality continues to be vitally important because of ethical, medical, social and legal implications.

Medical transcriptionists must be responsible in transcribing accurate medical records and maintaining patient confidentiality regarding those records. What is input into today's record will become a permanent part of the patient's chart, and the code of medical ethics must be upheld. If this is not done, the patient's right to confidentiality has been violated.

A patient's trust in the physician, a factor that is important to the patient's physical and emotional well-being, is directly affected by all personnel involved in that patient's care. Medical transcriptionists, because of our relationship with patient records, are in a particularly sensitive position. In the course of our work, we learn myriad intimate details about patients — more details than some members of the hands-on health care team learn. It is our responsibility to respect and protect that knowledge because of its privileged nature and its importance to patients.

AAMT CODE OF ETHICS

The American Association for Medical Transcription has adopted a strict code of ethics and, like other health care professionals, medical transcriptionists conduct their business in accordance with this medical/legal code. Noncompliance with this code of ethics can result in loss of professional credibility, loss of clients, and litigation.

> "Protect the privacy and confidentiality of the individual medical record to avoid disclosure of personally identifiable medical and social information and professional medical judgments."
>
> - Point 9, Code of Ethics
> American Association for Medical Transcription

Hospital accounts may require that you sign a nondisclosure agreement, which in effect states that if the confidentiality of a report is violated, you or your service will be terminated immediately. See a generic copy of a nondisclosure statement at the end of this chapter.

By California law, all health care professionals are required to maintain confidentiality of patients' personal and medical records. Legally, discussion of medical record information is allowed only in "legally privileged" medical/

legal situations. Casual conversation with family and/or friends about a patient's condition is not legal.

The patient is *". . . to be assured confidential treatment of personal and medical records . . ."*

-72527 Administrative Code, Section 9

To adequately ensure confidentiality of the patient record within the medical transcription office, purchase a paper shredder. Shredders range in price from $49 to as high as several hundred dollars. Nothing should be put into your wastebasket that contains any identifying information (i.e., patient name, age, address, etc.). All documents should be shredded so patients' rights are protected and you are not at risk for a lawsuit.

Keep your lips sealed where patient information is concerned. Derogatory comments about the patient — or even idle conversation you consider harmless — could be interpreted as slanderous if it gets back to the patient. And if his attorney is convinced that your comments have indeed resulted in "defamation of character," you may be sued.

*"**Slander** is a false and unprivileged publication, orally uttered . . ."* which results in *"injuries"* to the patient *"in respect to his office, profession, trade or business . . ."* or *". . . which, by natural consequence, causes actual damage."*

-46 Civil Code

Written communication regarding patient medical records, except for legally privileged situations, is also illegal if it results in harm to reputation or income. In this case, the injured patient may sue you for libel.

*"**Libel** . . . exposes any person to hatred, contempt, ridicule, or obloquy, or which causes him to be shunned or avoided, or which has a tendency to injure him in his occupation . . ."*

-44 Civil Code

UNETHICAL TRANSCRIPTIONISTS

There are no ethical shortcuts through the forest of professional medical transcription. Those who are lured along the path of unethical practices usually regret their action sooner or later. UTs (unethical transcriptionists), who do not adhere to generally accepted transcription profession standards, face a number of risks.

Unethical transcriptionists who fail to maintain confidentiality of the medical record or refuse to comply with other quality assurance guidelines that result in patient injury may face legal action. Even if they are not sued, they risk losing their professional reputation, the friendship of their work associates, and their livelihood. The ethical breach will be recognized by peers, who will not sanction the unethical behavior nor support this transcriptionist professionally.

Unethical behavior can have far-reaching effects. Some UTs attempt to build their businesses "the quick and easy way," by "stealing" accounts from other transcriptionists. Eventually, the truth catches up with them and they lose all professional credibility, along with all their purloined accounts. Unfortunately, innocent individuals may be hurt in the process. Patients, clients and other transcriptionists may be harmed, too.

Although most transcriptionists are ethical, public reports about even one unethical transcriptionist can damage the credibility of ethical transcriptionists, especially if they are self-employed. Be a professional. Honor the patient's right to privacy and the ethics of the American Association for Medical Transcription. You will never regret it.

NONDISCLOSURE AGREEMENT (SAMPLE)

By signing this Nondisclosure Agreement, I indicate my understanding that:

Patients, physicians and other health care providers furnish confidential information to obtain or carry out medical services, and medical service information and records are confidential.

Patients depend on the providers of medical services to keep patient information confidential. The provider's reputation depends on this confidentiality.

If medical information has been used or disclosed inappropriately, patients or providers who have suffered loss or injury may seek legal action to recover damages from the person who used or disclosed the information. Specific violations of patient confidentiality resulting in economic loss or personal injury to a patient may be punishable by law.

Any breach of confidentiality will be considered serious and subject to investigation and possible discipline, including immediate termination of services.

Therefore, as a contract service provider, I agree that I will not at any time:

1. Disclose services given or information about patients.

2. Allow anyone else to examine or copy any records or documents having to do with patients, physicians, or other health care providers and services.

_____   _____

Independent Contractor   Date

Business Operations

" . . . it either is or ought to be evident to everyone
that business has to prosper before anybody
can get any benefit from it. "

—Theodore Roosevelt

You decided to become an independent medical transcriptionist and have completed your homework. You have spent a great deal of time and energy accumulating information that will prove invaluable not only now, but in the future.

Now you must organize your business and make that organized system work for you.

GETTING STARTED —
STUDYING THE FACTS AND ORGANIZING

You now have at your fingertips a base of information that will be the foundation of your business. You have files on medical facilities available for your marketing, who and where your competition is, what transcription methods are being used in your area and in the transcription profession at large, and you have determined your target market as you review the following information.

- Set up specific reference files for the clinic, hospital, and physician reference lists you have obtained.

- Provide space for any journals or publications you may subscribe to for quick and easy reference.

- Set up a file (or files) of information you may have on other services in your area.

- Set up a "people" file in which you gather names, addresses, and notes on people you meet and may wish to contact in the future.

All of the above files, and others you may need in the future, can easily be updated as your business progresses.

By this time you have determined your specific market. You are ready for the next step.

CHOOSING A BUSINESS NAME

It is perfectly all right to name the business after yourself (e.g., Ima Mazing Medical Transcription Service). For you more creative people, let your imagination take charge. A business name, however, should be selected with great care. Here are some key guidelines to follow:

- Choose a name that is pleasant and easy to pronounce. If your client regurgitates your name every time it is mentioned, it is not likely to be repeated and people will not hear about your business.

- Choose a name that will do a little advertising for you, telling people what you do (e.g., Medi-Scribe, Healthline).

- Choose a name that will not severely limit you, a name that will stand up to the passage of time.

> *"A business name should be selected with great care. It should stand up to the passage of time and do a little advertising for you along the way."*

BUILDING A BIG IMAGE

Most home-based businesses are relatively small operations — but the smart ones don't advertise it or think of themselves as small. If you think small you'll be perceived as small, and chances are your results will be small. A major factor in establishing your professional image is your business name. In general, names should sound professional and tell something about the company. Avoid using the word "enterprises" as this is a name that has become synonymous with an amateur.

LEGALIZING THE NAME

If you select a name for your business other than your own, you should file a Fictitious Name Statement, called a DBA (Doing Business As).

There are several ways to handle this. The first and easiest is to go to your local newspaper and file a Fictitious Name Statement with them. They will then record the information with the city or county clerk's office and publish the DBA in their newspaper for the period of time required by law. Shop around for the cheapest newspaper prices as some newspapers charge $50; others, $100 or more.

You may go to your city hall or county clerk's office and review the alphabetical list of registered fictitious names. If you live in a small city and have no plans to expand, you may not need to search further.

However, if you live in a large city and plan to expand, consider utilizing the services of companies that specialize in name searches. Using computer data banks, they will review the millions of registered fictitious names in the United States.

If you live in a large urban area, you may discover your first, second and perhaps even third business-name choices are already registered.

You may wish to contact the person who owns the business name and find out if the business is still in existence. If it isn't, and if the owner of the name consents, an Abandonment of Fictitious Name Statement can be filed, whereby the previous owner gives up all rights to the name. You can then simultaneously file a Fictitious Name Statement for the name.

The Abandonment of Fictitious Name Statement procedures are identical to the Fictitious Name Statement procedures, including the requirement to publish the statement in the newspaper. The former owner will probably ask you to pay the cost of filing the statement of abandonment and may even want you to pay a fee for abandonment.

Avoid choosing a business name that is already in use by an out-of-county or out-of-state business. Corporations are usually granted exclusive statewide use of a business name, assuming they were the first in the state to choose the name.

Your state's secretary of state maintains a list of business names claimed by in-state corporations and by out-of-state corporations licensed to do business in your state. Check your state website for a list of registered and trademarked business names and products. Contact your state's secretary of state to determine if your proposed business name will conflict with one already in use.

An even greater potential problem involves federal trademarks of business names and products. Most large and even some very small businesses obtain trademarks from the U.S. Patent and Trademark Office. Trademark law basically states that a business with a federally registered trademark sometimes has exclusive use of that name throughout the United States.

Public libraries usually have a copy of the current *Federal Trademark Register*, in which you can look up your proposed business name. If you discover that it is the same as, or very similar to, a trademarked name, you may avoid future problems by not using that name.

What happens if you start your business and discover later that some other business has prior claim to your business name? You may receive a letter from an attorney telling you that you are in violation of the law and that you must cease using that business name or they will sue you.

If you receive such a letter and believe you were not in violation of the law, you must then decide whether or not to fight for your business name in court, which can be an incredibly expensive and time-consuming process.

Another way to avoid infringing on someone else's business trademark is to check your local telephone directories and review national trade directories for your type of business. Trademark or no trademark, avoid a business name already in use.

Once again, if you use your own personal name for your transcription service, you are not required to file a Fictitious Name Statement.

In summary, do your homework before selecting a business name to minimize any future liability. Be bold, brave, and daring when selecting a name, but don't be too cute. "Frenetic Fingertips" may be a delightfully creative name for a medical transcription service, but it does not promote a very professional image.

LICENSES AND PERMITS

Studies show that among self-employed individuals, 95% of those who succeed in business have obtained business licenses. Entrepreneurial consultants are not surprised by this pattern. They believe that obtaining a business license is a primary indicator of the commitment and planning necessary for career success.

In California, you will probably be required by town, county, or state to have a business license. However, some rural areas are excluded from this requirement. Required or not, a business license may be helpful to you. Many banks will not open a business account without verification of licensing and, in addition, operating a business without a required license can result in fines and business closure.

The first step in acquiring your business license is to investigate your city and county codes and zoning restrictions. If you are in a residential neighborhood there may be stricter policies than in commercial zones. Check on rules and regulations at the zoning department at your city hall or county administration office.

If you live in a small town, you may only need to go to the city hall, fill out a request to operate a home-based personal service and obtain a business license. This license must be renewed each year.

On the application, you will probably be asked whether or not your business operation will create additional pedestrian/auto traffic. If yours is a personal service in which you provide pick up and delivery with no clients coming in and out, your business should easily meet legal requirements. On the other hand, if your business will increase traffic, you may face restrictions. Standards vary so check with your city, county, or state on local zoning regulations before opening your doors to business.

When processing your business license, double check your assigned business classification and the fee rate. Most city clerks do not understand the work of a medical transcriptionist so they may classify you incorrectly and charge you an excessive license fee. We have found that business license fees generally average $50 to $75. If you are charged over that amount, don't hesitate to question the licensing clerk.

INCORPORATION

If you are considering incorporating your business, investigate the costs in your state or region. Attorneys' fees for incorporation vary, but many attorneys discount their legal fees in hopes it will generate future business.

The incorporation fees you are charged should include all filing fees, a corporation kit with a seal and a set of bylaws, and at least two hours of consultation time with your attorney, during which you can discuss your business and ask questions. You will receive a corporation tax ID number and in some cases, a DBA (Doing Business As) certificate if the corporation will be conducting business in a name other than its corporate name.

Some lawyers charge "a la carte" for their services, and some will recommend that you buy your own do-it-yourself incorporation kit and seal. Shop around, and ask what is and is not included in the fees you are quoted. The total cost of incorporation should be less than $500.

Some attorneys recommend against incorporation if they think your benefits from incorporating will be outweighed by the added expenses and time required to maintain and administer the corporation, which will include additional record keeping, tax returns, and corporate filings.

FINDING A MENTOR

Home-based medical transcriptionists experience an isolated career world, especially those who work for services that pick up and deliver work materials to the transcriptionist's home.

The transcriptionist is plugged into a machine all day, listening to others' voices, having little or no personal contact with anyone but the mail man and delivery person. In earlier chapters of this book, we explained why networking with other transcriptionists is essential to a successful transcription business. For those new to the field of medical transcription, it is also a good idea to seek a mentor. There is no substitute for an experienced eye checking your work.

MENTOR

A wise and trusted counselor.

—Random House Dictionary

How does one find a mentor? Probably the most efficient way is to network with other medical transcriptionists and determine who inspires you, shares your philosophy, and has qualities you wish to emulate.

This admirable professional is someone who, if willing and able, will advise you and nurture you as you establish your career. Your mentor will have in-depth knowledge and experience as a medical transcription business person and will help you with specific questions and provide you with a wealth of emotional support.

Be sure to thank your mentor. There are givers and takers in every profession, and medical transcription is certainly not an exception. Some of my dearest friends have acted as mentors for ten or more years and while 99% of the medical transcriptionists they have helped have been extremely grateful, there have been a few who have turned around and stolen accounts from them. Unethical? Yes! You don't have to give your mentor your first born child; a pretty bouquet of spring flowers, a nice leisurely lunch or just a pretty thank-you card will suffice. Remember, these people have taken time away from their lives and work to help you and have asked nothing in return. Let them know how much they are appreciated.

The authors of this book have served as mentors for many novice transcriptionists. It has been a pleasure helping them solve problems we have faced, nurturing their professional development, and seeing their businesses succeed. More often than not, mentors and those they nurture become close friends and confidants in their personal and professional lives.

THE WINNING ATTITUDE

"Be enthusiastic and positive about your medical transcription service, and others will be enthusiastic, too."

Most men and women who are successful set goals for themselves. Setting goals consciously moves them toward those goals and nurtures a positive attitude. So, set goals for yourself. Make them measurable goals so you can monitor your progress, make adjustments as needed, and reward success points.

Be enthusiastic and positive about your medical transcription service, and others will be enthusiastic, too. With excellent knowledge and skills, you should radiate the exhilaration you feel about the services you provide the medical industry and the patients it serves. When meeting a potential client, remember that the client has a need and your service will fill that need.

When results don't turn out as planned, a winning attitude helps you look ahead to the next opportunity. People only fail when they give up. Trying again means they have learned one way in which their goal cannot be achieved.

SETTING BOUNDARIES IN YOUR BUSINESS

For better or for worse, we are now living in a world without boundaries, in an era in which we are frequently dealing with issues that are no longer crisp black and white but hazy gray. Often it seems that no one is certain what rules to follow, and rules can change from one day to the next. Regrettably, in this fluctuating setting, instead of working together for the greater good, we frequently find ourselves working against one another.

For the most part, doctors are really fun to work with. Most of them are undemanding and are grateful to have their work completed in a timely fashion. When giving doctors excellent quality at a fair price, a transcriptionist will usually have them eating out of his or her hand. Unfortunately, dealing with office personnel is usually not as simple. Issuing a title to some people gives them delusions of grandeur.

It has been our experience that when contracting with a new client, the proposal is usually made to the office manager, not the physician. In fact, most physicians delegate all office decisions to the office manager, and sometimes, the office manager begins acting like the GREAT AND POWERFUL WIZARD OF OZ. The GREAT AND POWERFUL WIZARD OF OZ (or G-WOZ) begins to make decisions about how we should conduct businesses and, feeling great and powerful, has no qualms about telling us how to run our businesses even though he or she may have no idea precisely what we do. The G-WOZ is condescending and demanding. Out of the blue we receive a phone call demanding 24-hour turnaround instead of the agreed-upon 48 hours. The contract provides for the original work only; now the G-WOZ demands two copies. And the format is all wrong. Instead of block style, she now wants indented style; instead of 10 point, 12 point is required. Next, morning pickup and delivery is changed to afternoon.

COMMUNICATION AND ASSERTIVENESS SKILLS

It is important to have solid, clearly defined personal boundaries when facing the likes of a G-WOZ. Every independent transcriptionist must believe and act upon the knowledge that no one can dictate to us how we should run our businesses. Only we, as highly trained medical transcription professionals, can judge what works best for us and what doesn't.

If you do not have a firm grasp on your strengths as well as your limitations and weaknesses, do some personal analysis and list your qualities in writing. This way you will be able to set healthy boundaries for yourself and make decisions based on your own knowledge about what you will or will not accept.

Fear is the biggest drawback to healthy communication and assertiveness when conducting business. Often, we devalue ourselves by acquiescing to another's demands even though deep down we know that decisions should not be made for us but by us. To overcome the fear of speaking up for yourself, develop a stronger, more rooted sense of who you are and what you believe in. That is why making a list is so important.

In every relationship, especially business relationships, give and take is essential. Any type of relationship that is one-sided will only lead to resentment, anger and cessation of all communication. The following are some keys to open the doors to communication and negotiation.

1. **Be a good listener:** The first and most important step is to learn to be a good listener. All of us *hear*, especially in our particular line of work, but few of

us truly *listen*. Listening is a normal physiological process. Sound is transmitted to the ear and is transported to the brain for interpretation. However, listening is a more complex psychological process requiring us to interpret and understand what we just heard.

Skilled communicators know that they need to listen first to persuade or negotiate later. They do not make requests or plead their case until they have paid close attention to others. The single biggest mistake made by poor negotiators is their tendency to rush ahead of themselves and start talking before making an effort to understand their audience. If you want to assert yourself more forcefully in your business relationships, make a commitment never to speak unless and until you have prepared and listened first. Resist the temptation to interrupt, daydream, jump to a conclusion or change the topic abruptly.

2. **Assess ideas and viewpoints:** Do not dwell on whether you agree or disagree. Listening does not oblige you to pick a side. Keep your mind focused on the message itself, not on judgments of right-wrong or good-bad. Don't feel pressured to respond immediately to every comment made; it's better not to. Rather than talk back, assess the speaker's ideas and viewpoints in a clearheaded, unbiased frame of mind. Let the message hang out there, in beautiful silence, without the static that so often turns a conversation into a contest.

3. **Set your boundaries:** After listening to the speaker without any bias, then you and only you will have to decide what you will and will not accept (setting your boundaries).

4. **Be persistent:** To be effective in your assertiveness, you must be persistent. Continue repeating what you want again and again without getting angry, irritated or loud. More often than not, to communicate in a conflict situation, you have to be persistent and stick to your point. By practicing speaking as if you were a "broken record" you will learn to be persistent, keeping your focus on the point of the discussion and saying what you want to say while ignoring all side issues brought up by the person you are negotiating with. Continue in this manner in a calm, repetitive voice until the other person accedes to your request or agrees to a compromise.

5. **Offer a workable compromise:** You may find it practical to offer your prospective client a workable compromise. This should be done, of course,

only after you have determined that the compromise will not have a detrimental impact on your business or negatively affect your sense of personal and professional self-respect. A successful compromise results in a win-win situation for both negotiating parties. It should also help you move closer to your material goals.

TAMING THE GREAT AND POWERFUL WOZ

Imagine you are negotiating with the GREAT AND POWERFUL WIZARD OF OZ, who suddenly demands 24-hour delivery after having accepted the conditions set by you for 48-hour delivery. After listening very carefully ask, "Is this being done at the physician's request?" If you determine that the physician knows nothing about this and that the new demands have been initiated by the G-WOZ, take some time to evaluate the situation. Calmly but firmly tell Oz you will return shortly with an answer.

If, after having looked at your schedule, you realize that 24-hour turnaround is impossible, call the G-WOZ and state that as much as you might like to, you cannot comply with that request because of time constraints. If the G-WOZ becomes angry, hostile and will not take "no" for an answer, keep repeating your message in a very matter-of-fact, firm voice, reiterating that you cannot possibly comply with the demand. Say it as many times as necessary until the G-WOZ accedes and accepts your answer.

What if the G-WOZ does not accede after your broken-record method? Try another tactic! If you feel you could comfortably return the work within a 36-hour time frame, offer that option as a workable compromise. Nine times out of ten, the situation can be remedied without you or the G-WOZ feeling manipulated. A potentially harmful situation has been averted and you have both maintained your self-respect. It's a win-win situation.

COMPLAINTS

No matter how hard you try, you will not be able to avoid a few complaints . . . even if you and your service are excellent. Some complaints will be anticipated. Other complaints will appear unexpectedly, perhaps about something you never considered a potential problem. How do you solve problems, keep clients happy, and maintain your personal integrity?

- When a complaint arises, allow the client to ventilate, expressing his or her feelings.

- Verify the problem. Listen carefully. When you feel you understand the problem, repeat it back to the client for verification.

- Suggest a resolution to the problem. In a calm, matter-of-fact, professional manner, explain what you can and cannot do. Suggest a solution to the problem or give the client a choice of solutions.

- Be willing to compromise. If initial suggestions don't solve the problem, consider alternatives.

- Accept the outcome and move ahead. Solutions that result positively for both transcriptionist and client are ideal, but occasionally a client cannot, or will not, be satisfied regardless of how hard the transcriptionist tries to accommodate. In these situations, don't berate yourself, acquiesce to guilt, or dissolve in feelings of failure. You've done your best, so get on with your work.

WHY CLIENTS WILL STOP DOING BUSINESS WITH YOU

- 9% die, move away or develop other friendships.

- 91% leave for competitive reasons.

- 14% are dissatisfied with the service provided.

- 68% quit because of the service owner's attitude of indifference toward the client.

Medical transcription is a service-oriented business. We must offer quality service without jeopardizing our integrity. Speak with clients on a regular basis about their interpretation of the services you are offering. Remember, many accounts are lost due to indifference or a laissez-faire attitude on the part of the service.

Remember the days of old when you walked into a department store, a bank, grocery store, library, post office, restaurant or gas station and were greeted with a smile, a "hello" and "please let me know if I can be of assistance?"

Remember the old adage, "The customer is always right?" Today, too many businesses have an attitude of disdain and sometimes even contempt toward a customer who asks for assistance. From time to time, each of us needs to look into the mirror and ask if we have developed the same posture.

One of the best ways to judge the quality of your service is to prepare a questionnaire asking clients to rate your services in a variety of areas including turnaround time, quality and completeness of work received, as well as your working relationship with them. Ask for input regarding how you might improve service, and leave plenty of room for answers. You might discover that what you thought was an excellent relationship is only rated fair or good by the client. Just as we were given employee evaluations when we belonged to the 9-5 work world, we must take it upon ourselves as micro-businesses to make sure we are offering the best service possible. We alone are responsible for our mistakes, and we certainly can't remedy problems if we don't know they exist.

Remember, in many respects you are in competition with yourself.

THE THEORY OF NEGATIVITY

There are times when we long for the not-so-long-ago days when people treated one another with respect and dignity, the office of the President of the United States was looked upon with awe and reverence, our lives were centered around families, friends and communities, the work day lasted from 9 a.m. to 5 p.m., job loyalty was a reality and not a myth, and life was more gentle, secure, peaceful and relaxed. In that atmosphere, our country grew by leaps and bounds, because individuals were nurtured, new ideas were encouraged, creativity was applauded and ingenuity was revered. People had hope, rose above fear, welcomed change, and pursued their dreams.

In contrast, as we leap into a complex new millennium, it sometimes seems as though we're living in a lost world. A whirlpool of negativity surrounds us. We see it in every facet of our lives — home, personal relationships, workplace, entertainment, and government. Many politicians no longer confront issues directly, and they use character assassination as a routine and acceptable political tactic. American corporations have grown greedy at the expense of the people who made them great — their employees — with corporate energies focused on reorganizing, downsizing, outsourcing, and decreasing employee benefits to keep stockholders happy and the CEO assured of a job for the coming year.

People are frustrated, angry and, most of all, tired. There is never enough time, especially for our families and communities. Our children are no longer sustained by traditional values and are often overwhelmed with a sense of hopelessness. We blame one another for our misfortunes, and America appears to be at war with itself. Citizens are arming themselves to drive the freeways and hostile confrontations are increasing.

We find it easier to talk to one another through our computers than to spend personal time over a cup of coffee. Some of our professional associations are instilling fear in us by giving us no hope for the future. We are told that outsourcing medical transcription will replace us, especially work being done overseas, or that we are going to be replaced by speech recognition technology. We are being fed a daily diet of doom and gloom and now the ultimate insult . . . negativity on the NET. The NET, a forum meant for exchange of new ideas, problem solving and promotion of our profession, has become infatuated with itself and thrives on the unhappiness it spreads through negativity.

Being negative is a nonproductive waste of time, and it eats at our souls. In our negative world, it seems that people are no longer responsible for their words or actions. They blame bad childhoods, bad people, gender discrimination, racial discrimination, bad marriages, people they work for, addiction problems, and so on ad infinitum. The US versus THEM mentality results in blaming everything and everybody else for the sorry lot of one's life. If you doubt this, read any newspaper, magazine, or watch one of the regular daytime talk programs on TV. It's time we take charge of our lives and make healthy decisions about ourselves, putting the responsibility where it belongs . . . on our own shoulders!

Negativity feeds on itself like a cancer. It rears its ugly head with one comment or one diatribe and before you know it, we are all feeling sorry for ourselves. It is making us sicker and sicker in our thinking, and the sickness increases as negative people gravitate to one another, finding comfort and encouragement in their misery. How did this happen in our industry?

MEDICAL TRANSCRIPTION AGE OF INNOCENCE

When we began our careers as medical transcriptionists, collectively 65-plus years ago, there were no schools of medical transcription and no reference books, but there were people willing to mentor us and answer our sometimes silly and mundane questions.

During that era, some great and wonderful people in our profession had a vision: They would form an organization to introduce us to the world and to our peers, to provide us with education and instill pride in what we do. The dream became reality. The early years of that organization were wonderful. Members were encouraged to share in the vision, to network with one another and solve problems, to broaden our horizons and, as the U.S. Army's slogan says, "be all that you can be," and more.

There was a whirlwind of activity. Policies and bylaws were written, committees formed, conventions planned and leaders elected. The organization prided itself on its membership and began working for the betterment of all. People who had never belonged to an organization were invited to participate, to become members and leaders. Nurturing souls encouraged others to get out of their comfort zone and expand their horizons, to not be afraid, to take risks and to accept challenge. It was an exciting time for all involved. The members became a part of the dream and worked long, tedious hours without compensation and without complaint because they had hope for a brighter tomorrow.

The incredible minds — ours! — behind the machines were acknowledged. Suddenly there were reference books — tons of them — and abundant educational opportunities. Seminars and symposiums offered presentations by, and direct interaction with, the greater medical community, satisfying our never-ending thirst for knowledge. We began calling ourselves professionals and believed we deserved that title. A certification program was established that validated our knowledge and skills and instilled pride in our accomplishments. We were empowered because we were part of something greater than ourselves. We felt there were no boundaries, no barriers, and the sky was the limit for all who participated.

Then FEAR raised its ugly, foreboding head and before long, medical transcriptionists began feeling less confident. Lawyers sprang out of every crevice, talking authoritatively about "risks," "liabilities," and "lawsuits." We had to be careful, we were warned. If we said or did the wrong thing we could be sued . . . even by fellow members of our own professional organizations. We could be discredited; we could lose something called "face."

Faced with such dire warnings, transcriptionists grew overly cautious about expressing new ideas or discussing professional issues with peers. It seemed safer to say nothing at all and to warn others to say nothing, too. Fear began to replace the old joyous feelings of freedom and hope. Distrust and paranoia followed, preventing much meaningful communication, positive networking, mentoring, and professional growth.

Regrettably, fear has also crossed the borders of the Internet as transcriptionists talk endlessly about professional problems and negatively rehash old issues without working toward solutions. Instead, we should be brainstorming for workable solutions and make our feelings known through positive statements. If we are to take charge of our future, we must toss aside paralyzing fear and negativity, empower ourselves as a group and work together for the good of all.

The face we are presenting to the world on the Internet is sometimes ugly and unbecoming to our profession. Imagine physicians, hospital administrators, and even legislators coming on the Medical Transcription Bulletin Board at any given time. What must they think?

Let's quit dwelling on problems — perceived or real — and together welcome change and diversity, find and implement solutions, and pioneer new territories. Then and only then will fear and distrust disappear because they are cowards in an environment of positive thinking.

FACING OUR FEARS

Fear can be bold or subtle. It can come in millimeters or centimeters, inches or feet, years or decades. Fear instills insecurity, anger, self-loathing, and negativity. It tells us that we must be afraid of change, off-site transcription, large medical transcription services and independent medical transcriptionists, because they might take our jobs. It tells us to fear medical transcription teaching programs, which may produce too many MTs and dilute our job market. It tells us to fear independent thinkers who advocate change and visionaries who look with hope to the future. It tells us to fear even our thoughts, actions, and words — even when they are correct — because we might be sued.

Be clear about this: Fear is powerful. It keeps people in line, keeps them quiet, and keeps them inactive. Fearful people are not dynamic entrepreneurs, innovators, trend-setters or leaders. And, generally, fearful people are not happy.

- **Should we be afraid of overseas competition?** No. Like so many other businesses, we will soon be a part of the global economic scene. Think of the potential opportunities! Those wishing to travel and perhaps live in another part of the world may someday be able to do so as new businesses evolve or by working via the Internet, using new technology that offers worldwide phone lines for telecommunication and new software, which is now being developed, that will bypass the telephone companies.

- **Should we be afraid of large medical transcription companies?** Absolutely not. There will always be a need for experienced independent medical transcriptionists, especially for smaller hospitals, clinics and physician office accounts. If during the next few years standardized health care becomes a reality, and when 100% of this country's population will have free access to medical care, just think how much work will be available. We must learn to work together and not be divided.

- **Should we be afraid of medical transcription teaching programs?** Of course not. Most of the old guard medical transcriptionists are getting very tired, and some are even retiring. We need to encourage new people to enter the field to carry on our noble work. We must be willing to look at teaching programs, however, to see which are offering students the most for their money and time. We should praise the ones that are excellent and discourage students from taking classes that we know will only familiarize them with medical transcription equipment and a few medical terms. Many of you could start your own medical transcription schools to ensure quality education. Who better to teach medical transcription than an experienced MT?

Mentoring is another aspect of teaching. We must all be willing to mentor people new to the field and serve as their guides, not discouraging them with horror stories of impossibly hard medical transcription work. Remember, most of us were once mentored by experienced medical transcriptionists, to whom we owe a debt of gratitude. Experience the joy of helping another who is following a dream to be self-employed. It's a satisfying pleasure no one should miss.

Mentoring is needed for non-novice, transitioning professionals, too. These are the displaced, the wounded and the courageous, following their dreams to be self-supporting business owners. They come to our field with all the hopes and dreams many of our ancestors carried with them to the Promised Land. We might even learn from them as a majority bring expertise from their previous work lives. Before choosing medical transcription as a career alternative, they were accountants, nurses, computer technobots, marketing professionals, business executives, and others. They have much to teach us.

- **What purpose is served by fearing speech recognition technology?** None at all. Instead, let's analyze how we can use this technology to our benefit? We all know that physicians are not likely to spend weeks teaching their computers to speak for them. So why not form our own companies singularly or collectively to offer this technology to the medical community, edit reports and charge for our services as we do now? Can you imagine not having to keyboard 8 to 14 hours a day. Hallelujah and sing a joyful song!

We must not let the world of technology pass us by. In preparation for the future, we must continue to educate ourselves about new technology by taking computer courses, learning more about telecommunication, and maybe even taking coding classes to increase our marketable skills. Just as in any field going through transition, we must learn as much as we possibly can to stay current, because only the most knowledgeable and skilled will survive.

- **Should we fear our medical transcription peers?** No. Fear stifles professional communication and relationships which should nurture and sustain us. Fear also incites negative behavior as people who feel threatened lash out in defense of their territory or against someone they perceive as "different" or "wrong." No one is a winner in those situations.

Let's not hurt one another by being cruel and spiteful. Instead, let's treat others with the respect and dignity that we wish for ourselves. Helping strengthen our peers also strengthens us and our profession. Maligning another's character only drags us down. Diverse personalities — yours, mine and theirs — make this country great. We must learn to listen to others, welcoming all ideas with vigor and enthusiasm even if we don't always agree with them. In other words, agree to disagree, but do it with kind words and statements.

If we are going to survive as a profession and succeed as individual business people, we must step out of our comfort zone, embolden each other to be the best at what we do, and encourage everyone to bring to the table their own special talents and expertise. Otherwise, we will become as extinct as T. Rex.

SHOW ME THE MONEY! TAKING CHARGE

Your attitude can affect how much you earn, too. Do you feel that you, a skilled independent medical transcriptionist, are not making as much money as you deserve? Well, adopt a positive attitude and tackle the problem. The solution is in your hands. If you haven't raised your fees for awhile, do so immediately. Charge for extra copies, faxed reports, and extra trips for picking up work if you aren't telecommuting. Factor in your expenses for the most modern equipment demanded by your clients, telephone charges, utilities, car expenses, retirement and health care benefits. Look for more lucrative accounts.

We know many IMTs who are extremely happy and satisfied with their businesses. They are making more money than they ever dreamed possible, and it has nothing to do with the part of the country in which they live. Their success is a direct result of having positive attitudes and being willing to learn all they can about themselves as well as the world around them.

TRIUMPH OVER NEGATIVITY — A PERSONAL STORY

For forty years, one of the authors went through life mired in negativity. Nothing was ever good enough. How pitiful! She was never good enough, smart enough, thin enough, pretty enough. And, she kept telling herself — and others who would listen — that life was a living hell. You work and then you die! was her philosophy. She wouldn't let herself see the beauty around her and experience joy. Nor did she have hope or find ready solutions to her life's dilemmas. She did not realize that things could get better if only she would move away from her negative way of thinking. In other words, she was afraid and insecure.

Ten years ago, she had had enough. Her negativity had created a big hole inside her that nothing and no one could fill. She could feel herself dying from within and when she was finally ready to listen and willing to change, teachers appeared everywhere. They told her she had to take responsibility for her life; and, for every negative feeling or observation she experienced, there was also a positive side. If she practiced every day, she was assured, she too would find those positives in her life. You must be kidding, she thought to herself; but deep down she knew they were right. They had been practicing this way of life for some time, and she could see that they were much happier, more grounded, filled with self-assurance, patient and understanding and doing great things with their lives. She took on the challenge of a lifetime.

It was hard not being miserable all the time, blaming other people and circumstances for her troubles. It was equally hard allowing herself the freedom to be happy, to look for and expect the best outcome in every life situation. But she did it, and soon she began seeing significant changes in her life. By being positive, she found herself surrounded by like-minded people; people who were trusting and caring; people who taught her how to take chances and risk disappointments, how to learn from her experiences — good or bad — and how to be willing to help others facing negativity in their lives. In other words, her new acquaintances became her cheerleaders. For every success in her life, she was given kudos and a multitude of "Attagirls!" For every disappointment, she received a patient and understanding ear, someone who listened and did not judge her or her actions. When she stumbled, they picked her up, dusted her off and set her off in a different direction. In short, she was given hope.

Hope minimizes negativity, allowing us to walk through and beyond fear with the realization that nothing we do is a failure but rather a life lesson. And when we have overcome negativity and are filled with self-confidence and joy, we are eager to share what we have learned and foster this same inspiring hope and joy in others. This is definitely a better way to live, and we recommend it for everyone.

HOME-BASED TEMPTATIONS

As an independent medical transcriptionist, you will face myriad temptations: sleeping late, daytime television, the urge to "kick back" in sweats, personal telephone chats, browsing through favorite magazines, shopping sprees, and other nonproductive and nonprofessional enticements so subtle you'll scarcely be aware of them until your business suffers.

PLANNING FOR SUCCESS

If you plan to succeed, and we assume you will, structure your workday as if you were employed in a standard office setting. One successful independent explained her action plan this way:

"At the beginning of my home-based career, I set short-term career goals and gave myself one year's probation. I made up my mind that if I didn't reach my goals by the end of that year, I would have to get a 'real' job.

Since I really wanted to remain independent, I made sure I was at my desk promptly on schedule each morning. At year's end, I had exceeded my goals."

One of the authors of this book accomplishes optimum productivity with an unorthodox 2:00 a.m.-10:00 a.m. transcription schedule. After 10:00 a.m., business calls are returned and priority business items completed. The rest of the day is filled with personal activities, including horseback riding regularly.

Some professionals begin work at 9:00 p.m. or midnight or work early in the morning, break for the afternoon, and work again at night. You probably know your most productive hours and will schedule your workday in that time period. On the other hand, you may have to experiment until you find what works best. This flexibility is fantastic and one of the primary benefits of being an IMT.

COPING WITH DISTRACTIONS

Medical transcription requires great concentration. Little interruptions can create big problems. Take control of your home-based career at its beginning and don't allow distractions to erode your business.

- **People:** Immediate family, knowing you are readily accessible, will seek your personal touch and attention in a wide variety of situations. Establish your home-based-career ground rules immediately and adhere to them.

  Extended family and friends will undoubtedly be delighted to learn that you are home-based and may drop by unexpectedly for visits. "It's okay to interrupt," they reason. "Working at home isn't a **real** job."

  Be gentle but firm as you explain schedules, deadlines, and entrepreneurial responsibilities. Make it clear that although you look forward to having coffee, lunch, or a visit with them, you must do it around your work schedule.

  Generally speaking, people who are unemployed during the day don't intentionally wreak havoc with home-based career schedules. They simply do not understand your responsibilities.

> "As the owner of your home-based business, you have the right to determine the working environment in your home office."
> —Norm Ray, CPA, *Smart Tax Write-offs*

- **Telephones:** An answering machine is a must! During peak work hours, let the machine take your calls until you have met your deadlines, then call back. One home-based acquaintance, whose work routine is very specific, announces on her machine, " . . . Lori isn't available right now, but she will be returning calls this afternoon at 3:30 . . . " If your work schedule is very regular, you may find that this system, or a variation of it, will work well for you.

- **Doorbells:** Salesmen, political activists, religious promoters, and youthful fundraisers are just a few of the uninvited people who will knock at your front door during the work day. You are not obligated to answer their summons, rushing to the door and wasting time on their pitch and your response. Such unexpected interruptions are inconvenient and detrimental to your work. Besides, you can always review the handouts they leave and contact them later if you wish. Some home-based professionals post a "No Solicitors" sign at the front door. Others install a two-way speaker system so they can easily determine who is at the door without leaving their desk.

- **Food:** Your desk is not a deli counter or a snack bar so save snacking for breaks and meals. Nora Nibbler not only slows her productivity but gains weight, too.

- **Internet:** Online Olivia is captivated by websites and chat rooms, wasting precious hours she could be transcribing. If she isn't careful, her life and her career will be lost in cyberspace.

- **Television:** Game Show Gertie finds herself consistently lured by fun and laughter. Soap Opera Sally is drawn to tears and trauma. Too much of either will result in poor transcription career ratings.

- **Housework:** If you are a Nelly Neatnik, you will be tempted by dozens of household projects. If you take time to do them on a daily basis, you will scuttle your transcription work schedule. Instead, set aside blocks of time for housework. Train yourself to ignore noncareer tasks during transcription hours.

MAINTAINING THE MOTIVATION

Successful home-based professionals are masters of self-motivation and utilize a variety of techniques to recharge and maintain their professional enthusiasm. We hope the following suggestions help motivate you personally and professionally, and we encourage you to modify and add creative inspirations to meet your needs.

- Believe and be proud that you are a professional. As frequently as necessary, remind yourself that YOU ARE A PROFESSIONAL.

- Look on the light side. Post inspiring verses and humorous cartoons around your work station and on your calendar. Smile frequently.

- Remember praises. Keep an "ego file" of letters of commendation, positive press/newsletter coverage, thank-you notes for transcription work, brief notations about verbal praises, and any other item that lifts your spirit.

- Dress for success daily. Not only will the drop-by client be favorably impressed, but you will feel better about yourself.

- Take breaks. Take regular ten or fifteen minute breaks and lunch during your work day. Also schedule occasional leisure activities with acquaintances. All work and no play makes Trish a dull transcriptionist.

- Exercise. Make it a regular part of each day, even if it's only twenty minutes per workout. Get outside when possible, away from your desk.

- Network. Professional communication and interaction is stimulating.

- Surprise yourself. Keep a list of intriguing things you haven't tried — massage, exotic clothing shop, museum tour, Indonesian food, skydiving — and try one.

- Volunteer time and talents to your children's school, your professional organization, or a community activity. This is a real "perker-upper."

- Reward yourself. For work well-done, pamper yourself with favorite things — bubble bath, movie, an afternoon at the beach, a round of golf, new shoes, facial, pedicure, mini-vacation, or time with a favorite book.

> *"You are an independent professional.*
> *Take time to enjoy the perks."*

THE WORKPLACE

In order to make a full professional commitment and provide optimum opportunity for success, you must establish a proper workplace or office. A suitable workplace provides essential professional elements: tools capable of producing quality medical transcription and an environment that nurtures physical, mental, and psychological health, with all elements designed to meet client and government agency criteria.

AVOIDING ISOLATION AT HOME — DON'T GO THERE!

When working for someone else, you spend most of your time in a *reactive* mode, responding to other people's requests for action. As an IMT or business owner/operator, you must switch that mode to *proactive*, which means that you think through situations, anticipate potential difficulties, and take positive action in advance. By being proactive, you become the in-charge person. For many, it is difficult to change from a reactive to a proactive mind-set, but it is essential if you are to avoid the negative impacts of work-at-home isolation.

There are several work-at-home websites that contain useful information about telecommuting, freelance work, contracting and much more. There is also information on MT job opportunities. Some sites offer free trial memberships. We recommend that you investigate these sites, which will be useful in helping you build your home-based career.

- **Independent Homeworkers Alliance**
  www.homeworkers.org

- **Work from Home Digest**
  www.intlhomeworkers.com

- **Homeworkers Union and Small Business Association** (H.U.S.B.A.)
  www.telecommuting-jobs.org

- **Homeworkers**
  www.homeworkers.com

There are also a number of public forums and chat rooms specific to medical transcription, such as MT Daily and M-TEC.

- **MT Daily**
  www.mtdaily.com/Chat/freechat

- **M-TEC Message Board for Students**
  www.mtecinc.com/wwwboard/wwwboard
  www.mtdaily.com/mentors/leaders/francis

SELECTING HOME-BASED BUSINESS SPACE

It is extremely important for your office to be comfortable and located in an area where you will have the fewest distractions.

A work environment that is light and airy is physically and psychologically healthy, so try to locate in an area that is open and has windows. Use draperies or mini blinds to cut down on computer screen glare. If you have worked for services, hospitals, or clinics, you know that it is very depressing to work in the basement or in dark, dank rooms in which you develop hidrosis in the winter and frostbite in the summer. Don't re-create that scene.

Since you now have control over where you will spend the majority of your day, make it great — or near-great. Establish a work area where you will not be disturbed by children, husbands, wives, pets, and the incessant ringing/chatter of nonbusiness telephones.

Establishing a separate work area is important for another reason. Internal Revenue Service guidelines for home businesses stipulate that the home office be separate from the living quarters of the home and used only for business-related activities.

If you are planning to cordon off a section of the living room for a home office, it should be separated by a partition from the rest of the living space. This can be done very simply and inexpensively. Use your imagination.

> *"[Studies show that]. . . behavior changes start becoming permanent after the twenty-first day."*
> —"Captain Bob" Smith
> *Eat Stress for Breakfast*

PRICING YOUR TRANSCRIPTION SERVICES

> *"He is well paid that's well satisfied."*
> —William Shakespeare
> *The Merchant of Venice*

Transcriptionists who began self-employment careers during the early days of transcription's modern era found pricing very difficult. Because the large majority of us were female, novices in the field, and working without benefit of adequate peer communication, we often set prices too low and sold ourselves short.

For many years, there was no professional organization (AAMT) and no networking between transcriptionists. When transcriptionists did discuss "business," we talked about improving our output, workplace, or equipment — rarely, if ever, about dollars-and-cents issues.

Back then, women accepted many less-than-ideal conditions without question. We generally fulfilled society's expectation that we be "grateful" for income-producing opportunities, and we avoided discussing issues considered inappropriate for females. Unfortunately, that lack of significant professional communication became a breeding ground for paranoia. We transcriptionists, fearing others might take our business, avoided asking questions and sharing professional facts regarding pay rates and income. While our silence may have protected us from others, it also impeded significant professional progress. Today, transcriptionists take a more realistic view of career communication, are more confident and assertive in the workplace, and are reaping the professional benefits.

PRICING RESEARCH

Pricing research helps decrease the frustration many transcriptionists experience as they struggle to establish initial transcription rates. If you are a newcomer to transcription, we recommend immediate networking with other home-based transcriptionists in your area to determine the "going rate" for transcription and whether the price is by the line or by the page.

As a professional, you should charge professional fees, setting rates that correspond fairly and competitively with those of other transcription professionals.

Don't ever hesitate to find out what your competition is charging. It's good for you and your business. By being aware of current transcription rates, you will be able to set your own rates appropriately in the beginning and in the future. Never, never ask anyone what they charge their clients. That really is none of your business, and most people are offended by that question. Instead, ask about the range of rates charged in the area (e.g., 12 to 16 cents per line).

> *"A desk is a dangerous place*
> *from which to view the world."*
> —John LeCarre

John LeCarre said, "A desk is a dangerous place from which to view the world." He's right. It is impossible to keep track of the competition with your eyes fixed constantly on the computer screen. Look beyond your office, stay on top of fluctuations in the transcription marketplace, and adjust your rates accordingly.

Ask yourself two basic questions when deciding how to generate income from your professional services:

- What should my fee be?

- How will I command that fee?

Your fee should reflect your professional competence as a medical transcriptionist who has extensive training, experience, and successfully manages a bona fide business. YOU ARE AN EXPERT IN YOUR FIELD. Your fee should be commensurate with your expertise. Clients who value your quality service will not hesitate to pay an appropriate professional fee.

THE EFFECTS OF CAPITATION AND MANAGED CARE

Today, Managed Care Organizations (MCOs) are responsible for establishing protocols to ensure that quality care is provided in a cost-efficient manner leading to positive medical outcomes. To achieve their goal, MCOs work through vehicles such as provider review, utilization review, case management, formularies, primary care gatekeepers, and concurrent review.

In order to provide necessary services to its members while remaining financially solvent, an MCO must enter into reduced-cost contracts with providers. A simple method of reducing costs is to establish a contract through which the MCO pays the provider at a discount from normally billed charges. Similarly, MCOs may contract with providers on a procedural fee schedule or on a Diagnostic Related Group (DRG) basis. Using this method, the provider and the MCO essentially share financial risk and cost.

Another method is full shifting of financial responsibility to the provider, which many MCOs perceive as the most cost-effective method of providing care. The most common vehicle used to shift financial risk from the MCO to the provider is through a capitation contract. Capitation represents a fixed negotiated amount that the MCO pays to the provider on a per member/per month basis. By receiving the capitation amount, the provider is obligated to deliver or arrange for the delivery of the service required by the MCO member as designated in the contract between the provider and the MCO.

How do we medical transcriptionists fit into this equation? Simple. Since the doctor is receiving a set amount of money to care for each patient during a specific month, the doctor's volume will unquestionably be affected. The key word here is "volume." Physicians will be receiving less for each patient but, because of the added volume of patients they will be seeing, their income may remain the same or even decrease. The medical transcriptionist's income is predicated upon the number of lines/pages/bytes transcribed and is variable from month to month, season to season, and solely dependent upon the physician. When physicians receive capitated fees, they are able to control the amount of time spent with each patient. The independent medical transcriptionist does not have that luxury. We are totally at the mercy of the dictator and his or her workload. If the physician's practice balloons because of participation in an MCO, it is reasonable to assume we might be transcribing more and receiving less!

Let me give you an example. While negotiating a new contract with your client, you must establish a monthly capitated or flat fee for transcription services. Using standard medical transcription methods, you determine your monthly fee by averaging the total past year's income from that account. If the physician enrolls in an MCO and his or her volume doubles because of increased access to patients, you will find yourself transcribing double the volume and not benefitting monetarily from that increase. In fact, you will probably be losing money on that account.

If you have been approached by a client to enter into a relationship to provide services for a capitated fee, do your homework. There are several factors you must consider before agreeing to a flat fee for service:

- Number of physicians in the group

- Volume of dictation and patterns (including level of technical difficulty)

- Current turnaround time (TAT) and expected turnaround time (ETAT)

- Projected increase in patient volume

- Your level of expertise in handling the account

- Sufficient staffing to handle the volume

We know of one independent medical transcriptionist who contracted for a capitated rate with seven orthopedists. This was a new account and a fee was agreed upon, which initially seemed like a handsome sum to the transcriptionist. Unfortunately, there was lack of communication between the medical transcriptionist and the office staff and the physicians in the medical practice. In addition, the IMT had not considered all factors that might negatively impact her work for this client and, as a result, did not negotiate her contract wisely.

While picking up work on the first day, the IMT was shocked to be presented with work not only from the previous day, but two weeks of backlog work, too! Do we hear a collective gasp?

Who is to blame, you ask? Obviously, the independent medical transcriptionist, who should have done her homework, asked more questions, and communicated more effectively with the client. Regrettably in this situation, all communication was controlled by the office staff, who, as the medical transcriptionist later discovered, were deeply opposed to the physicians' decision to contract work out.

Significant information was not communicated by the office staff to the physicians. They were not told about the two-week backlog of dictation, nor that additional time should have been allowed for formatting adjustments. The doctors simply expected to receive **all** transcribed reports within 24 hours.

This account turned out to be a nightmare for the IMT — Physicians calling demanding their transcription, office staff faxing back document "corrections" for which they had not provided correct formatting instructions or client information, and so on. After several days dealing with the "office staff from hell," the IMT determined that this account was not worth all the money in the world, and she fired the client.

Fortunately, this story has a happy ending. Although the account turned out to be a monumental disaster, the transcriptionist was able to extricate herself with little effort. Although terms of the contract had been verbally discussed, the office manager had never gotten around to typing the contract and obtaining signatures from the parties involved. For this, the MT thanked her lucky stars, and never again made the same mistakes when evaluating potential new clients.

CHARGING BY LINE, CHARACTER, OR PAGE

> *"Not everything that counts can be counted and not everything that can be counted counts."*
>
> —Albert Einstein

Most independent MTs prefer to be paid by the line or by the page. Others, however, prefer charging by the character, establishing a set fee for a fixed number of characters. Please note that when using a character count, the rates are generally 10-15% less than when using a gross line count. This is important when computing your fees.

Line counts are more widely used because of their simplicity. What constitutes a line? Most independent medical transcriptionists charge for each and every line, whether there is one word or several. There is no standard for what constitutes a line. It is what you negotiate with your client. For some accounts, a line may consist of sixty characters; for another, eighty characters.

What constitutes a page? Whatever standard you set is acceptable, as long as the fee is within the normal fee range for your area. It is not uncommon to charge half the fixed-page rate for a page that is only a quarter- or half-page. However, charging the entire page rate for half pages is also an acceptable practice.

When interviewing a prospective client, ask for samples of past transcription so you can judge the size of the line. This will help determine your pricing for services. Certainly an 80 character line would be worth more price-wise than a 60 character line.

Whether you count every line or half-line is not really important. What is important is to be consistent with your client from the beginning in order to avoid later confusion. Develop and maintain confidence about what your terms are. Then, when negotiating your service contract, be clear and concise regarding how your lines will be counted, and stipulate your terms for line counting in your contract.

COUNTING CALCULATIONS

In addition to determining how you are going to price your services — by cost, demand, competition, or going rate — you must also consider your pricing strategy. Are you going to base your fees on the word, line, page, keystroke, byte or character?

Submitting bids to your clients for your transcription services is very important. You must convince clients that you are offering them a cost-effective rate, but also take into consideration that you must incorporate your costs into your fees. Clients, on the other hand, must determine which service is the most cost-effective, and they will solicit bids from several services to do this. They will take into consideration that bids are based on factors such as varying units of work measure.

WHAT IS A UNIT OF MEASURE?

There has been much discussion within the medical transcription industry regarding units of measure — byte, character, line, minutes of dictation, reports by page, etc. — and more specifically, how they should be defined. Currently, there are no inclusive unit-of-measure definitions that are recognized and accepted as standards within the medical transcription industry. As a result, numerous definitions abound, which often lead to confusion, inefficiency, and an unprofessional image.

At the present time, there are too many variables in measurements to standardize them. For instance, standardizing charges by minutes of dictation is difficult, if not impossible, because dictation speeds vary from dictator to dictator and from region to region. A minute of dictation in slower-paced Georgia, even though it may contain the same number of words, is likely to be very different from dictation in fast-paced New York.

Currently within the medical transcription industry, as transcriptionists seek logical solutions to transcription measurement confusion, increasing numbers of transcriptionists are accepting *character*, *word* and *line* as the standard units of work.

There are those in our industry who believe that clearly defined and easily verifiable units of measure would improve communication between health-information professionals, service owners and transcriptionists, as well as support work measurement across the industry. Without doubt, the issue will continue to be discussed, and perhaps units-of-measure standardization will occur within the next decade.

WHAT IS A STANDARD?

An established measure of weight, length, quality or the like, especially one serving as a model by which the accuracy of others may be determined; any type, example or model generally accepted as correct.

Suggested standard units of measure are the following:

- **Character:** Letters, numbers, symbols and function keys including but not limited to the space bar, carriage return, underscore and all characters contained within a macro, headers and footers.

- **Word-five characters:** Total character count can be converted to words by dividing the total character count by the specified number of characters in a word.

- **Line, 65 characters:** The total number of lines for reporting purposes is determined by dividing total characters by the specified number of characters in a line. Margins may vary resulting in gross lines of varying numbers of characters.

- **Keystroke:** Strike of a single key. Measures the input only, reducing a macro to entry strokes rather than meaningful output terms.

- **Gross line:** Any line of print with one or more printed characters.

- **Minute of dictation:** Measure of access time to a dictation unit or system.

- **Page:** One side of any sheet of paper with one or more printed characters on it.

As technology continues to change, so will the needs of the our industry and units of measurement. Even those that are standardized will require periodic review and updating.

In 1998 The American Association for Medical Transcription issued a "Position Statement" addressing the need for full disclosure of any method used to measure medical transcription productivity. This position statement reversed their previous position published in 1993, recommending that the unit of measure for transcription be the character count.

In summary, in today's medical transcription industry there is no standard for what constitutes a line. It is still what you negotiate with your client. If you are currently successfully using a measurement other than those recommended by the authors, continue with it. There is no reason to change a system that's working for you and your client.

LINE- AND CHARACTER-COUNT SOFTWARE

There are several utility line-counting programs you can purchase that work with WordPerfect and Word. One is *Sylcount* by Sylvan Software, which has a version for DOS and for Windows. It counts lines, words, pages and characters, keeps a log and is priced around $79.00. A second is *WPCount* for WordPerfect by Productive Performance. For more information, see the product reference list in the back of this book.

- **Sylvan Software**
  800-235-9455
  fax 719-495-8119
  www.sylvansoft.com

- **Productive Performance**
  206-788-8300

- **Productive Performance**
  425-788-8300
  www.foxcomm.net/productive/WPCOUNT.htm

- **ATS Software (DocuCount)**
  www.flash.net/ ~ actrsrv/

Many clients remain confused about the character count; they find it easier to understand charges by straight line count or page-rate methods.

If you are defining your unit of measure by the character, there are several software programs available on the market to help you. Some of these are described as line count utilities. They are designed to produce line and word counts for documents. The macros in these utilities allow the user to decide the character length of the line and character length of a word. In other words, you can revise the macros to change the count options. For example, if you negotiate with your client a 55-character line and the macro is set at 65 character, you can revise the macro and set it at 55 characters per line. It can also be revised to skip spaces, skip or add hard returns, count merge codes, skip or count headers and footers, etc.

With these software programs, character counts are easily converted into words and lines. You can count a block of text, a document or directory file. You can generate line count reports by directory or by report, which can then be printed and incorporated in your client billing. If you are using a program like WordPerfect you can build a character count macro.

Whether you count every line or half line is not really important. What is important is that you be consistent with your client. Be clear on how your documents will be counted and stipulate your terms for line counting in your contract, thereby avoiding confusion between the client and yourself.

> *"Your primary activity should be in generating profitable business operations."*
> —Norm Ray, CPA, *Easy Financials for Your Home-based Business*

SAMPLE LINE COUNT DOCUMENT

Document Name	Words	Lines	Date Counted
22.06	10	0	6-24-2002 00:11
Brooks.H 06	344	31	6-24-2002 00:11
Bruce.D 06	562	51	6-24-2002 00:11
Cann.O 06	524	47	6-24-2002 00:11
Cristoph.H 06	582	52	6-24-2002 00:11
Croswait.O 06	417	37	6-24-2002 00:11
Fausto.D 06	584	53	6-24-2002 00:11
Goozee.O 06	457	41	6-24-2002 00:11
Hall.O 06	422	38	6-24-2002 00:11
Hamilton,O 06	467	42	6-24-2002 00:11
Kinlock.O 06	752	68	6-24-2002 00:11
Lewis.H 06	660	60	6-24-2002 00:11
Macgrego.D 06	749	68	6-24-2002 00:11
Total words/lines	6530	588	

UNDERPRICING

"Underpricing can lead to an MT's undoing."

When setting up a medical transcription business, it is sometimes tempting to attract clients by cutting your fees and underpricing competitors, but that strategy could very well backfire on you. If a client spreads the word that you do great work for seven cents a line while others in your area are charging twelve cents, you may acquire a reputation that is hard to shake and that you will grow to regret. Granted, your underpricing strategy may result in enormous quantities of work as people clamor for your low-priced service, but you will have to work twice as hard to earn an adequate income. Is that really what you want? Wasn't the idea of becoming home-based to work smarter, not harder?

DOING BUSINESS AT ANY PRICE

Anyone who has been an MT for more than a year has probably experienced the service that undercuts transcription prices charged by other local services. Whether you are a sole proprietor or a service owner, there is nothing more depressing than receiving a call from a long-established client telling you they have decided to do business with someone who has undercut your price. Undercutting is not unique to the field of medical transcription; in our free market society, it often occurs in service-related fields.

Based on our experience in the medical transcription industry, we believe the primary culprit for underpricing is ignorance. Very few people who enter the medical transcription field take time to do the necessary homework. Not realizing what it takes to run a financially sound business, they undervalue themselves by undercutting local competition with misguided hopes of getting into the game quickly and painlessly. They don't network with local medical transcriptionists to discuss going rates for transcription. Most important, they don't realize how greatly they hurt others as well as themselves by taking the edge off competition. Yes, they are swamped with work for a period of time, but because they have charged too little, they have to make it up in volume. Within a short time, they burn themselves out and move on to less exacting careers, leaving their transcription peers and clients feeling cheated, angry, and bitter.

Some naively believe they should charge less because they are home-based. Well, where is it written in stone that a sole proprietor must charge less than a large service? Independent transcriptionists offer the same high-quality services, only on a smaller scale, and our overhead and expenses are much the same. There is absolutely no reason to charge (or accept) less for our work.

Several years ago at an AAMT convention, I attended a lecture given by an attorney who had been employed by a large medical transcription service. His job was to conduct medical transcription studies and to talk with prospective clients regarding how much the service would be saving them. After much research, the attorney concluded that in most cases a full-time, in-house medical transcriptionist with a full benefit package cost the employer between 45-75 cents per line. Considering that the going rate for a line of transcription nationwide ranges from 10-16 cents, we should never apologize for our rates.

In a cost comparison presented with a transcription service proposal, the following was noted:

MEDICAL TRANSCRIPTION EMPLOYEE COST COMPARISON

Base salary level transcriptionist $ 11.50
Benefit package provided by hospital 18% 2.07
$13.57 x 2080 hrs. $ 28,226

Vacation/holiday replacement cost
($13.57 x 80 hrs., 1 week vacation, 5 holidays) $ 1,086

Cost of transcription station space, equipment,
service contracts, supervisory expense, personnel
department expense $ 2,000/yr.

Total cost of FTE $ 31,312

Shift differential of 15% $ 15.30/hr.

TOTAL COST OF FTE PER YEAR** **$ 35,048**

**Transcription service output based on
1000 lines per day @ .12 = $120/day x 260 days
(52 x 5) per year = $31,200

The **Association of Business Support Services International, Inc. (ABSSI)** **—formerly National Association for Secretarial Services (NASS)**—serves member owners of business support services through a variety of benefits. A partial list includes its monthly 16-page *Industry Focus* magazine, unlimited free consultation, and 15 discounted industry-specific manuals. One of these manuals is a 120-page blueprint for starting a business support service; another provides industry production standards which, when combined with your own unique hourly rate, is a useful estimating and billing tool.

- **ABSSI**
  714-695-9398
  800-237-1462

If an MT in your area is undercutting your service, don't be intimidated and think you have to lower your prices to match your competitor's. Find out as much as you can about your competition, his or her background and the services offered. Then, compare this with the positive aspects of your service that give you the edge over their lower-priced business. Do you have more experience? Are your skills specialized? If so, then your services are worth more because you are a specialist. Plastic surgeons with skills beyond those of the family practitioner, athletes whose track records are outstanding, and attorneys who consistently win court cases are adequately compensated for their skills and professional attributes. Then why not the professional medical language specialist?

HIGHER FEES SUCCEED

Professionals who charge fees in the upper market range are generally the most successful, according to Howard Shenson, author of *Contract and Fee-Setting Guide for Consultants and Professionals* ($39.95; John Wiley & Sons, 1990).

Shenson, who heads his own Woodland, California consulting firm and gives popular seminars and lectures on consulting and practice management, has also written the *Consulting Handbook and How to Strategically Negotiate the Consulting Contract*.

According to Shenson, you must ask yourself two basic questions when deciding how to generate income from your professional services:

• What should my fee be?

• How will I command that fee?

Your fee should reflect your professional competence. As a medical transcriptionist who has extensive training, experience, and successfully manages a bona fide business, you are an expert in your field. Your fee should be commensurate with your expertise. Clients who value your quality service will not hesitate to pay an appropriate professional fee.

> *"Your home-based business must be profitable to survive in the long run."*
> —Norm Ray, CPA, *Easy Financials*
> *for Your Home-based Business*

LINE RATE FACTORS

To our knowledge there has never been a book, newsletter or journal published for medical transcriptionists in which specific fee ranges were discussed. As stated earlier, people new to the field of medical transcription have a tendency to undercharge for their services because they are unaware of the fee range in their area. Some surveys have been conducted via the Internet to determine what transcriptionists are charging, how they count lines, equipment, etc. The surveys have been published on some webpages and are available upon request. For more information on these rates/surveys, hop on the Worldwide Web and browse the MT sites referred to throughout this book. You will pick up lots of information about rates.

Pricing ranges have been recorded according to regions by postmark on the survey. Range is based on **cents per line** as follows:

UNITED STATES REGION	LINE RATE RANGE LOW	HIGH
Northwest	10-12	17-19
West	8-11	12-17
Midwest	8-9.5	16-17
East	10	12-15
South	10-12	13-16

Within the United States, subcontractors' fees ranged from 6.5-9 cents in the East; 8-10 cents in the West; 7 cents in the South; and 8 cents in the Midwest. Fees for telecommuters working for services ranged from 8-10 cents. There were also respondents who reported they were paid a flat page rate.

Although these prices vary from city to city, we feel this survey is an accurate representation of fees being charged by independent medical transcriptionists. Consider these factors when setting your price:

- **Geographical differences.** Rates vary from area to area.

- **Availability and competition.** If there is little competition and large consumer demand, you can charge whatever the market will bear. It is a matter of supply and demand.

- **Current market prices.** Like all economic factors in our free market system, transcription prices fluctuate. Generally, these fluctuations are not great but should be monitored regularly because they do affect individual transcription fee schedules.

- **Your experience.** If you have specialized skills you may be justified in charging higher rates.

- **Special services.** If you are offering unique or specialized services such as rush turnaround, after 5:00 p.m., curriculum vitae forms for a physician undergoing board certification, or medical manuscripts, consider incremental charges for the additional services you provide.

- **Overhead expenses.** Be sure to include your overhead expenses when arriving at a price for your services. New business owners often forget to include many expenses of self-employment when setting prices. These expenses include your transcription equipment, telephone, gasoline, electricity, rent, transportation, advertising and many other items. You can obtain a list of write-off expenses from your tax accountant, or from one of the references provided in this book.

> *"Look around your home office. Just about everything there that is used in your business is deductible."*
> —Norm Ray, CPA, *Smart Tax Write-offs*

- **Management time.** Do not underestimate the hours you spend managing your business. It takes time to pick up and deliver, count lines, do quality checks, produce statements, set up formats, purchase supplies and update books, to name a few responsibilities. Be sure you have incorporated your administrative expansion into your fees.

COUNT CALCULATIONS

Before deciding how much to bill for your services you must know your transcription production capabilities — by the line, page and hour. Do not *underprice* your services, which will hurt not only you, but your competition and the transcription profession as a whole. And do not *overprice* your services, which will make it difficult for you to attract clients.

Be sure to accurately determine your production capabilities. In other words, are you fast enough and efficient enough to make a profit while charging the going rate?

Here are some simple formulas to calculate by lines or pages transcribed per hour:

- **Lines transcribed per hour.** Divide the total number of lines or pages transcribed by the total number of hours worked.

- **Entire job, total lines or pages.** Multiply the total number of lines or pages by your rate per line or page.

- **Dictation transcribed per hour.** Divide the total minutes of dictation by the total hours worked.

- **Hourly rate.** Divide the total amount charged for the job by the total hours worked.

NOTE

It is important to remember that **hourly rates are looked at critically by the IRS** and could jeopardize your independent contractor status. It is wise to set your fees based on production or job, not by the hour.

COMPUTER LITERATE PHYSICIANS AND PRICING SERVICES

Computers have been a part of the American scene long enough for many physicians, especially those who are younger, to become computer literate. They use computers and understand the basics of word processing, boiler-plating and templating. Sometimes this presents a problem for medical transcriptionists.

Some physicians are now calling home-based medical transcriptionists to ask about their services and to request or demand that boiler-plate and macro work not be charged at the same line rate as work that is typed word for word.

This has happened to me four times in the past two years. Recently a local dermatologist called seeking information about my service and my line rate. She then stated that many of her reports could be standardized and put into macros and that she didn't feel it fair that I charge her the same line rate for that transcription because I wasn't physically entering the data.

I reminded the doctor that I had invested a significant amount in purchasing the equipment and had also invested considerable time learning the technology so I would have the capability to put that information into macros and store it. Then I presented a hypothetical scenario and asked her a question. Our conversation went something like this:

"Doctor, from typing your reports I know that you do quite a bit of laser surgery in your office. One procedure takes approximately thirty minutes to complete, and the patient is charged a set fee for your work. If you bought a new adaptor for your laser machine that would cut the surgery time in half, would you pass the savings on to your patients and only charge them half the previous charge?"

As you probably anticipated, the doctor responded with a resounding NO! I then asked her why she was asking me to do something that she herself would not consider doing. She had no answer and did not complain further about my billing rates.

I believe it is important that medical transcriptionists — not physicians — determine how we enter and price medical data. This is a personal, professional choice, and if we have the technology to store information in macros, then so be it. We should charge physicians no less than if that information were entered repetitively.

SPECIAL CHARGES

At times, clients will ask for services above and beyond the call of duty. As with any other business, it is appropriate to charge special fees for these specialized services.

- **Lost Reports.** Clients, especially hospitals, are notorious for losing transcribed reports. There is no fixed charge rate for reprints; some services charge the original line count; others, half that amount, while some charge a flat page rate.

- **Stat Work.** Work requested in a short turnaround time, which obliges you to reprioritize your work schedule to accommodate the rush job, should be charged a higher rate (e.g., two to three cents a line more).

- **Faxed Reports.** Most clients have fax machines and as a result, some may request that you fax copies of each and every report and deliver the original copy as well. Although you do not pay a direct fee to send a fax from your machine, it does take time from your busy schedule, and your time is a valuable commodity. It is not uncommon, nor is it inappropriate, for independent medical transcriptionists to charge a fee for each page faxed (e.g., one to two dollars per page).

- **Copies.** When setting rates, most clients request only one copy — the original. However, some clients want more than one copy and this should also be factored into your pricing. Your final price should cover the additional printing supplies and the additional time you spend duplicating the requested material.

- **Special Deliveries.** If you have to take time away from your transcription during a work day to hand-deliver a report, you should charge a fee for this special service. You can determine your fee by the amount of time it takes to deliver the report and what it cost you time-wise in transcribing. For example, if the trip took you an hour and you consistently earn $20 an hour transcribing, then a $20 fee should be charged for special service.

NOTE

Regular pickup and delivery charges are usually factored into your line rate when negotiating with a new client and should not be charged separately from the contracted line/page/character rate. Unless your contract indicates otherwise, a delivery fee should be charged for **special deliveries only**.

QUESTIONS FOR PROSPECTIVE CLIENTS

When talking with prospective clients, and before quoting a price, there are some key questions you should ask. For instance, what length of line do they require — 60, 65, 70 characters — and what kind of turnaround time are they seeking? Also ask if they have written policies for quality. If they don't have quality standards, tell them about your quality standards and describe the various services you can provide.

Define what constitutes an error, and set standards for editing and reprinting. Find out if there are penalties for failing to meet deadlines.

Ask the medical records director or medical transcription supervisor (when you are talking to hospital or clinic accounts) to specify the in-house cost per line.

If charging by the page, you may want to charge a minimum page rate and/or establish a minimum number of lines (perhaps 20) for each page. Both are frequently used, acceptable practices among home-based medical transcriptionists.

RAISING RATES

For most transcriptionists, there comes a time when they must charge more for their services. There are several ways to manage this. Some transcriptionists charge a lower rate until they are well established and have a comfortable working relationship with clients — usually within six months to one year. At this point, a rate increase is generally not difficult. For your first as well as future clients, also consider negotiating a contract for a low rate for perhaps 90-120 days, after which the rate automatically increases.

When you become more established and take on new clients — again, usually within 6-12 months — you might decide to raise rates for new clients while maintaining lower rates for older clients. By this time you will have established credibility with existing clients and you should feel comfortable taking on and successfully managing more work.

For existing clients it is acceptable to raise rates every 12-18 months with a 30-day written notice. Make sure your rate increase policy is clearly defined in the client's contract when you negotiate. You could provide a 30-day notice at the time of submitting your monthly invoice, perhaps at the end of the year, by stating "As of January 31, 2003 there will be a rate increase to XXX per line."

RULES OF ENGAGEMENT

If you think "Rules of Engagement" refers only to warfare, think again. With any relationship, whether it's professional or personal, ground rules must be established at the outset for it to be a rewarding and satisfying experience for all parties. Nothing is more devastating to an old-timer or a neophyte in the independent medical transcription arena than to have a new or an established account do a 180-degree turn and become an unhappy client. What causes such a breakdown? Lack of communication.

It is extremely important when speaking to a client for the first time to clarify not only what the client expects of you, the IMT, but also what you expect of the client. Are you crazy? you say. I cannot be so audacious as to dictate my expectations to the client! Let us assure you, if you are to succeed professionally, you will do it.

Give some thought to the following: When hiring an attorney, you are given a page or two of his or her practice standards before signing the contract. When taking your VCR for repair, you are given a contract specifying what type work will be done and when the work will be completed. When having clothes altered, specifications are written down, and you are asked to sign a contract. This is standard professional procedure. Why should our medical transcription businesses be run differently?

Rule #1 — Communication

Communication is critically important to business success. The cumulative effect of everything you say and do affects your clients' perceptions of you and your business, ultimately determining whether or not they continue with your service and refer others to you.

"Professionals with valuable skills should be adequately compensated for their work."

145

Rule #2 — Proposal

Before meeting with a potential client, draw up a proposal. A proposal is your sales presentation, your effort to persuade a prospective client to award you the contract or use your service. The proposal should include a description of the specific attributes of your service and working terms.

Rule #3 — Presentation

When meeting with a prospective client, you present not only your proposal but yourself as well, and both should convey professionalism. Your dress should be tasteful; your demeanor, confident and warm. Your proposal should be thorough, concise and accurate.

The first meeting with your prospective client can be held with the office manager, but to avoid misunderstandings and potential future problems, subsequent meetings should include both the physician and the office manager. Remember, physicians are very busy and you should be prepared to be flexible, adjusting your time schedule to meet with the physician at a time that is convenient for him or her.

This is the time to sell your medical transcription services on a personal level. With enthusiasm and energy, but without monopolizing the meeting, describe what you can offer the client: knowledge, skills, quality service, experience, prompt turnaround, direct phone-in line and other benefits. Answer questions at the meeting, and make yourself available for any questions that may come up later. Provide a resume upon request.

Rule #4 — Put it in writing

Gone are the days when a verbal agreement and a handshake were acceptable contracting practices. Today when dealing with a new client, make sure to put everything in writing.

WRITING A SUCCESSFUL PROPOSAL

Your proposal is the written document you prepare for a potential client in which you describe specific attributes of your service and the proposed working terms between you and the client.

Following are methods we have found successful in developing effective proposals.

- **Introduction:** Begin with a brief statement of who you are, your general qualifications, and a brief abstract of your approach to providing service to the client (you can be more specific in later sections of the proposal).

- **Discussion:** Discuss the benefits of using your service, how it could provide an alternative for staffing, overload, and other problem areas. Make it clear that you are aware of and committed to quality transcription and maintaining confidentiality of transcribed records and reports.

- **Defining Specifics:** List specific services you will provide the client, and the terms. Describe your transcription equipment, staff availability, method of pick up and delivery (by modem, etc.), quality, confidentiality, schedules and prices. When preparing a proposal, discuss tailoring your services to meet the client's needs and include special services in the contract.

- **Putting It In Writing:** Misunderstandings about agreements can occur so don't depend on verbal agreements alone. **Put everything in writing.** If you and the client later agree to changes in the original agreement, write a letter to the client, confirming the changes and outlining the new terms, and file that letter with the original agreement.

CONTRACTS

A written agreement — a contract — should be negotiated with all new clients. In this agreement, the contracting parties commit to specific professional responsibilities. At the start of any professional relationship in which a contract is to be negotiated, it is important to discuss policies and procedures and to reach agreement on items to be included in the contract.

A contract clarifies how work is to be done. It should spell out what services the client is to receive, provide adequate information on processing reports, specify the price of transcription and for how long the rate is guaranteed. In general, rate increases occur every 12-18 months, with a 30-day notice given. The contract should also indicate when billing will be sent and when payment is due.

Specify in the contract when work will be delivered — 24, 48, or 72 hours — and stick to that schedule. One of the authors once contracted for a 48-hour turnaround time, but during a prolonged lull in her work schedule, actually completed work within 24 hours. That was a major mistake! When business picked up again and the transcriptionist resumed the original 48-hour schedule, the client was displeased and demanded that the 24-hour schedule continue.

In general, deviations from contractual terms usually result in unpleasant complications. Prior to negotiating a contract, all factors relating to the business relationship should be considered carefully. When the agreement is finally set down in writing, it should be followed consistently.

Other important items to consider in contract negotiations include: Nondisclosure agreement (confidentiality policy). Information on required transcription material to be provided by the client. Method of access and delivery. Schedules. Quality procedures. Error definition. Pricing policy, which should include line or page lengths and rate. Editing and reprint policy. Missing deadline penalty. Termination date or renegotiation date and waivers of liability.

OPEN-ENDED CONTRACTS

An open-ended contract is one that does not specify a time frame for service. In this case, if an account does not want to use your service any longer, it simply provides no work for you. You might consider inserting a clause in your contract regarding the volume of work you will receive (minimum/maximum) and a termination or renegotiation date. Many hospitals use open-ended contracts so they can utilize the services of IMTs on an as-needed basis.

VERBAL CONTRACTS

No contract business should be concluded on a handshake alone; it is always best to have your contract agreements printed out and approved with signatures from negotiating parties. However, it should be understood that although we do not recommend them, there are legal verbal contracts, and courts of law sometimes find them as binding as written contracts.

A verbal agreement may constitute an "implied contract." That is, if a client verbally agrees to pay you a certain rate per line, a contract is clearly implied. Should a legal dispute occur, a judge could conclude that an implied contract was in force.

Settling verbal contract disputes is usually problematic because it is difficult to establish exactly what the contract provided. It's one person's word against another's. Such problems are avoided with a written contract. In a well-written, detailed, signed contract, the parties are protected in the event of subsequent disagreements or misunderstandings.

If you have only verbal agreements with some of your clients, follow up with a letter to the client summarizing the terms of the verbal agreement and asking for acknowledgment. Send this registered mail with "return receipt requested" or just ask the client to sign a copy of the letter if he or she is in agreement and mail it back to you.

FINE-TUNING THE CONTRACT

If the contract is entered into in good faith with complete understanding and agreement by both parties, it is considered to be binding. If the contract lacks these qualifications, a court could declare it invalid. Contracts are often overturned because they are defective in some respect. Since contract laws are not always crystal clear and straightforward, caution in writing and signing contracts is always advisable.

To fine-tune your contract, avoid misunderstandings during contract negotiations, and to avoid future legal problems, you should always review contracts with your attorney. Your attorney will evaluate contract details, advise you on contractual requirements and procedures, answer any questions you may have, and recommend changes that should be made prior to your contract negotiations.

If an attorney reviews and approves the contract for your first two or three clients, you probably won't need an attorney to review it each time you get a new client. Use the same contract unless there are major changes.

NOTE

It is important to remember that the Internal Revenue Service does not recognize a written agreement as verification of your status as an independent contractor. Contracts and agreements only provide details and terms of your services with the client. Even if your contract states that you are acting and operating as an independent contractor in providing your services to the client, this has no effect on IRS determining whether you are an independent contractor or an employee.

Important items to consider in contract negotiations include the following:

- Nondisclosure agreement (confidentiality policy)

- Information on required transcription material to be provided by the client

- Method of access and delivery

- Schedules

- Quality management guidelines

- Special services, policies and procedures

- Error definition

- Pricing policy, which will include line or page lengths and rate

- Billing policy

- Length-of-time guaranteed rates and rate increase policy

- Editing and reprint policy

- Missing deadline penalty

- Termination date or renegotiation date

- Waivers of liability

To review a sample contract, refer to the appendix of this book.

BILLING FOR SERVICES

Semimonthly billing is more cost-effective than monthly billing, especially for larger accounts, and will improve cash flow throughout the month. Although you will spend somewhat more time on semimonthly billing, the accelerated cash inflow will decrease your stress level immeasurably. Ask your clients about their payment policies. Some large companies and institutions insist on paying invoices according to their policy. Therefore, understand their payment policy so you can decide if you want to accept the account.

Ask who is the contact person for billing inquiries. Generally if your client is a hospital or large clinic it will be someone in the accounts payable department.

Be sure to record your invoices in your software accounting systems or in your bookkeeping ledgers by invoice number, date and when submitted to the client. (You should submit your line count logs with your invoice. Most clients and services require that you do this). Then record when it is paid and record the check number. Once your invoice is submitted to the medical records director or transcription supervisor, it is authorized and forwarded to the accounts payable department. It is then out of the hands of the transcription department. It is keyed into their computer according to your business or vendor name and invoice number.

When designing your invoice, be sure to include the company name, your name and title, business address and phone number. Include the invoice number and invoice date; client's name and address; date and time frame of services delivered; total number of lines calculated at rate charged (e.g., 1520 lines @13 cents per line — 3360 lines @ 15 cents per line; total lines and total amount due). If appropriate, add any past due penalties or payment discount policies on your invoice. Finally, be sure to add a closing remark such as "Thank you." (See sample invoice on the following page.)

TIP

Clearly explain your billing policies and procedures and payment terms to your client, and also include them in your contract.

SAMPLE INVOICE / BILLING STATEMENT

INVOICE #XXXXXX

HEALTHLINE HAWAII
(street address)
(city, state, zip code)
FAX: xxx-xxx-xxxx; PH: xxx-xxx-xxxx

ACCOUNT:　　　　Anytown Hospital - Medical Transcription

BILLING PERIOD: October 15, 2002, through October 31, 2002

Transcription Date	Number Of Lines	Rate Per Line	Daily Total
10/17/02	1743	0.135	235.30
10/18/02	1167	0.135	157.60
10/20/02	1530	0.135	206.58
10/22/02	561	0.135	75.68
10/23/02	1328	0.135	179.31
10/26/02	1438	0.135	194.15
10/28/02	1088	0.135	146.88
10/30/02	897	0.135	121.15

TOTAL LINES:　　　　　　　SUBTOTAL: $1316.65
GENERAL EXCISE TAX (0.04167):　　　54.87

TOTAL DUE: $1371.52

Thank you.

REMIT TO:　　　Donna Avila-Weil, RHIT/HealthLine, Hawaii
　　　　　　　(business address)
　　　　　　　Waikoloa, HI 96738
　　　　　　　FAX: 808-xxx-xxxx　PH: 808-xxx-xxxx
　　　　　　　E-MAIL: ontomaui@netscape.net

TWELVE WAYS TO GUARANTEE PAYMENT

1. **Call it a bill.** Your form should carry the title BILL or INVOICE in large letters at the top of the page. Never call it a statement. Always number your invoices sequentially.

2. **Include your terms.** Make invoices payable on presentation or due on receipt.

3. **Submit bills quickly.** If you have a major account, bill it bimonthly (i.e., 1st and 15th). Never allow more than two weeks to go by without invoicing. Remember, the payment clock does not start ticking until your customer opens the envelope.

4. **Follow up firmly.** Most accounts will pay on time. However, there are always slackers, especially with new accounts. Don't be afraid to follow up with a phone call if you have not received payment within 35 days. If an account refuses to pay, don't hesitate to use collection agencies or small claims court to collect what is owed.

5. **Accommodate where you can.** Ask your clients when they would like to receive their monthly invoices. If they say never, you know you have a problem.

6. **Offer incentives.** Many business owners report they get paid faster by offering a 5-10% discount to clients who pay invoices immediately. Many companies respond to a "2%-10"discount, which means they can take a 2% discount if they pay the invoice within 10 days of the invoice date.

7. **Carry a big stick.** On the bottom of every invoice, post a monthly rebilling charge of $15 if payment is received after 30 days. You may not get paid immediately, but you can be assured you will receive payment shortly after sending the second bill with the $15 charge added.

8. **Consider color.** The Xerox Corporation, which has studied every aspect of document design, reports that when color is used to highlight the all-important "balance due" section, invoices are paid up to 30% more quickly than when boring old black-and-white bills are sent.

9. **Pick a format and stay with it.** It's most helpful if the last line of your invoice showing the amount owed is clearly identified with words or phrases such as PLEASE REMIT.

10. **Curtail details.** The more details you give, the more questions you get. Include date of service, the line count total, and amount due.

11. **Find software solutions.** Decide what works best for you, whether it is a macro with your present word processing program or a specialized billing and bookkeeping program.

12. **Keep good records.** Use a system that works for you. For example, an invoice record keeping system can be as simple as one file of unpaid copies of invoices you've mailed and another file of paid invoices with PAID scrawled across the top.

MAINTAINING CLIENTS

As an independent medical transcriptionist, you will face the challenge of deciding what you are willing to do to keep clients. This is not an easy task. For instance, a client may want to negotiate a flat fee for your services such as XXXX dollars for each billing period. This is called *capitation*. The offer may seem appealingly simple, but it's risky because you could be bombarded with dictation far beyond what you are prepared to process. We do not recommend this. Tell clients you prefer to be paid for what you do. If you do a lot in a month, you should be paid for it. If you do little, compensation should reflect that, too.

Occasionally, a client whose contract demands have not been accepted will take the account and go elsewhere. Stick to your guns, but don't burn any bridges. Three months later the client may call you again, admitting they need you because they can't find a skilled transcriptionist capable of completing their work on a regular and dependable basis.

CLIENTS WHO DEPART UNEXPECTEDLY

It is a painful fact of medical transcription life that few physicians let you know when they are leaving town temporarily, making a practice change, closing their practice, moving away, or have decided not to use your service any longer. They just DO IT — without informing you verbally or giving you written notice. Our advice is, be prepared for this. Once you are psychologically and physically prepared, you will find it easier to make necessary business adjustments and maintain a happy balance in your professional and personal life.

We have come to the conclusion that doctors probably erroneously compare your business to theirs. Their patients usually don't notify them when transferring health care to another doctor so why should your doctor notify you regarding his or her life changes? Perhaps doctors believe their account doesn't make any significant difference to you because they think you have numerous accounts and a long waiting list of potential clients.

Some transcriptionists take the initiative and meet with the physician or office staff to discuss future scheduling. You might consider inserting a clause in your contract regarding the volume of work you will be receive (minimum/maximum) and a termination or renegotiation date.

There are very few situations where the client actually informs the independent medical transcriptionist that he or she is having someone else do work for them. This problem is a frequent topic of conversation in transcription networking circles. Perhaps we need to change our thinking and avoid the employer/employee mode; that is, expecting to be told if we are going to be fired. No matter what, don't get discouraged. There will always be another client needing your services if you consistently increase your networking contacts and continually market your services.

GIFTS FOR CLIENTS

We all need to know that we are appreciated, and clients are no exception. I have always given gifts to my clients during major holidays, and will continue to do so. In past years I have received especially positive feedback about gifts sent which the entire office can enjoy, such as food items. If your clients are physicians, you probably have very little contact with them during the year. However, their staff is, and will continue to be, your lifeline in the office, and they should be acknowledged.

If you know that your client enjoys a hobby, consider a gift related to that hobby. Donations, dinner or theater tickets, also make great gifts. Donations are wonderful, especially if your client has a favorite charity or is on the board of a charity. A donation to a charity in the client's name is also beneficial from the standpoint of tax deductibility, because you can include it on your Schedule A along with other personal contributions which are fully tax deductible. If you decide to take a client to dinner or a show as a gift, you'll only be able to deduct 50% of the cost on your federal taxes.

Gourmet fruit baskets such as those from Harry and David are fun to receive and can be shared with the whole office. Gourmet coffee baskets which include teas, scones, hot chocolates, flavored coffees and specialty cookies also make terrific gifts. Since many people are now becoming vegetarians or have dietary restrictions, these are gifts that can be enjoyed by all.

Keep all of your business-related receipts organized and itemized, and for tax references, it's a good idea to note the purpose of the purchase on the back of the appropriate receipt.

CHARGING INTEREST ON ACCOUNTS

Some businesses charge a 1.5% service charge if a bill is not paid within 15 days; others give a 1% or 2% discount for payments made within 10 days of the billing. Such policies must be explained to your accounts when discussing terms and must be clearly printed on each invoice.

GOVERNMENT CONTRACT PAYMENT

Government clients can offer lucrative contracts, but beware of the fine print. Many of these facilities will not send a vendor payment for 90-120 days. You must ask yourself if you are prepared to wait that long for payment. If not, then a government contract is not for you.

COLLECTING FROM POOR PAYING ACCOUNTS

> *"It has been said that debt enslaves, so I feel it is my duty to free as many slaves as possible by promptly collecting all money owed me."*
> — attributed to Isaac M. Tarcher

If you are in business for any length of time, you will probably confront the unpleasant task of collecting payments from overdue accounts. This can be a problem not only with hospital accounts but with single physician accounts, too. As stated earlier, when discussing your contract with a new account, be sure to stipulate terms of payment with your client. Small vendors are among the last to be paid by some hospital accounts; at times, checks may be held for an unacceptable length of time.

If you have a problem with a client not paying on time, there are several steps you can take:

- Call the client and discuss the matter.

- Agree on a payment date and payment plan (which you should have done at the beginning of the relationship).

- Follow up the phone conversation with a letter outlining the agreement and payment arrangement.

If you have a question about a past-due invoice, contact the accounts payable department, not the medical records department. Be sure to identify your business name, the invoice number and amount of billing. It is very important when submitting billing statements that you include an invoice number. Most of these are keyed in by computer and your billings are tracked by invoice number.

If payments continue to drag out, communicate your displeasure to the medical records director or transcription supervisor. If they think highly of you and your service, they will probably do everything in their power to expedite payment.

Several years ago at a transcription convention, this author sat with a group of home-based medical transcriptionists and their husbands who were discussing slow-paying accounts. One man told about a psychiatrist his wife had once worked for — a doctor who had a tremendously large volume of work and was consistently late in paying for services rendered. Although the psychiatrist insisted he was very satisfied with transcription produced, he always had some excuse for delaying payment.

One day the husband reached his limit of frustration. He marched into the psychiatrist's office, picked up the office copier, told the receptionist that he was taking the machine hostage and would return it when payment was made. Within two hours, the copier was back in the office and payment was made in full. Needless to say, from that point on, the psychiatrist made sure the medical transcriptionist was paid within five days of billing. Most of us will not go to such extremes to force payment, but this story demonstrates potential frustration in attempting to collect overdue accounts.

157

I have never withheld work from an account that was slow in paying, but I have refused to pick up additional work until payment was made. This seems to work well with smaller physician accounts. Fortunately, since I let my first hospital account go due to slow pay, I have not had a problem collecting from my other hospital accounts. I work with a delightful transcription supervisor, who is very conscientious about payment. On the few occasions when checks have been delayed, she has marched directly into the hospital controller's office and made sure the check was promptly mailed.

Remember, you do have options in pursuing nonpaying accounts. You can engage the services of a collection agent. For a nominal filing fee, you can file a petition in small claims court where the dispute can be settled in front of a judge. Never hesitate to use these avenues if the need arises.

Some clients refuse to pay medical transcriptionists until they have received payments from their own accounts. If you have the cash reserve to see you through this period, which may be as long as three months, you can probably afford to work for them. This is a matter of personal choice. Working with services that pay every two weeks, regardless of when they are paid, is preferable.

If you are subcontracting for another service, you may run into a situation where there are no funds to pay you. As an independent, you have the choice of not taking any more work from them until you are paid or continuing to work not knowing when you will be paid.

It still amazes us that some transcription services demand that you turn their work around in 24 hours or less but feel they are only obligated to pay you when they get paid. We have also met transcriptionists who have not been paid for their services at all because the companies they worked for went bankrupt. Investigate services you are considering working with, and be on the lookout for fly-by-night companies soliciting your services.

If you have to hire a collection agency to collect an account, don't feel badly. It is part of being self-employed. In the real business world, professionals sometimes have to be aggressive to collect what is owed them. After all, you did do the work!

In summary, be patient and persistent. Use all appropriate means to collect payments, always remaining calm. If you find that an account is unreliable about payment, network with other medical transcriptionists in your area so they won't fall into the same trap. If the reputation of slow-pay gets around, the physician or hospital will have a problem finding qualified MTs to take their work. That can be very effective collection leverage.

DEALING WITH A CHRONIC COMPLAINER

Few things are worse than unjust verbal assaults from an unhappy office manager who has decided you are fair game for his or her fury. Often, the physician is totally unaware of staff game playing and one-upmanship. If you find yourself in this situation, immediately make an appointment to meet with the physician or medical record director. At that meeting express your concerns and ask if there is anything you can do to help turn this negative situation into a positive one for all concerned. If you have given this client the best service possible and they cannot or will not be satisfied, then rest contented knowing that you have done all you can. If the situation cannot be resolved positively and you continue to receive unjust criticism, then cut your losses and fire the account. Yes, we said fire the account. There is nothing to be gained by continuing in an abusive relationship.

Michael LeBouef, a management consultant and author of *How to Win Customers and Keep Them for Life* (BERKELY) says you have to be careful with an unsatisfied client. "When you get a client who is never satisfied, you need to go along with them initially. But if you find that it's a recurring problem, you have to remember that you're not in business to lose money." LeBouef says it is a good idea to remind the client in subtle ways that you are taking special care of him or her. You might try pointing out that you are providing a variety of services tailored to his needs, more extensive than those for the average account, and that while you are happy to do this for him, there is only so much you can do.

BOUNCED CHECKS

No matter how long you are in business, you will occasionally get a returned check marked in big, bold letters NSF (nonsufficient funds). Most retail businesses charge clients for returned checks, and it is appropriate for professional medical transcriptionists to charge for returned checks, too. You may charge only what your bank charges you or add an additional fee for your time and trouble.

159

FIRING AN ACCOUNT

Transcriptionists rarely fire accounts although they sometimes should. Instead, they needlessly endure poor tape quality, inefficiency, rude behavior, slow payment, and a host of other torments. Why?

Within recent years, this author has terminated two accounts and has suffered no regrets. The first account demanded, and received, 12-hour turnaround time but refused to pay until three months later. It took almost a year of increasing frustration and resentment to propel me into severing the relationship.

I terminated the second account because the rules kept changing. One week after agreeing upon transcription specifications which included copies of all reports and establishing what I believed was excellent rapport with the office manager, she announced that only some reports required copying. Two days later, she once again ordered copies of all reports. Two days after that, she demanded 24- instead of 48-hour turnaround. Two days after that, she decided afternoon delivery was preferable to morning delivery. The account's front office staff was disagreeable and inefficient; hours were wasted waiting for tapes and transmit logs. In an attempt to solve the problem I met with the manager. We discussed the issues; she praised my work and continued to change the rules. Finally, I ended the relationship.

Transcriptionists should never sacrifice their integrity. Loyalty to an ethical account is admirable, but not all accounts are ethical. If you find yourself in an unpleasant and unproductive work situation, take action. Acquire and nurture accounts that are professionally rewarding.

ENDING A CLIENT RELATIONSHIP

Always leave an account with professional dignity and decorum. If you are informed that your services will no longer be needed, it is appropriate to inquire why. It is important for you to know if the quality of your service has been unsatisfactory. Do not, however, withhold work or refuse to finish work in progress simply to be vindictive.

Being released from an account is not necessarily a negative reflection on you or your work, and the separation may be only temporary. In a few weeks or months, you may receive a call from the client who discharged you, once again requesting your services. Always leave clients with a memory of your smile and professional demeanor. It may result in future business when you least expect it.

SCANNED WORK

"Scanned work" refers to taped dictation the client has listened to and about which he or she has documented certain facts. This is called "scanning." These facts are recorded on a transcript log sheet which serves as proof of what is actually on the tape. This should always accompany the untranscribed tapes and should include the following:

- Name of patient

- Date dictated

- Type of report

- Dictating physician

When the transcription is returned to the client, a copy of the transmit log sheet should accompany the work. Be sure to keep a copy in your files.

There may also be occasions when there will be dictation on scanned tapes that is not recorded on the log sheet submitted to you. If this happens, be sure to transcribe these reports and add the names of additional patients dictated on to the log sheet before returning it to your client, making a note that these were additional unscanned dictations that were found on the tape.

UNSCANNED WORK

We recommend never taking unscanned work because it frequently results in problems for the transcriptionist. Often, when a client is not sure what work is being sent out and material disappears, the outside transcription service is blamed for the loss. To avoid this situation, make sure you always have completed log sheets to refute any unfounded allegations regarding missing material.

If a client is not inclined to scan work, explain that you require it in order to maintain professional quality assurance standards established for patient medical records. Also emphasize that scanned tapes help prevent errors and delays that might impact the client's work schedule.

As a professional transcriptionist and a member of the health care team, your goal is to provide prompt and accurate transcription to enhance patient care. A transmit log sheet helps you reach this goal.

DETERMINING TURNAROUND TIME

In order to accurately estimate hours required to transcribe dictated tapes, you will need to know how much dictation is on the tapes. A tape containing 15 minutes of dictation may take 30 minutes to transcribe; a 60-minute tape may require 1½ hours to transcribe. Knowing dictation time will eliminate much frustration and improve work flow.

There are varying sizes and types of tapes. The most commonly used are tapes that hold 30 minutes, 60 minutes, 90 minutes and 120 minutes of dictation (this includes both sides). It is important when making a work commitment that you know how much dictation is on a tape and how many minutes the tape will hold. The average transcriptionist can transcribe approximately 20 minutes of dictation per hour. This includes time spent spellchecking, proofing, transmitting and counting the documents.

If you are transcribing physician accounts, which is the case for 75% of independent medical transcriptionists, it is important to know specific facts about the tapes being used so that you can more accurately determine your potential work load.

It is easy for a transcription supervisor to assign minutes of dictation off a digital system. If you take 80 minutes of dictation, which is assigned to you in minutes and rerecorded on tapes, it will result in approximately four hours of transcription.

The worst nightmare for any home-based medical transcriptionist is to request a certain number of minutes, be assured by the client that the 25 tapes contain only one dictation per tape, and later discover that each dictation is 25-30 minutes long (750 minutes of dictation = 37.5 hours of transcription). Hope you didn't guarantee 24-hour turnaround because this job will probably take you a week!

PRIORITIZING TAPES

It is important to ask your accounts to prioritize work in order to maximize work flow. If they do not, handle all dictation with the same consideration.

"STAT" WORK

"Stat" is a marvelous, and sometimes confusing, word. Derived from the Latin *statim*, which means *immediately*, stat is used frequently in medical settings to indicate activities requiring immediate follow up. In medical transcription, deadlines on stat work vary.

In a recent hospital survey of over 150 physicians, the following definitions of "STAT" and "ASAP" were given:

STAT

- Unstable patient or serious change in the patient's condition. Results affect therapy for the patient and results are required quickly. Critical findings are expected.

- Systems in the diagnostic service will be interrupted to work quickly on the stat order.

- Stat orders must be verbally communicated to the nurse and written in the MD's orders.

- Turnaround: 30 minutes during regular hours; one hour after regular hours.

ASAP (AS SOON AS POSSIBLE)

- Unstable patient or serious change in the patient's condition. Results affect therapy for the patient and results are required soon. Critical findings are **not** expected.

ASAP continued on page 164

ASAP *continued from page 163*

- Systems in the diagnostic service will **not** be interrupted. At the next possible break in sequence, the report will be done.

- ASAP orders must be verbally communicated to the nurse and written in the MD orders.

- Turnaround: 1½ hours for completed report.

As you can see from the above study results, the definition of "stat" varies remarkably. When stat work is requested, communicate with your clients to determine precisely what they mean by "stat" and when the work is **really** needed. For many hospitals, stat means one- to two-hour turnaround. On the other hand, a medical office may expect completion of stat work within 24 hours.

FORMATS

A format is a blueprint or arrangement of, in this case, the medical document. Each health care facility will have its own type of preferred format, so it is important that you consult with the client to assure proper format use.

HOSPITAL FORMAT

There are many types of medical documents that may be entered in the hospital record, but the most basic reports, which are included for **every** patient, are the following:

- History and Physical Examination (H&P)
- Consultation Report
- Operative Report
- Pathology Report
- Medical Imaging Report
- Discharge Summary

These reports generally have specific subheadings, and it is important for the medical transcriptionist to be able to identify these sections because the dictating physician does not always break down a report into the correct sections.

MEDICAL OFFICE FORMATS

Office and clinic formats can be quite different from hospital formats. Medical offices generally use a chart-note format, and a format for consultation and referral letters. As 75% of independent transcriptionists do medical office transcription, it is important to be familiar with these formats.

Chart notes can be transcribed in paragraph form with the patient's name and date seen on the top of the entry. The most common chart-note format is the SOAP format:

S: Subjective — chief complaint
O: Objective — physician or clinician's findings
A: Assessment — diagnosis
P: Plan — goals and direction of treatment

Another common format is HPIP:

H: History
P: Physical exam
I: Impression
P: Plan

Often, physicians will combine both the above formats by dictating: Subject, History, Impression, Plan, etc. In any case, they will have standard styles they prefer, some of which may be their own designs.

Letter formats vary from full-block to a modified-block style. Some physicians have no preference regarding formats and allow transcriptionists to use whatever style they prefer.

Sample history and physical (H&P) format, operative format, and discharge summary format are included on pages 167-169 of this reference book. The consultation format may be similar to the H&P format, but in some cases a subheading will not be included and, often, the physical examination portion of the format is requested in paragraph form.

An excellent reference that provides medical basics and format guidelines for 27 medical specialties is *Manual of Medical Transcription*, published by W. B. Saunders.

DIGITAL DICTATION

Home-based transcriptionists who utilize digital transcription units and transcribe directly off digital dictation systems will find their turnaround time greatly decreased because they are eliminating pickup time entirely.

This transcriptionist's clients are long distance — anywhere from 75 miles to the other side of the United States. Transcribing from a digital dictation system can be done directly real-time or done by downloading off a digital system and rerecording onto cassette tapes. Technology is ever changing and continuously upgrading, offering better and faster methods for completing transcription work. It's an exciting time to be a transcriptionist!

Transcribing directly off the transcribe unit is like working right in the client's office. You do not handle tapes at all. Patient demographics and ID information are shown on an LCD screen on the digital dictation unit in front of you, which includes the medical record (MR) number, physician, date, length and time of dictation and other statistics. When transcription is completed, the transcriptionist signs off the job with the push of a button and another report comes onto the system.

After spellchecking and proofing documents, they are printed out and downloaded onto a disk for delivery to the client; or they are sent via modem back to your client. These very efficient digital dictation systems save transcriptionists vast amounts of time.

> *"Home-based transcriptionists who utilize digital transcription units and transcribe directly off digital dictation systems will find their turnaround times greatly decreased."*

HISTORY & PHYSICAL EXAMINATION (SAMPLE)

Attending Physician: Date of Admission:

CHIEF COMPLAINT:
HISTORY OF PRESENT ILLNESS:
PAST MEDICAL HISTORY:
Illnesses:
Surgery:
Injuries:
Allergies:
Medications:
Habits:

SOCIAL HISTORY:
FAMILY HISTORY:
REVIEW OF SYSTEMS:
HEENT:
Cardiopulmonary:
Gastrointestinal:
Genitourinary:
Neurological:
Musculoskeletal:

PHYSICAL EXAMINATION:
HEENT:
Neck:
Chest:
Heart:
Breasts:

> **NOTE:** Each dictating physician or clinician will have a specific style. In many cases you will be asked to follow not only institutional formats, but individual physician formats as well.

IMPRESSION (or ADMISSION DIAGNOSIS):
1.
2.
3.

/
d
t

ANY TOWN HOSPITAL
Any Town U.S.A
HISTORY AND PHYSICAL EXAMINATION

PATIENT NAME:

MEDICAL RECORD #:

167

OPERATION RECORD (SAMPLE)

Date:
Surgeons:
Anesthesia:

PREOPERATIVE DIAGNOSIS:

POSTOPERATIVE DIAGNOSIS:

OPERATION PERFORMED:

> **NOTE:** All operative reports must indicate the preoperative diagnosis, postoperative diagnosis and name of operation as well as anesthesia and operating surgeons. Some facilities prefer the surgeon and the assistant surgeons be listed separately; others prefer anesthesiologist and anesthesia be listed separately, and they will also request the operation start and stop times. In any case, the basic headings above must be on every operative report.

_____

ANY TOWN HOSPITAL
   Any Town U.S.A
OPERATION RECORD

DISCHARGE SUMMARY (SAMPLE)

Date of Admit: **Date of Discharge:**

ADMISSION DIAGNOSIS:
1.
2.

DISCHARGE DIAGNOSIS:
1.
2.
3.

HISTORY OF PRESENT ILLNESS:

HOSPITAL COURSE:

DIAGNOSTIC STUDIES:

DISCHARGE INSTRUCTIONS:
Diet:
Activity:
Medications:
Follow up:

CONDITIONS ON DISCHARGE:

_____

ANY TOWN HOSPITAL
Any Town U.S.A
DISCHARGE SUMMARY

PIRACY OVER THE AIRWAYS

Digital dictating and transcribing equipment is wonderful! Imagine having a desk telephone that includes a simple headset and foot pedal; and with one stroke of your finger, the telephone will patch itself directly into the transcription pool of any hospital, allowing you to work at any time of the day or night.

Ten years ago I attended a workshop on the **new** digital technology and swore under my breath "they will never be able to do the impossible." Little did I know that four years later, I would have that *impossible* technology installed in my office.

As with all new technology, digital wizardry requires safeguards to foil unscrupulous services or unscrupulous MTs. I had such an experience with airwave piracy not long ago. The hospital with which I contract bought a digital system and everything seemed to be working just fine. Then one Sunday around 9:30 p.m. I received a phone call from the hospital's transcription department. I was asked when I was going to finish transcribing, and the caller commented that I had been on the system since 8:00 a.m. Well, I had just stepped out of the shower, and I hadn't worked in my office all day so I knew something was terribly wrong!

I explained my situation to the hospital representative, but she insisted **my number** was showing up on their board. Short of having her send the transcription police to make sure my machine wasn't on, I didn't know what else to do. She simply refused to believe me. The next evening I was again asked if I was on the digital line. At that particular time I was, and had been since mid-morning. Again I was asked about the work I had supposedly completed the day before. I assured her that if I had worked 14 hours the day before, I would have made sure the 5000+ lines of dictation were delivered on time so I would be paid!

The next day I was informed that a service that had been contracted to work weekends only had used my number — as well as those of every other medical transcriptionist using the system — and had drained all work from the system over the weekend. Needless to say, I was extremely angry as the service had **stolen** my work. I realized then why there had never been work on the system early Monday mornings for the previous four months. This unscrupulous service had found a way to break the code and had taken work from everybody. The hospital fired the service and is now implementing passwords to gain access to the transcription pool.

If you are using a digital system and your client has not begun to use some kind of password system, please inform them that in order to protect themselves and you, they should implement one ASAP. The password system is simple and consists of either a four letter word or a set of four numbers. Each medical transcriptionist, whether an employee or an outside contractor, is assigned a different password that only they can use.

SETTING UP YOUR HOME-BASED OFFICE

Thoroughly research office equipment before establishing your business. It does not take professional marketing research to obtain the information you need. You can easily do this research on your own through a variety of methods including phone surveys, mailing questionnaires, and facts obtained from published materials.

You can work anywhere that is private, comfortable, has good lighting and minimal distractions. To avoid distractions, separate your work space as much as possible from your other living space. To separate work space from living space, you must use partitions if walls are not present. If your work space is clearly separated from your living space, either by walls or partitions, the work space can be written off as a tax deductible business expense. Check with your accountant.

You must establish a true office if you are serious about being self-employed. Create a working atmosphere — a room furnished with a desk, a good ergonomic chair, telephone, typewriter, file cabinet, computer, printer, phone, transcribing equipment, and answering machine. Adequate lighting and ventilation are also essential.

Don't settle for a part-time office on the kitchen table or for temporarily borrowed space elsewhere in your home. An established office space is very important. Creating your work environment will help you learn to take your work more seriously. If your office is home-based, you must create a separate environment from your residence, despite being located physically within it. You must feel as if you are truly "at work."

Your home-based office must be in legal compliance with local laws. Most municipalities restrict certain types of home-based businesses so check on local zoning laws. Businesses that generate heavy traffic are often prohibited from operating within certain areas. Generally speaking, one-person transcription businesses located in private homes face no restrictions.

For specific information, contact your town or county clerk and request pamphlets or other materials on ordinances related to home occupations.

Also check with your homeowners association and examine your house deed for possible restrictions. Zoning is probably the only legal barrier to starting your home business.

THE MEDICAL TRANSCRIPTION OFFICE — EQUIPMENT

COMPUTER

- 400 MHz, 64 MB 100 MHz SDRAM
  15" to 17" Monitor

  Most computers purchased new come with some software included such as Microsoft Word or WordPerfect.

PRINTER

- Good quality, inexpensive laser or inkjet printer Companies such as NEC, Epson, Hewlett Packard have some great products on the market.

MODEM

- Get at least a 56K bps modem, internal or external.

FAX MACHINE

- Plain paper fax machines use cheaper paper but are more costly than thermal fax machines.

- An automatic paper cutter will help you avoid wasting paper.

- An anti-curl feature keeps paper flat, especially helpful when filing.

- Fax-Tel switch routes call for fax or voice communication.

- You can also get all-in-one fax, copier, scanner and printer products.

FAX MODEM

- On the plus side, it is cheaper and lets you send faxes directly from your computer. Saves paper, and the quality is better because the document doesn't have to be scanned.

- On the minus side, it cannot be used to send printed documents such as newspaper clippings.

SOFTWARE

- WordPerfect

- DOS

- MS Word

- Norton Utilities or equivalent

- Word abbreviation program such as PRD + or Instant Text

- ProComm Plus — Enables you to telecommute

- Quicken — Bookkeeping software

- Line Count Programs — Sylcount II by Sylvan Software, WP Count by Productive Performance

- Medical Dictionaries — Dorland's and Stedman's (Book and computer disk/CD-ROM formats are available)

- Spellcheckers — Stedman's Plus

- PCAnywhere — file transfer program

- Backup Systems

REFERENCE BOOKS

- *DOS For Dummies* — IDG

- *Windows For Dummies* — IDG

- *ABCs of WordPerfect* — Sybex

- *Word for Windows* — Microsoft

- *WordPerfect Instant Reference* — Sybex

- *WordPerfect Made Easy* — Osborne

- *Modems Made Easy* — Osborne

PLACES TO EVALUATE COMPUTERS

- Best Buy

- Circuit City

- CompUSA

- Computer City

- Costco

- Sam's Club

- Internet resources such as CDW, Dell, etc.

When buying a computer, make certain you will get the technical support you need should your equipment malfunction. Most computers come with a 90-day warranty, but companies such as Dell offer a one-year, at-your-home-or-office warranty, which can be extended an additional two years. If they cannot tell you how to solve the problem over the phone, they will send a technician out the next business day. All this is included in the purchase price. So shop, compare . . . and shop some more.

If you use your American Express card to purchase equipment, AMEX automatically doubles the manufacturer's warranty on the product. This means that if you buy a computer with a one-year warranty, it will be extended to two years.

THE DESK

After selecting a work space, you will be ready to furnish your office. Your desk will probably be your first purchase.

When selecting a desk, make sure it is the right height for you. One that is too high could result in physical difficulties such as carpal tunnel syndrome or back and neck problems.

It is not necessary to purchase an expensive desk. Some very fine computer desks with shelves and drawers can be purchased for as little as $50, if you are willing to expend the time and energy to assemble them yourself. Watch the newspaper for businesses that are liquidating their furniture. You can save a tremendous amount of money this way.

THE CHAIR

Carefully select the proper chair. Every fiber of your body will thank you.

Most experienced MTs have worked in offices where they endured THE CHAIR FROM HELL, which is a modern-day torture device with two square wheels and a back that flips you into abduction and external rotation every time you lean back too far. Avoid buying such a chair. If you do buy the chair from hell, we guarantee you a future of prolonged discomfort and many physical complaints.

If you live in or near a metropolitan area, go to a furniture manufacturing company and test-sit as many different chairs as possible until you find the one that is right for you. If you don't have access to furniture manufacturers, do your research in stores that sell office equipment.

The most important factor in selecting a good chair is adjustability. When seated, you should be able to plant your feet firmly on the floor. The height of the seat back should correspond to your lower back, where you need support for your spine. Arm rests should not interfere with free movement. Your typewriter or computer keyboard should be low enough so that you can hold your wrists straight without tiring your arms.

State-of-the-art chairs have 10-15 adjustment settings. The most convenient chair has pneumatic adjustments, allowing the user to pump the chair up and down without getting up. Pneumatic chairs can be expensive but many transcriptionists believe this investment is money well spent.

COMPUTER TECHNOLOGY

Small companies are a significant driving force in our national economy. In such a setting, opportunities for independents will abound. To take advantage of those opportunities, you need a powerful computer.

Years ago, correcting selectric typewriters were state of the art for self-employed transcriptionists. There are some people who still manage their business without a computer, but their numbers are few and dwindling. Today's smart transcriptionists use state-of-the-art computers.

Since the first personal computers appeared in the late 1970s, our economy and lifestyle have undergone dramatic transitions. In the blink of an eye an "information highway" has appeared, redefining our personal and professional lives, the workplace, and the way we work. It has also been a catalyst for the independent medical transcriptionist movement. Home computers, sophisticated software, modems, and digital dictation systems have opened many new doors for independent transcriptionists, allowing them to operate small businesses as efficiently as large services. Many are operating the "paperless office" and servicing clients entirely through telecommunication. The future promises more exciting innovations in the realms of speech recognition and optical imaging. We can't imagine running a home-based business today without the aid of a computer. To remain professionally competitive, you must be computer-competent.

CHOOSING A COMPUTER

You may be surprised to discover that you can afford a powerful computer with sophisticated capabilities. Computer prices have dropped significantly within the last few years, to the point where some computers are now less expensive than typewriters.

If you feel hesitant to use a computer, you are not alone. Most people who have no experience using a computer are initially fearful, but it doesn't take long to feel comfortable with this great technology, and once you do, you'll wonder how you lived without it. And if you think computers have too many capabilities that you'll never use, think again. You will soon be using most or all of them, adding memory to increase your computer capabilities, and looking forward to new technological innovations.

Because there are so many types of computer hardware available, it's a good idea to network with peers and research industry standards thoroughly to determine precisely what you need. Keeping in mind that the computer industry is an extremely competitive market, be a smart shopper. Buying quality brand name components is the key to a reliable PC, and larger companies invest big dollars in research and development of their products to assure reliability and performance. They offer warranties to consumers and also have dedicated, well-trained technicians to support their products.

Frequently, computer salespersons don't understand the type of work medical transcriptionists do nor do they comprehend how much capacity we need in our computers for document storage. Determine what your computer needs are and, when shopping, be prepared to inform salespersons of the facts. Don't settle for less than a computer system with a storage capacity that will meet your needs.

Computer consultants recommend that you have a Windows environment loaded. You can still run WordPerfect from DOS (or Windows) but with a windowed machine, you will also have multi-tasking or background processing capabilities. This will give additional flexibility, allowing you to work in several different environments at one time.

Effectively, this means that you can send or receive files or faxes while you are processing documents, spreadsheets or other items. Without a doubt, multi-tasking is one of the greatest timesavers ever invented. Even if you aren't interested in windows and think you won't run WordPerfect in it, we recommend getting it anyway with the thought of learning it when you have the opportunity. Future software developments will certainly continue to utilize the Windows environment, offering exciting possibilities.

LEARNING ABOUT COMPUTER EQUIPMENT

If you have had little or no experience with computers, it is important to do some networking. Ask fellow transcriptionists in your area where they bought their computers and, more specifically, about the best prices they found and the quality of any follow-up service they are receiving.

Visit a local college that offers computer courses. Talk with the instructors, especially those who teach word processing, and ask for advice concerning the type of computer they recommend for your work application.

Attend computer swap meets and small business shows. Review the many excellent computer magazines such as *P.C. Computing* and *Home Office Computing*, which can be purchased through newsstands and book stores. After you have completed your fact finding, it is time to visit the dreaded "C.S." — the Computer Store. We **do** recommend purchasing from a computer store or dealer — especially for first-time buyers — rather than from discount or department stores.

Computer dealers are specialists and generally provide more prompt and skilled service when you need help. They are invaluable for initial training, ongoing guidance, and computer repairs. Remember, if your machine is down, so is your business.

Small, independent computer manufacturing companies can also be helpful in initial computer purchases. They are usually eager to work with you and their prices may be lower than those of some larger computer franchises. It has been our experience that small, independent stores usually provide excellent in-house service, which shortens a transcriptionist's downtime. In addition, many of these small firms loan backup units while machines are being repaired.

Computer downtime is not common, but when it happens, it may take five to ten working days to get the required service performed. As a professional, you probably won't be able to delay work for that long. Therefore, when computer shopping, find out about the system's guaranty or warranty, whether repairs will be done in-house or sent out, and about the company's policy regarding computer "loaners."

BUYING A USED COMPUTER

Consider buying a used computer. There are many computer "techies," also known as computer "nerds," who frequently upgrade their computer systems. They then sell the older computer model, which is generally in excellent condition, throwing in software, disks and accessories at no extra charge. You may find a terrific bargain!

However, if the seller gives you used software, make sure that he gives you all the original diskettes and manuals and agrees to help you get the software license transferred into your name.

COMPUTER SERIAL NUMBER

Do not buy a used computer that lacks the manufacturer's serial number. Serial numbers are printed on adhesive labels, which are peeled off when the equipment changes hands illegally. If you can't find a serial number on the equipment, it may be stolen property, which could cause you problems. Remember, if there is no serial number, beware!

Look for computer bargains in your local newspaper's classified ads or on the bulletin board at computer stores.

An important feature to look for in a computer is how much available software the machine will accept. Don't limit yourself in your software capabilities. Your software is your computer's real power. Be sure you buy a machine that can be upgraded as your business expands.

KEYBOARDS

There are two major keyboards available for personal computers — the standard keyboard and the enhanced keyboard. We recommend the enhanced keyboard because it has more keys than the standard model, and it is the preferred model sold with most personal computers (PCs) today.

In addition to the keys found on standard typewriters, all PC keyboards include a few keys not found on typewriters. These are keys that move the characters around the screen — error and cursor control keys, keys that let you page through entire screens in a single keystroke, page up and page down keys, home keys, end keys, and function keys that will perform special actions and help access the systems in many programs.

Personal computer keyboards also have caps lock keys, which shift keyboards into capital letters, number lock keys, and more. There are also insert keys, delete keys, and keys that let you print screen contents. Most keyboards for desktop PCs have both standard numbers and separate number keys in ten-key-format for quick entry. Finally, all keyboards have **ESC**, **CTRL** and **ALT** keys, which, when pressed with other keys, access special program operations.

Most newer keyboards have function keys at the top of the keyboard, and some special keyboards have function keys at both the side and top. There are also *kinetic* or contour fit keyboards of various types. These are designed to prevent repetitive strain injuries such as carpal tunnel syndrome. Some are quite unusual so try them out before you make a final selection.

Selecting your keyboard will be one of your most important decisions, because when your hands feel comfortable and the keys feel "right," your productivity will soar. Each keyboard has a different fit and feel. You may try out dozens before you find one that feels good to your touch. Also evaluate a "nonclick" keyboard, which eliminates that constant, potentially annoying, keyboard clicking. If you prefer a quiet office setting, you'll probably find the nonclick keyboard more efficacious for you. It is for me!

THE KINESIS ERGONOMIC KEYBOARD

Unlike the traditional flat computer keyboard, the kinesis key system is contoured to fit the shape and movements of the human body and has integral palm supports. The design puts less stress and strain on muscles, reduces the user's risk for fatigue in hands, wrists and arms as well as identified risk factors for developing or compounding painful injuries such as carpal tunnel syndrome, tendinitis or other cumulative trauma disorders (CTDs).

Results from a pilot study have demonstrated that keyboard users adapted quickly to the kinesis ergonomic keyboards. Participants in the study acclimated quickly to its unique contours and most equalled or exceeded their speed and accuracy as measured on the traditional computer keyboard after only eight hours of use on the kinesis keyboard.

The kinesis keyboard is available directly from Kinesis Corporation at a suggested retail price of $390. It has a 30-day money back guarantee and a three-year warranty. To order the keyboard or for additional information, contact Kinesis.

- **Kinesis Corporation**
  800-454-6374 (orders)
  206-455-9220 (office)
  fax 206-455-9223

COMPUTER PRINTERS

The computer printer is an important purchase. Clients demand professional looking documents, and many transcription services suffer because they lack quality printers.

Some clients require that their reports be printed on a laser printer while others don't have a preference. By networking with other transcriptionists, you will discover which printers are most reliable.

When you begin your search for a computer printer, look for one that will best meet your professional needs and perform the functions your work demands. Use the following seven major criteria to evaluate your options:

1. Price

2. Print quality

3. Speed

4. Flexibility of paper handling

5. Software compatibility

6. Durability

7. Cost of operation

If you buy a dot matrix printer, which you will need for clients who have tractor-fed paper for chart notes or if you use roll stick-back paper, make sure it is a letter quality printer. It should have a 24-pin dot matrix with near letter quality and various font options. Dot matrix printers with two paper paths will save you considerable time.

> ## NOTE
> **Do not buy a used or rebuilt dot matrix printer, which may not function dependably and result in major problems.**

If your work requires a laser printer, Hewlett-Packard's are some of the most well-built and require very little maintenance. However, there are several other brands on the market that are also very good and cost 20% to 40% less than the Hewlett-Packard brand.

Purchasing a used or rebuilt laser printer may be a viable option for you depending upon how much you will be using the printer. If you need it only for your personal use and a few business items, a used model might be satisfactory. If, however, you are planning to print reams of reports, you will probably be better served by a new printer. Laser printer prices have decreased considerably in the last few years and there are now some very affordable models on the market — at prices we were paying for dot matrix printers not long ago!

Another major consideration in purchasing a laser printer is your day-to-day operating costs, which can run four to five times higher than a dot matrix printer. Replacing the toner/developer cartridge usually costs around $75 and must be repeated every 5000 to 6000 pages. Laser printer image drums cost from $100-$125 each and with heavy use, may have to be replaced two or three times a year. These figures will vary between printer types and models, so check details at your computer store.

Another aspect that makes laser printers somewhat less attractive than dot-matrix printers is their paper-handling limitations. The most popular laser models have a single paper tray that holds about 100-200 sheets of paper. If you want to print letterhead and second sheets, you will have to feed one paper type manually or look for a more expensive model with dual paper trays.

When print quality is your major concern, a laser printer usually is the way to go. Laser printers are wonderful and quality is unequaled, but if your major clients are going to be hospitals or large clinics, a laser printer probably won't be necessary. These facilities generally use impact printers or request that transcriptionists modem to their in-house printer. Impact printers use tractor fed NCR paper, which has an original and two or three copies.

Inkjet printers represent the smallest market segment of the three technologies, but for some, they are an adequate alternative to laser printers. Inkjet printers spray tightly controlled streams of ink onto paper to produce text and graphics, and print quality is only slightly less than a laser printer's high-quality output.

The primary difference between ink-jet and laser printers is price. If you need print quality and are on a budget, ink-jet is worth investigating. The trade-off, however, is operating speed. What you save in dollars you will make up for in waiting time. A single ink-jet page takes about a minute to print, which is extremely slow compared to laser printer output.

Two other important printer features are 1) tractor feed and 2) automatic single sheet feed. Some accounts use continuous paper and others use single sheets, so it's best to be prepared for both.

Ribbons are another consideration. Ask your computer dealer for information about ribbon types, features, and costs. A printer may look desirable because of its cost, but the cost to replace ribbons may be excessive.

If the printer you are considering is not a name-brand, ask the dealer to recommend other ribbons that are compatible with it. You can then shop for ribbons under that compatible name-brand and may get a better price.

If you plan to print graphics — designing your own fliers, brochures and letterhead — we recommend purchasing a Post-Script™ compatible laser printer or one with Post-Script upgradability.

Purchasing additional printer memory at the time of the initial purchase is more economical than adding it later. Check with your computer dealer for more information regarding this and other upgrades.

You will save money in the long run if you buy a quality printer in the beginning. And, ALWAYS plug your printer into a surge protector.

DICTATION AND TRANSCRIBE UNITS

A dictation unit is a small machine with a built-in microphone into which a person dictates for recording purposes. As a transcriptionist, you will not need a dictation unit; your clients will use these. You will soon discover, however, that the better the dictation unit, the better the clarity of dictation and ease of transcribing.

As an MT who learns as much as possible about the medical transcription industry, you will find it useful to have a basic understanding of dictation units. Spend some time with sales representative and learn about the various types of dictation equipment currently available. This information will help you speak more informatively with clients about their dictation units and their needs. Also, a new client may ask you to recommend a dictation unit he or she should purchase, and given such a golden opportunity, you will want to recommend the best unit available.

A transcriber is a machine with a headset and foot pedal attached, so that it plays a dictation tape back for listening and typing purposes. You must have a transcriber to do your job as a transcriptionist. There are four types of transcribe units: standard, micro, mini and digital.

At the present time, standard and micro transcriber units are used most often in the medical transcription industry. However, digital dictation units are rapidly growing in popularity. *(See page 187 for more information on digital dictation units.)* Occasionally you will run across an account still using a mini cassette, or God forbid! an old Grundig Stenorette (a reel-to-reel unit as old as Methuselah).

No matter what system your clients use, you must be prepared to accommodate them. If a client uses micro dictation, you must have a micro transcriber available or purchase one. Some transcriptionists purchase a standard transcriber with micro and mini adapters. In today's market, these adapters are not as readily available as they were ten years ago. Product representatives rarely, if ever, offer them. They prefer you buy a separate unit for standard, mini, and micro transcriber (which they have in ample supply and which provide them greater profits). If you are interested in acquiring adapters, ask about their availability for mini or micro tapes when purchasing your standard unit. Remember, however, if you purchase a Lanier transcriber, **only** a Lanier adapter will work. Mismatched brands won't work together.

Although transcribers sold in office supply stores sometimes appear to be considerably less expensive than those sold by authorized dealers of dictation and transcribe equipment, they may cost you more in the long run. Equipment purchased from non-authorized dealers is sometimes lower quality and may break down more easily. Also, you may not have local service available when you need it. The non-authorized store may have to send your machine to the manufacturer to get it repaired.

Quality is the key here. Dictation and transcribe equipment sold in office supply stores are generally not commercial quality but rather consumer grade equipment; therefore, stores set prices so it is more economical and easier to replace broken equipment than to repair it. We recommend splurging a little and buying commercial-quality equipment from an authorized dealer.

To save money, consider buying a used, rebuilt, or reconditioned unit from a dealer. These usually carry a 90-day warranty on parts and labor, and a maintenance agreement for future repairs can be obtained at the time of the purchase or any time thereafter.

WARNING

If you decide to buy a used transcriber, be sure you don't get an obsolete machine for which obtaining replacement parts will be difficult, if not impossible.

Besides equipment quality, the most important factor to consider when shopping for transcription equipment is future personal service. Will you be able to get immediate service and loaner equipment when needed? If you don't get an affirmative answer to this question, buy your equipment elsewhere. Don't hesitate to ask what type maintenance service is available and find out how quickly the store responds to breakdowns. Service should be provided on the same day you make the call for assistance. Eliminating downtime is crucial to your work.

Whether you buy, rent or lease equipment, you can test reliability by using equipment for a short period of time on a free trial basis. Equipment should also come with a 30- to 90-day warranty, and you should have the option of returning any item that does not meet your professional needs. Among other things, watch out for dirty or faulty equipment, which can keep you from hearing dictation clearly. Be sure to test transcribers and dictation units sold at office supply stores; you will be amazed at the differences in the quality of transcribe machines. Again, as a safety precaution, **always** plug your transcriber into a surge protector.

Plan on spending more for a transcribe unit from an authorized dealer such as Lanier, Dictaphone, Sony, Phillips, or VDI than from a local office supply store. Exactly how much more depends on whether the unit is new or used and how great a negotiator you are. Yes . . . dealers **will** negotiate. Whether purchasing, leasing or renting, begin by looking at what each vendor has to offer to meet your needs. Get quotes. It's better not to buy the machine on your first visit. Take time to research and shop around before you make your final decision.

When working with an authorized sales representative, it is usually possible to negotiate an equipment price reduction — sometimes as much as 30%-45% off the list price. Therefore, take 30%-45% off the lowest list price and consider this amount the price you will accept. Tell the sales rep that this amount is the maximum your budget will allow. He or she may not meet your price but may make a counter offer. And, it never hurts to let salespeople know you plan to purchase additional equipment and supplies from them in the future.

After writing down the sales representative's lowest offer for the equipment, call other vendors and repeat the scenario. Once you have all the quotes, take the lowest quote, call the higher priced vendors and tell them that XXX company will do business at XX price, and ask if they can beat the price. Continue your negotiations until you believe you have the lowest quote. At this point, make your actual purchasing decision based on the best quoted price **and** services offered **and** attributes of the sales representative.

When evaluating equipment or other products with a sales representative, most transcriptionists logically and intuitively know whether or not they would enjoy working with this person and the company they represent. In addition to personal rapport, you should determine the company's average response time to service calls, their loaner policy in case your equipment breaks down, warranty and maintenance agreements, number of free cassettes you will receive, other freebies or benefits they may offer, and the price.

If you are considering purchasing a digital dictation system, be prepared to pay considerably more than you would for a regular transcribe unit. This is because digital dictation systems **cost** more to produce as a result of sophisticated technology used in their manufacture. As a transcriptionist, you benefit from this technology, which allows you to directly access dictation without downloading onto cassettes, handling tapes, pickup, etc.

There are several companies that offer digital dictation systems. If you are considering this investment, be certain it is compatible with your clients' transcription system. Lanier will not work with Dictaphone, and vice versa.

DIAL-AND-DICTATE TRANSCRIPTION

Another option for the home-based transcriptionist is the call-in dictation system. This is also known as a "dial-and-dictate" system, which allows your clients to dial in and dictate on your unit. There are also new products that can be installed in your PC that allow clients to phone in and dictate. You can transcribe dictation as they are dictating. Some of these systems cost over $1000 so you may want to forego this added expense, especially in the early stages of your business.

Phone-in dictation systems cost $3000-$5000, which is admittedly pricey but may be well worth the investment because this system eliminates pickup of tapes, which cuts delivery time in half instantly. Transcribed documents can then be sent electronically to the client, be hand-delivered, or sent by express mail. If you transmit electronically, you save almost 100% of normal delivery time, which greatly facilitates turnaround commitments.

Phone-in dictation systems are very effective for physician office clients. Doctors are often reluctant to invest in expensive dictation and transcription equipment. They prefer the option of calling right into the transcriptionist's dictation system. Phone-in dictation systems are available in digital and tape systems that hold several cassette tapes.

DIGITAL DICTATION

Over the past ten to fifteen years, computerization has touched all facets of our personal and professional lives. Home computerization has changed everything from alarm clocks to video cassette recorders. In the workplace, computers have revolutionized the way medical documents are transcribed through the use of word processing systems. Just as we have become proficient with word processing systems, the computer has changed the way physicians and transcriptionists dictate and transcribe reports.

WHAT DOES "DIGITAL" MEAN?

Digital means conversion of analog voice wave forms into a series of numbers (usually 0s and 1s) that can be understood by a computer. Within the computer, the numbers go through a digital-to-analog conversion, and a very high-quality replica of the original dictation voice is audible.

HOW DOES DIGITAL DICTATION WORK?

"Using modern technology and telecommunication, it takes me three hours to do what it took me eight hours to do ten years ago!"

Physicians dictate into telephone or specialized dictation stations. The procedure is much the same as it would be with an analog tape system except that the dictator must enter certain identifying information — author ID#, work type ID, or patient ID — through a telephone key pad or bar code scanner. Physicians benefit from a number of special control options unique to digital systems. They can mark the spot where they start dictating the impression, jump instantly to the beginning or end of their dictation, and take advantage of numerous other exciting options.

All dictation stations or telephones are connected to a central computer by direct wire or standard phone line. Both the ID codes and dictator's voice are received by the port board, which digitizes the voice and transfers it to the systems disk to be stored along the code, thereby providing instant selective access by any user who needs to listen to the report — just like data with text retrieval on a more traditional computer system.

Currently, reports can be dictated, digitized and listened to, but they still have to be typed. It is difficult to predict how long it will be before speech recognition technology is sufficiently advanced to be truly user friendly and unambiguous, but we think it is safe to say that most medical reports will require human transcription for at least several more years.

Digital dictation systems facilitate the transcriptionist's work by eliminating cassettes and providing instant selective access to any dictation. These jobs can be routed by supervisors, who assign a number of jobs to each transcriptionist through a management terminal. For self-selection, jobs can be accessed through the digital keypad controlling the type of report to be transcribed. Selection is by author, work type, and patient ID. Standard earphones and foot pedals are complemented by special controls on the transcription station. There are systems which offer undistorted speed control. These have LCD screens that display report type, length, patient ID, author ID, and other necessary information.

Prices of digital dictation units vary widely, so comparison shop and find the best system for your needs. It's also a good idea to attend transcription conventions and seminars to evaluate and test various products and systems that vendors exhibit.

Digital dictation equipment maximizes productivity by providing the transcriptionist with many timesaving features including instantaneous playback, digital audio voice quality and easy location of dictated reports. Digital sound quality is unparalleled, and there are no tapes to lose or damage. A digital dictation system will provide a crystal-clear recording without static.

The digital dictation system is a computer with very few moving parts and therefore it is very reliable. Problems such as tape breakage, battery failure and poor sound quality no longer occur. Digital systems can be accessed remotely from literally any location that has access to a telephone line, including cellular phone lines. Dictated reports are transcribed through telephone lines by use of a telephone transcribe station.

Once you have accessed a digital dictation system through a telephone line, reports can be transcribed online or actually rerecorded to a desktop cassette unit for transcription at a later time. This latter method is very cost effective for long-distance clients because you avoid transcribing "online" long distance, which can be very expensive. Work can be downloaded via virtually any touch-tone telephone with an inexpensive telephone coupler and a basic cassette recorder, either standard or micro.

The cost of a telephone record coupler is approximately $75. The cost of a desktop recorder ranges from $50-$600. In addition, if you are purchasing a digital dictation system — a specific unit such as Lanier or Dictaphone — the cost for your digital transcribe unit will range from $800-$1750.

THE VIRTUAL REALITY OF
SPEECH RECOGNITION TECHNOLOGY

> *"That great, growling engine of change — technology."*
> —Alvin Toffler, *Future Shock*, 1970

Fifteen years ago, I attended a workshop on speech recognition technology that left me feeling very unimpressed. The dictator spoke in a very slow, monotonous tone (which is not the real world of transcription) and spent much time editing and correcting text. We medical transcriptionists were told that within five years our jobs would be in jeopardy as a result of speech recognition technology, but, after seeing the demonstration, none of us felt the least bit threatened.

Every transcriptionist in that room knew that few doctors would be willing to spend the time and the money (at that time the system cost $50,000) to train a system to accept their dictation. Doctors are busy people and most would not have the patience to speak at a rate of 30-50 words per minute, let alone clearly and succinctly. Doctors love to dictate on the run, especially while eating breakfast, lunch and dinner, enjoying quality time with the children and assorted pets at night, calling from their car phones on the way to an emergency or dictating late at night when narcolepsy overtakes them. Sometimes while dictating, they also chomp on snacks, drink, belch, yawn, snore or follow ambulances with sirens screaming.

Some doctors have a phobia about dictating and even though they may be the most articulate member on staff, when faced with a microphone their natural speaking skills disappear. I once worked for a physician who was the worst dictator I had ever heard, which surprised me because he was normally a very engaging and happy man. When he dictated, however, he stuttered, slurred his words and spoke as if having a panic attack.

One day this doctor told me his story. As a young intern, he had worked in a large metropolitan hospital. He'd been there about seven months when one morning the chief resident grabbed him in the hallway and took him to the medical records department. The chief resident stood the baffled intern in front of a mountain of medical charts and asked why he had not dictated his reports. Try as he might, the intern couldn't recall ever having been told that this was his responsibility. That, he said, was his initiation into dictating and from that day forward, every time he picked up a microphone to dictate, he broke out in a cold sweat and envisioned that endless stack of charts.

WHAT IS SPEECH RECOGNITION TECHNOLOGY?

Speech recognition technology was developed to recognize the spoken word, which activates computer input on the screen. This ability to interact with a computer system in the same fashion that we communicate with one another is almost universally appealing, and during the last fifteen to twenty years, the technology has been researched extensively by many firms. During that time, major technological advances have occurred.

The earliest speech recognition systems depended on the user to chop their utterances into distinct words, which is an unnatural, robotic way to speak. Even then, reliability of spoken-word recognition was poor. The 95% accuracy rate sounds impressive until one realizes that 5% inaccuracy means the system missed one word out of 20. Most people would find it frustrating to speak to someone who misunderstood 5% of their speech. We think they would reach their boiling point even sooner if they were talking to something as impersonal as a computer.

Eventually speech recognition will be a standard feature of new personal computers. It will be the ultimate in user-friendliness. In the not too distant future, this exciting technology will allow us to use voice commands to operate our front door locks, turn lights on and off and operate televisions and stereo systems.

The latest speech recognition technology can now accept continuous speech as opposed to discrete speech. Discrete speech required a distinct pause of 1/10 of a second between words, which required the operator to learn an unnatural speech pattern. Under no circumstance should you consider an older discrete-speech version. Modern Pentium computer processors now permit acquisition of continuous speech patterns and the necessary wave-form comparative analysis to be performed in an acceptable time frame — a five-second delay. This means that as you dictate in your normal voice, about five seconds go by before the words appear on the screen, already checked for spelling and grammar context. The newest 300 MHz and 400 MHz CPUs combined with 96 MB of RAM virtually eliminate the time lag, though this consideration is less important than you might think since one should be dictating without looking at the computer's monitor. Some physicians such as radiologists and pathologists, who benefit most from this technology, already use speech recognition dictation equipment while viewing X-ray charts, biopsies and client records.

191

HOW SPEECH RECOGNITION TECHNOLOGY WORKS

A microphone and personal computer sound card are used to produce a digital waveform from analog human speech. Complex algorithmic equations are used to isolate, identify and interpret the individual phonemic components of each spoken word. Each user enrolls by speaking a defined and known-in-advance text that creates a voice model. Enrollment produces a personalized collection of user files that statistically model how the phonemes of a word correspond to the data produced by the acoustic processor. The system uses a speech engine that updates or averages new speech data with existing voice model files. If the user clicking on an improperly recognized word or phrase indicates an error, alternate statistical choices are presented to the user for correction by selection and substitution. This step is very important to the continued improvement of the recognition system, which learns from these mistakes.

According to some experts, speech recognition technology has advanced more in the last three years than it had in the previous decade. As processors get faster, many products enable the user to bypass keyboards and dictate directly into their computers.

Until a 686 computer is built, continuous speech will not exist. With systems available today, current technology can only process speech in discrete utterance, requiring a pause between every two to three words. However, it can be modified by building voice macros and single word commands that represent larger groups of words or keystrokes, thus speeding up the process. Such modifications are similar to our methods in using PRD+ and other abbreviation programs.

In any speech recognition system, speed and accuracy of the system is affected by vocabulary size and the number of users recognized. At this time, many highly skilled MTs are keyboarding in a continuous speech mode, using faster computers, ergonomic keyboards and abbreviation programs.

There are three major speech recognition programs currently available: IBM's ViaVoice Gold, Dragon System's NaturallySpeaking and Lernout & Hauspie Speech Products' Voice Xpress Plus. Each of these programs combines text formatting commands with continuous speech (natural speech) text recognition. Some of the above vendors offer varying degrees of hands-free abilities depending upon the make and model, which are invaluable to pathologists and other professionals who are accustomed to tape recording dictation while working with both hands.

The **IBM Personal Dictation System** is designed to be used in the OS/2, DOS or Windows configuration and can be used with either Microsoft for Windows, WordPerfect or Lotus Notes. It provides a 20,000-word standard vocabulary that includes a 30,000-word journalism vocabulary, 16,000-word emergency medicine vocabulary and 19,000 word radiology vocabulary. The system transfers text to an application by cut-and-paste or by keyboard emulation. Instead of continuous mode, it works in a discrete speech recognition program, requiring a short break before and after each word. Accuracy is rated at 90%. Contact IBM for more information.

- **IBM**
  800-426-2968

Dragon Dictate works with DOS or Windows and includes a 110,000 word backup dictionary as well as a vocabulary optimizer. Unlike other systems, it is phonetically based and requires a pause between words. A unique feature of the software is that it "learns" as you dictate by moving the most frequently used terms into a priority scale. Call Dragon Dictate for more information.

- **Dragon Dictate**
  800-825-5897

The **Phillips SP6000** is a digital dictating system that is currently limited to radiology reporting. A 45-minute to two-hour setup period is required per author. The system offers continuous speech recognition and can be used with WordPerfect for Windows or Microsoft Word.

To whom are these systems being marketed? Mainly to the keyboard illiterate, the disabled, doctors, nurses, reporters, loan officers, lawyers, auditors, insurance personnel and researchers. The Kurzweil system is being primarily used in emergency rooms, and radiology and pathology departments. The IBM Personal Dictation System is being marketed to physicians, lawyers, and word processors while the Dragon Dictate is being marketed to anyone who uses a computer.

How well do these systems work? Well, I was given a private demonstration of the Dragon Dictate system by an attorney who had been using it for 1-1/2 years, and, frankly, I was not very impressed. This lawyer was exceedingly articulate but even so, in the one paragraph he dictated, the system made four glaring mistakes.

I was more impressed with Barbara Grow, a medical transcriptionist from York, Pennsylvania, who has been using Dragon Dictate since October 1993 and is a true believer in the system. Through a series of unfortunate mishaps and a multitude of surgeries including bilateral carpal tunnel releases, two cervical fusions, a laminectomy, biceps tendinitis, adhesive neuritis in her neck and entrapped ulnar nerves, she found it impossible even to hold a hair brush.

Barbara's chances for employment were slim to none. She was rated permanently and totally disabled as an MT. The thought of sitting home and collecting SSI was not appealing so, with the help of her vocational rehabilitation program, she looked into retraining for another career path. Vocational Rehab thought she should be able to operate a computer with a stick taped to her forehead, until she reminded them about the wires in her neck from the fusion and expressed her concern that they might break. She also explained to the rehab counselors that by typing this way, she would probably earn no more than $19.00 a day, not even enough to pay for her electricity and telephone charges.

One day someone mentioned the Dragon Dictate System and Barbara set out on her own to find out about this technology. After gathering information and convincing the Voc Rehab people that she could work full-time with such a system, they agreed to pay for it. Barbara spent three weeks full-time mastering and training her program before accepting any work and another three months getting up to speed. Her biggest adaptation was synchronizing her voice with the physicians' voice for system input. Currently, Barbara is "typing" between 1800-2000 lines a day and working full-time as an IMT. These days instead of contending with "typos," Barbara must deal with "mouthos." With modest pride, she reports she has never had work returned because of mistakes.

Using speech recognition technology, Barbara Grow is now able to work faster and with much less physical stress. Instead of carpal tunnel, her only work hazard is hoarseness. She's tackling new projects, too. Recently, in addition to her daily transcription, she worked with Dragon Dictate to develop an updated medical dictionary for their systems. Barbara Grow is a remarkable person who has shown us not to be afraid of new technology but to use it to our advantage.

TAKING ADVANTAGE OF TECHNOLOGICAL TRANSITIONS

Who will survive technology's many transitions? Those with excellent skills. Excellent computer skills. Excellent medical transcription listening skills — for accents, in multi-specialties, etc. Excellent grammar, punctuation and editing skills. In the future, all will be in great demand.

It is predicted that within the next two decades, the number of acute care hospitals, both rural and urban, will be reduced by at least 20%. Hospitals, especially smaller ones with fewer than 200 beds, will increasingly outsource a wide variety of services in an effort to reduce operating expenses in favor of a more "variable cost" management philosophy. Outside contractors will provide services now covered by ancillary departments and specialty care units, including their costly high-tech equipment.

Physicians will continue to consolidate their practices and hospital corporations will continue to form alliances with one another. Hospitals that survive beyond the year 2010 will be run without the current departmental system, with less management and more technology. The future will favor managers who can manage resources, particularly human resources.

The future will also favor those who are flexible and stay alert for new opportunities. Each of us must take charge of our life, beginning today to prepare for the future. In large part, future employment opportunities will be determined by how we prepare ourselves right now, during the next decade and beyond. The era of the dedicated word processing system has come to an end. These systems can no longer meet the needs of the changing and evolving health care environment.

Since longer than most of us can remember, other professionals (and the general public, as well) have viewed medical transcriptionists as merely typists. Fortunately, thanks in large part to today's excellent communication and networking systems, that attitude is changing. People are learning about our specialized education and skills. We have no doubt that once consistent emphasis is placed on our true skills instead of just keyboarding, transcriptionists will become highly respected health care professionals, and we will be in greater demand. Imagine our future opportunities and benefits. The demand for our advanced skills will open doors not accessible to those with only limited medical language training. New and exciting medical language careers unheard of today will evolve. And, we will be able to work faster with less physical strain.

We can empower ourselves by working with, not against, new technology. Perhaps we will provide speech recognition technology to our clients. Perhaps we will work with companies developing speech recognition and other technology, not only for MDs but for MTs. Perhaps we'll develop our own new technology. In the future, medical transcriptionists will no longer be the invisible profession, but a very visible and a vocal one.

OTHER EXCELLENT COMPUTER SOFTWARE

A few years ago, WordPerfect Corporation and Williams & Wilkins Electronic Media, a division of Waverly, a leading independent publisher of medical reference books and electronic media, teamed up to produce the most comprehensive electronic medical/pharmaceutical spellchecker. The latest version is *Stedman's Plus* and *Stedman's Electronic Medical Dictionary*, a complete pop-up electronic medical dictionary.

Stedman's Plus spellchecker contains more than 500,000 medical, pharmaceutical, and bioscience terms from 57 major medical specialties, over 100,000 abbreviations, acronyms, symbols and eponyms and current terms related to diseases, treatments, procedures, lab tests, equipment, and more. It is compatible with all versions of WordPerfect 5.1 and up, MS Word, Excel, Access, PowerPoint, and Outlook and is available on CD-ROM in DOS, Windows and MacIntosh platforms.

Stedman's Electronic Medical Dictionary contains more than 102,000 medical and pharmaceutical words with definitions and audio and written pronunciations, etymologies, hyphenations, tables, animations, over 1000 images, and more. You can instantly find any medical word, word part, phrase, or definition. Stedman's Electronic Medical Dictionary is available on CD-ROM in DOS, Windows and MacIntosh platforms.

OTHER COMPUTER HARDWARE AND SOFTWARE

You will want to invest in other office necessities, too, including computer cables, additional surge protectors (Surge protectors do wear out.), diskettes and diskette filing cases, antistatic computer cleaning cloths, chair mats, pads, monitor screens to reduce glare, foot rests, computer paper, additional toner cartridges, extra ribbons for dot matrix printers, printer paper, plastic covers for all components, and a switch/box if you are using more than one printer or computer. All of the above and more can be purchased at your local computer store.

SOFTWARE BY THE TRUCKLOADS

Today, there are countless software programs available, but the most popular by use and demand are the following:

- Microsoft DOS (MS DOS) — try to purchase the most recent version.

- WordPerfect (WP) for DOS is one of the most popular, but Word for Windows is being aggressively promoted. It is difficult convincing a die-hard DOS user to switch to a windows environment, but this appears to be what the future holds for our industry as well as many others. It's not as bad as it seems. Having worked in both environments, and as a former die-hard DOSsie, I have become spoiled by many windows enhancements.

- Utilities Program: *Norton Utilities*, *PC Tools*, and *Central Pointe* provide shell and data recovery utilities, hard disk backup and restore, disk compression and desk top organizers.

- Bookkeeping Software: *Quicken* or *Quick Books* by Intuit, *Peachtree Accounting*, and *ACCPack*. The latter two are more sophisticated and expensive accounting software programs.

- *Quicken*, which seems to be most popular, costs about $49 and will save you countless bookkeeping hours. It is very easy to learn and will make completing your tax return a breeze.

- Legal Software: *It's Legal* is a program that produces boilerplate legal agreements and contracts, which are useful in writing client agreements.

WORDPERFECT DOS VERSUS WINDOWS

WordPerfect and MS Word are currently the most popular word processing programs for medical transcription. The industry does seem to be moving toward MS Word, but many transcriptionists remain loyal to WordPerfect DOS, praising its reliable stability. I have run WP5.1 for more than ten years and it just keeps on going. Because Word is less expensive, however, many products are supporting that program. Although I still favor WordPerfect DOS, I feel comfortable with both.

REGISTER SOFTWARE

Fill out all registration and warranty cards that come with new equipment and software. As a registered software user (WordPerfect, Quicken, etc.) you will readily obtain online help and service. You will also be notified by the company when software upgrades are released, allowing you to upgrade your system at bargain prices.

You can spend a small fortune on computer software so shop wisely. It's a good idea to network with other transcriptionists and professionals in the business community to see what works well for them and their home computers. Read *Home Office Computing*, which lists best selling software in each issue, and research some of the other computer and software publications for updates on products.

NEVER, NEVER, NEVER!
BORROW SOMEONE ELSE'S SOFTWARE

Only buy new, unused software. It is against the law to copy software, because it is copyrighted. Some software is copy-protected, which makes it impossible or extremely difficult to copy. Additionally, according to the National Computer Security Association (NCSA), "borrowed" software sometimes contains a virus, which is put there by the manufacturer to deter copying. If a virus gets into your computer you will certainly have serious software problems. Use *Norton Utilities*, *DOS or PC Tools* to check for a virus.

COMPUTER AIDED TRANSCRIPTION (CAT) TECHNOLOGY — OR HOW YOU, TOO, CAN TYPE 225 WORDS A MINUTE

225 WORDS A MINUTE! This sounds like a sales pitch, doesn't it? Are you wondering how this is possible and thinking about how much you could earn if you could type this fast?

It's not a gimmick, and it is being done every day by court reporters all around the world. Now it is possible for medical transcriptionists to achieve the same typing speed by using machine shorthand and Computer Aided Transcription (CAT) technology.

Shorthand, of course, has been around for centuries. The mechanical device that is used to write shorthand is called the stenotype machine. It allows the simultaneous depression of multiple keys, and entire words can be written with one stroke. In machine shorthand theory, single letters and abbreviations are used to represent words; and students are taught to write words phonetically. For example, "Judge" is written J-U-J.

The keyboard of the stenotype machine has 23 keys. Since vowels come in the middle of words, the vowel keys are in the middle of the keyboard, and consonants are on either end. Letter combinations represent long and short vowels, and letters of the alphabet. Not all alphabet keys are present. There is no letter "C", for example. A "K" is used for the sound of the "C" in *car*; and an "S" for the soft "S" sound in *cease*.

Machine shorthand, as you probably surmise, is another language. The shorthand writer hears an English word, mentally and physically converts that word to shorthand, and presses the appropriate keys. When desired, the writer can read the shorthand, translate it, and either read or write it in English.

Computer Aided Translation software (CAT) does the same thing. After an electronic copy of the machine shorthand stroke is transferred to the computer, by modem connection or disk, the computer looks up each word in a shorthand-to-English dictionary and translates the words into English. The dictionary is created, a word at a time, by deliberately making dictionary entries from a list of words, or after the translation process, and untranslated words are translated and entered into the dictionary by the computer operator. As the dictionary grows, more and more complete translations are possible.

Some specialized CAT programs allow functions normally performed on a computer keyboard (block, move, delete, underline, etc.) to be performed on the stenotype keyboard, and most CAT programs also allow spellchecking with external medical/legal dictionaries. Generically described as "rapid text entry" programs, they are essentially high speed word-processing programs that use a stenotype keyboard instead of a computer keyboard. Medical transcriptionists will probably favor the program that uses WordPerfect for word processing.

Advantages of CAT technology: increased words-per-minute speeds; reduced misspellings because the dictionary converts "slop" shorthand strokes to correctly spelled English words; fewer repetitive motions because words can be written in one stroke; ergonomically satisfactory keyboard position because the shorthand machine sits on an adjustable tripod that can be positioned many ways.

Disadvantages of CAT technology: length of time required to become proficient at writing machine shorthand at high speeds; and equipment costs. CAT software prices average $3000-$5000; computerized shorthand machines average $2500 (although one CAT firm makes a $200 add-on device for the noncomputerized steno machine that would suffice for medical transcriptionists.

Most modern CAT systems will produce an ASCII transcript that can be imported into WordPerfect. The proficient WP user can then convert the document into the desired format. The most modern versions allow real-time translation, which can be used for captioning for the hearing impaired. This same capability allows for immediate onscreen correction or translation of the word just written.

CAT technology is made specifically to capture the spoken word, which is what court reporters and medical transcriptionists work with. Mispronunciations, inaudibles, bad grammar, and all other difficulties of transcribing the spoken word will still plague CAT users.

CAT technology is probably best suited to the many students of machine shorthand who are unable to achieve the 225 wpm speed required for court reporting jobs. (The dropout rate averages 95%). These students could use the skills and speeds they have acquired by using CAT technology for word processing and/or medical transcribing. (Of course, they would have to learn medical terminology and English skills as well.) Indeed, some court reporting schools are now teaching medical transcription using CAT technology. Call or write for more information on CAT technology.

- **Stenoware, Inc.** (makers of IntelliCat software)
  12337 Jones Road, Suite 200
  Houston, Texas 77070
  800-328-8220

TELEPHONE ANSWERING MACHINES

A telephone answering machine is vital to every home-based medical transcription business. It saves you time and money, because it is not time- or cost-effective for you to answer the telephone every time it rings. By having a telephone answering machine, you can monitor calls, immediately responding to those that are urgent or those from clients or potential clients. Non-urgent calls can be returned later.

There are a variety of answering machines on the market and brand-name should not be your main consideration. The key features to look for in answering machines are the following:

• A voice-activated, unlimited incoming message
   (This machine can also be used for stat dictation)

• Remote message retrieval capability

• Capability to change the outgoing message from a remote phone

• Recording of time, date, and number of calls

Low-end units cost as little as $50-$75 but lack voice activation, remote access, and some other features. Machines in the $75-$100 range usually include the extra features.

TELEPHONE COMPANY VOICE-MAIL SERVICE

Most local telephone companies now offer sophisticated voice mail that gives a small or home-based business the appearance of being a larger, more professional entity. The voice response sounds very professional, unlike some tinny-sounding tape-based answering units, and with this service, you also guarantee callers won't receive a busy signal. BellSouth's MemoryCall service handles up to six calls simultaneously even though you have only one phone number and one voice mailbox.

Some telephone companies charge a flat rate with unlimited usage for voice-mail service; others charge per minute beyond a fixed amount and for multiple mailboxes. For example, Bell Atlantic charges $8.50 per minute for a single mailbox with 45 minutes of storage and $10.50 per month for one mailbox that you can divide into eight submailboxes. This is an excellent alternative as the calling party never gets a busy signal and you don't have to interrupt one call to accept another as you do with call waiting.

If you already use local phone company voice mail, look into having the voice mailbox automatically notify your pager when a call comes in. For $10-20 per month you will be able to get back to your clients quickly. Your callers will appreciate being able to leave messages knowing you will pick them up and respond promptly.

If you only have one phone line, how can you tell if an incoming call is business or personal? With a distinctive ringing service, which you can purchase. Bell Atlantic offers *IdentaRing,* a system that allows you to add two additional dependent numbers to an existing phone line. Each phone number has a distinctive ring pattern — one long for the primary number, and a short-long-short or two shorts for the dependent numbers. With this system, it's easy to determine which number was dialed.

With the addition of a call-routing device, a switch that automatically identifies each ring pattern and directs the call to the appropriate telephone device, you can have a phone, answering machine, fax machine, or fax/data modem for a particular number. Call-routing devices are easy to install and cost from $50-$100. Contact your local phone company for information on this type service. The wonderful voice mail and fax-on-demand systems available today can make your home office sound like the corporate headquarters of YOU, INCORPORATED.

MODEMS

Consider purchasing a modem, either an internal modem or an external modem. Investigate the pros and cons of both to determine which you prefer. Both types connect to your computer via the telephone line and allow you to communicate with other computers and online data bases. In this age of telecommuting, and with the abundance of resources available to us via the Internet, a modem is a must.

SAFETY THROUGH SURGE PROTECTORS

Electrical surges can destroy valuable data, so take precautions to protect your computer system by installing surge protectors, which have electrical outlets that protect equipment plugged into them from power surges. It's a cost-effective way to prevent damage to your computer hardware and software.

When one of the authors of this book bought her first computer, she learned about surge protectors the hard way. One day during a lightning storm, the lights flickered for just a moment, but in that brief power surge an entire half-day's work — about thirty pages — was lost. It was a devastating and needless loss.

Surge protectors/surge suppressors protect your computer and peripherals from sudden variations in electrical current. Underwriters Laboratory has established an objective rating guide for surge protectors. Look for the UL 1449 sticker on any surge protector you plan to purchase.

Surge protectors are not totally fail-safe, however. Experts caution against relying on any surge protector during a thunderstorm, since "lightning can arc across open contacts and do extensive damage to your computer."

Surge protectors (or surge suppressors) protect your equipment from power shortages and outages (not enough power) and power surges (too much power). We recommend that you purchase the best surge protector you can afford, with a built-in AC filter, and we cannot overemphasize the importance of plugging all computer and office equipment into surge protectors.

If you have a modem, it is suggested that you disconnect either the incoming telephone line or cable during a thunder storm. A lightning strike to the telephone line will zap your computer.

In your home office, consider having an electric circuit dedicated to the computer and other electrical office equipment. Office electronics suffer from power ebbs when a dishwasher, oven or other appliance kicks on. It's best to have computers on a circuit used only for low power consumers such as lights.

COMPUTER BACKUP

Every home-based medical transcriptionist should have a computer backup in case his or her main machine breaks down. It isn't necessary to buy a new piece of equipment for this purpose. If you have upgraded your existing computer to a faster, higher-powered machine, save that older computer for your backup. Although it may be somewhat slower, you'll be able to continue working. Believe us, there is nothing worse than an office full of work and no equipment with which to transcribe it!

> ## TIP
>
> Make backup copies of new software and store original diskettes in your safe, in a fireproof file cabinet or in your safe-deposit box at the bank.

BACKUP SYSTEMS

It is simply good business sense to protect your files by copying or transferring them regularly to removable tape cartridges or zip disks that can be stored in a separate location outside the office or in a locked fireproof safe.

While most computers have a backup system on the hard drive, if the entire system crashes, you'll lose that too. Floppy disks provide some backup protection, but their storage capacity is limited.

The newest tape backup systems compress data so you can transfer an entire database onto a single cartridge. For under $200 you can buy a basic backup system to create a taped library of all your files. More sophisticated, higher-priced version let you make selective backups or schedule unattended backups automatically, perhaps while you are out of the office or at night.

A tape backup drive operates much like a tape recorder, reading your files and copying them onto a tape. A special cassette tape, which must be pre-formatted, is inserted into the drive's slot; onscreen programs offer several options to choose from, including automated daily backup, backing up only selected files, scheduling after-hours backup and backing up files in the background while you work on other applications.

Several easy-to-use, easy-to-install tape backup devices are available for small business budgets. The internal models are sold with mounting hardware to fit into one of the existing 3.5.-inch or 5.25-inch floppy disk bays in your computer. External, stand-alone models are about the size of a hardcover book and plug into either a printer port or a Small Computer System Interface (SCSI) port at the back of the computer.

Most external backup drives have extra ports so printers can be connected to them; this feature, called a "printer-pass-through," reduces extra cables and ports needed. External drives are also a good solution if you want to backup multiple PCs with a single drive or for laptop computer backup and file transfer.

If you have a PC, your backup drive will connect to a floppy bay disk or your parallel port. Tape backup systems come with Windows or DOS software that is easy to install.

The advantages of a tape backup drive are that you can archive data, leaving more space on your computer's hard drive or use the backup system as an extra hard drive. Files can be transferred easily from one computer to another, enabling you to share removable tapes or take them on the road to use with your laptop. Most backup systems not only record files but can also hold software programs, so rebuilding after a computer crash needn't mean refeeding dozens of separate disks.

When shopping for a tape backup system, make sure the drive and the tapes you purchase are fully compatible with your computer. If you are short on ports, get a system with a printer pass-through. If you have hundreds of documents, look for a device with a cataloging feature which allows you to create a directory of files for easy reference. Make sure the system has a "compare" feature so you can check data on your tape against data you have just copied. Be sure the storage capacity and speed are sufficient for your present and future needs. Most manufacturers offer several models with different storage and speed capacities.

INTERACTIVE TECHNICAL SUPPORT

Technology is great, but it is definitely more beneficial and user-friendly when it is backed up by that "human touch," which in this case translates to "technical support." There are a multitude of high-tech ways to find answers to technical questions, but, unfortunately, they are not always reliable. Often, techs don't understand the medical transcriptionist's needs. And sometimes trying to get a live technician on the phone can take more time than building your own computer from scratch! Calls to technical support lines often result in hours spent on hold or worse, nothing but busy signals. Still, for desperate occasions, interfacing with a computer technician can be a lifesaver.

Most major computer and software companies offer technical support — often for a fee — and provide toll-free numbers for customer calls. Check your computer or software users manual or call your computer/software distributor for tech support numbers for IBM, Compaq, Hewlett-Packard, ACER, Dell, Gateway 2000, Packard Bell and others.

FAX MACHINES

Almost all home-based medical transcription businesses have purchased or are in the process of purchasing fax machines. This terrific technology is now reasonably priced and has become a standard office feature. There are many advantages to investing in a fax machine for your office.

A fax machine increases efficiency and profitability by providing 24-hour access to your business. It saves time and money over express mail, postal services or courier while improving your response time. A fax machine allows you to transmit documents across the street or across the world, and it reduces miscommunication by immediately transmitting hard copies of important documents.

A fax machine also enhances your professional business image. Today, business and nonbusiness contacts alike expect professionals to have fax machines. When business associates have something to send to you, more often than not they'll want to send it immediately via fax machine.

To further enhance your professional image and prevent great frustration for others, get a fax that responds automatically to incoming fax signals. Other professionals do not enjoy making one phone call to ask you to turn on your fax machine and another phone call to send the fax. And, if you aren't home when the first call comes in, additional calls are required. Telephone tag is especially irritating when someone urgently needs to send a fax. We know some business people who, after experiencing much frustration with this type of system, simply stop sending faxes. That can hurt business!

If you don't own a fax machine, you should have ready access to one, perhaps through a local copy center or drug store. Sending and receiving documents at a public location usually costs $1-$2 per page and is an expense the transcriptionist must bear. However, copy-center faxing is not ideal, and we recommend investing in a fax machine. It will save you much time and many dollars.

To get the most out of your fax machine, include your fax number on your business cards, letterhead, stationery, purchase orders, invoices, print and

206

advertising. Use your fax for sending and receiving documents after hours, and encourage those who do business with you to fax rather than mail documents. For instance, you could have patient IDs, log sheets or tape logs faxed to you on a daily basis, which is especially helpful if your clients are long distance.

The fax has nothing to do with your computer, although it can be installed as a fax board in your computer or purchased as a stand-alone fax unit. There is now fax software that works on a dedicated PC with one fax board/one phone line and several network connections. Today's fax software allows you to convert and receive documents into files.

The issue of internal versus external fax modems parallels the advantages and disadvantages cited for internal and external data modems. In brief, an internal modem requires less space since it is placed in the computer. Due to its internal location it does not require a separate power supply. However, there are no visible indicator lights like those on an external modem, and for some transcriptionists, indicator lights provide a comfort zone they need. Techies even claim ability to *interpret* the indicator lights.

An external modem does require some desktop space and a power cord, but on the plus side, it is easy to install, is highly portable, and can be used with more than one computer. Ultimately, the internal versus the external issue is largely a matter of individual preference.

NOTE

Some computer consultants do not encourage installing a fax board in your computer but recommend getting a stand-alone fax because earlier modems have been known to damage PC hard drives.

Once you get a FAX machine, you'll wonder how you ever did without it.

ADVANTAGES OF OWNING A FAX MACHINE

- It can increase efficiency and profitability by providing 24-hour access.

- It saves time and money over express mail, postal service and courier while improving response time.

- It allows you to transmit documents across the street or across the world.

- It reduces miscommunication by having agreements/terms and other material in writing.

- It enhances the professional image of your business.

To get the most out of your fax machine:

- Include your fax number on your business cards, letterhead, stationery, purchase orders, invoices, print advertising, etc.

- Use your fax in place of first class or express mail.

- Use your fax for taking or sending documents after hours.

- Encourage those who do business with you to fax rather than mail documents.

PAPER SHREDDERS — THE GREAT PAPER CHASE

Although most independents now telecommute via modems and the Internet, confidentiality remains a serious concern. How can we protect ourselves from unscrupulous identity thieves or, even more important, protect sensitive medical information from falling into the wrong hands? No one wants his or her privacy invaded or leaked to curious ears, and public figures are especially at risk, for there are those who seek out and grasp opportunities to sell hot tips on the rich and famous to tabloid magazines. MTs must be conscientious in maintaining medical record privacy for all patients, famous and common alike.

For many decades paperwork that was not filed or mailed was simply thrown in the trash, but that action is no longer wise. We now know that some people make a profitable living sifting through dumpsters and landfills looking for personal information — social security and bank account numbers, mother's maiden name, physical and mental health, and relationships — which they can sell or use for dishonest purposes. We could burn sensitive papers, but that would put our offices at risk for a five-alarm fire. We could tear it up, but that still would not offer the protection we need as independents and responsible business owners.

Fortunately, the solution to protecting sensitive information is simple and affordable: the paper shredder. The electric paper shredder has a system of motorized blades that start rotating at a very high speed when a document is inserted into it. These blades shred the document into very thin strips which, even in the hands of a determined thief, are practically impossible to piece back together.

When choosing a paper shredder, there are several things to consider — type, size. and price. Paper shredders are available in various sizes and models, from tabletop versions for single sheet documents to large, heavy-duty models for multiple sheets or continuous paper rolls.

Shredder Type: Stripcut shredders are designed for a higher volume shredding capacity and require less maintenance. Crosscut shredders cut documents into small, confetti particles and reduce the shredded paper bulk by 80 percent. Shredders come in a variety of styles, from freestanding models to those that fit over waste baskets.

Shredder Size: The size of the shredder you buy is determined by how you will use it. If you intend to shred continuous-form documents wider than 12 inches, you should consider buying a shredder that has a 16-inch throat opening. This will allow the forms to continuously shred and provide unattended operation. Smaller throat openings will result in continuous-forms breaking as they enter the paper shredder and you will be forced to constantly refeed documents into the shredder.

Shredder Price: Shredders range in price from $49 to as high as several hundred dollars. For more information on shredders, visit your local office supply store or search the Internet.

MISCELLANEOUS SUPPLIES

Aside from your printed materials, equipment, computer hardware, software and furniture, you will need numerous miscellaneous items to bring your office to peak efficiency — a calculator, adding machine, copy paper, printer paper, postage scale, tape, sticky notes, file folders, labels, binders, telephone message pads, pens, pencils, paper clip, stapler, etc. You may be tempted to buy everything in the office supply store but remember, office supplies add up fast so don't overbuy.

CALENDARS

Scheduling and short-range planning are key elements of successful home-based businesses. Every transcriptionist needs an efficient calendar to organize her life. Month-at-a-glance or three-to-four month wall-mounted calendars are very effective time-management tools.

There are some great computer programs, such as *WordPerfect Office Timeslips*, that offer calendars and appointment setups.

Whatever type calendar you choose, review it frequently. Scan not only the day ahead, but the upcoming week as well. This will remind you of regular monthly meetings, appointments, holidays and vacation schedules (for those hiring outsourcers), as well as scheduled time off, business lunches, etc. With a chart of future activities, you are less likely to overcommit yourself or make promises you can't keep.

> *"Smart transcriptionists make professional decisions based on sound business practices."*

RESERVE CAPITAL

At the start-up of your business, you can anticipate that no money will come in for at least six weeks. We recommend having reserve capital for unexpected expenses during this time and shortly thereafter. Be prepared to cover payments for rent, gas, electricity and telephone, as well as money for supplies, for at least four months. Under-capitalization is one of the main reasons new businesses fail within the first year. If you do not have enough reserve capital, perhaps you should consider getting a business loan.

When you are the business owner and have financial obligations, everyone else gets paid first — the phone company, the landlord, subcontractors, and employees. If you are like most independents, there will be times when you won't even be able to take a salary. Work volumes will probably fluctuate and your business may go through slow periods. Monitor your situation regularly. If you are not making enough money during the "good times" to make ends meet, you are probably not charging enough.

THE COST OF RUNNING A PERSONAL COMPUTER

A recent study measuring the energy used by different systems under test conditions found the wattage listed on the nameplate of each component is conservative. Actual electricity use is much lower. Costs range from ½ to 3½ cents per hour, depending upon what kind of components you have and how hard they're working.

Of the personal computers with monitors studied, use ranged from 30-210 watts. In a standby mode, dot-matrix, daisy wheel, and ink-jet printers used 3-45 watts, while typical laser printers use 40-130 watts. The study also showed that printers may use two to three times this much when printing.

ESCAPING DATA DISASTER

Insurance companies may cover the restoration of lost files if disaster strikes your business, but they still haven't come up with a way to replace lost business while you're re-creating those files. Although there is no way to completely protect yourself from catastrophes, here are some strategies to safeguard valuable information.

- **Secure a second copy.** Backing up isn't hard to do, so make it part of your daily routine. Besides your database, creative works and billing records, other items that need duplication include investment documents, contracts, supplier lists and receipts.

- **Create an inventory list.** Most office components have visible serial numbers. Record them with such programs as Proof 2.0 (Fusion Software, 800-856-8566; Win; $9.95), print out two copies and store each in separate locations off-premises. For extra protection, videotape your office equipment.

- **Find a safe haven.** Stash your inventory lists and backup disks and videotapes in such places as a safe deposit box or your parents' home. However, avoid the basement to avoid possible flooding.

> *"Backing up computer-generated data frequently is good insurance against hardware or software malfunction."*

BACKING UP INPUT

Be sure to back up disks, copying material from your hard disk onto a floppy disk. One of your authors remembers an unfortunate early computer experience when an entire day's work was lost because she hit the wrong command. No one had told her about the importance of backing up input. Whether you operate from a floppy disk or a hard drive, back up your system every two or three reports.

Frequent backup of computer-generated data onto floppy disks, tape, or other media is insurance against hardware or software malfunction. Inexpensive backup software programs are fast and simple to use. Backup data is essential when you need to retrieve previous transcription.

Computer files are easily saved by patient name, medical record number, date of transcription, or any other system that works for you. Once your files are on backup disks, you can easily retrieve the information. No matter how far in the future clients may ask for records they cannot locate, you will be able to quickly review your computer-generated list of files and print out the old transcription.

A tape backup system is optional since you can purchase backup software such as PC Tools or DOS. You should have either hardware backup capabilities or software backup capabilities to prevent losing data in the event of a hard drive crash.

If you are going to invest in a tape backup system, consider programming it to update your data backup every evening or during the time when you are not active on your computer. The system can be set to automatically back up your data to the point of the last backup. Ideally, data backup should be done on a daily basis.

DISKETTE CARE AND MAINTENANCE

Handle backup diskettes, the duplicate copies of your programs and records, gently. Computer disks are very delicate and should always be used and stored carefully.

- Make backup disks of your software and replace disks after 50-100 hours of use.

- Protect disks from dust, dirt, fingerprints, and old age, which can make disks unreadable.

- Store disks upright, away from excessive heat, cold, and moisture.

- Store disks away from magnetic interferences such as transcribers, computer monitors, television and VCR, magnetic paper clip holders, bulk tape erasers, and other similar technology.

COMPUTER CARE AND MAINTENANCE

Despite their hearty constitutions, personal computers need care and attention if they are to have a long life of reliable performance. Dust and dirt are always hazardous to a computer's well-being and home-based computers are at even greater risk.

When you work at home, your computer is subject to a variety of household pollutants that can interfere with its performance. Computer threats include dust, cooking grease, pet hairs, aerosol sprays, soft drinks, food crumbs, smoke, erasure particles, and miscellaneous specks that float around our homes.

Just as there seems to be no way to avoid exposure to the common cold, there is no way to totally protect your computer from exposure to hazards. There are, however, several steps you can take to reduce harmful effects on your computer.

- Cover computer components when not in use.

- Periodically vacuum air intake vents. (Invest in a computer cleaning kit.)

- Vacuum and dust the computer area once a week, including the printer and keyboard.

- Keep disk drives closed when not in use.

- Keep the computer area free of smoke and food.

- Print copies of important files.

- Replace filters regularly on forced-air heating and cooling systems.

- Keep the area around your computer clean, including floors, baseboards, bookcases and books, lamps, decorative objects, furniture, and windowsills. Clean the computer itself gently. Do not use detergent or chemical solvents to clean computer casings. Use a soft, damp (but not wet) cloth for dusting, or buy a commercial computer cleaning kit. You can also buy a disk-drive cleaning kit. In addition to cleaning, don't let stray paper clips or staples pile up around your equipment.

COMPUTER "HOUSECLEANING"

To lower the odds of a hard disk crash, do some basic computer file housecleaning on a monthly basis. Files get shuffled around from one sector to another when added or deleted frequently.

It's easy to tell when your hard disk needs maintenance: Its speed will decrease during basic functions. Keep your hard disk uncluttered and organized by regularly compressing, moving, or deleting files. This greatly decreases the chances of your disk crashing. Compress your disk whenever your computer's speed begins to decrease. Use PC Tools or Norton Utilities to compress your hard disk.

TIP

During thunderstorms, disconnect your phone lines, cables and plugs, and make sure your computer is turned off. Never unplug your keyboard from your computer when the computer is on. This could "kill" your keyboard permanently and also do serious damage to the hardware.

FILE COMPRESSION PROGRAMS

File compression serves two important purposes. It can combine a number of files into one smaller, easily manageable file archive, and it can transport and copy these archives faster due to the compressed file size. If you are going to be downloading or uploading computer files on a regular basis, you definitely want to have a file compression tool on hand in order to make the process as painless as possible.

As most of my clients have required me to change to the Word program, I recently found a compression program called WinZip v8. I can "zip-up" a day's files into one archive and send it on its way in a matter of a few minutes.

There are a number of compression programs to choose from — ZipMagic, CuteZip, Zip Explorer Pro, WinPack Deluxe, and others. Incidentally, WinZip is a free download and there are other shareware products available as well. To download WinZip, go to www.goto.com.

Many of us are so busy with day-to-day activities of our business, most of which is keyboarding, that we have little free time to investigate alternatives that would make our tasks easier. When we discover timesaving products, it's very exciting. One great compression program called *PKZIP* is a real time saver. This wondrous little tool allows you to take a file or directory, or groups of files or directories, and compress them into a single file that is much smaller than the original.

Soon after I started using PKZIP, I discovered I was saving more than the cost of floppy disks because I used the "ZIP" to compress my old files. I can get five to ten times more on my floppy disks than I could with just the old move/copy procedure.

COMPUTER CONSULTANTS

Every medical transcriptionist, especially one who is new to the computer world, needs the help of a computer consultant or "techie." These are extremely warm and caring people, but they do have one flaw: They love computers more than life itself.

They eat, sleep, and breathe computers. They can be found in computer stores, or in the computer section of book stores, perusing the wonderful world of computers and the latest technology.

Computer consultants can take a computer apart and put it back together faster than the speed of light. Nothing excites them more than spending 24 hours (or more!) working nonstop on a computer glitch. If you don't have a computer consultant at home, shop around for one.

Join a computer club. Every area has at least one club, and they are loaded with computer techies. There are even computer clubs for singles. In fact, we have a friend who met and married a wonderful techie she found on a computer club's bulletin board.

Some clubs are for people who live in a geographic area, some are for people who have one specific type of computer or computer operating system, and some are for people who use a particular type of software. Whichever you choose, you might be bringing your very own computer techie to the next transcription convention.

Computer publications are also good resources for information on computers and specialists available to help you solve computer problems. You will find publication recommendations in the resources section at the back of this book.

UTILIZING VIDEO LIBRARIES AND AUDIOCASSETTES

Have you visited your public library's videotape section lately? If you haven't, you probably should. Public libraries have numerous computer applications videotapes that you can view at home simply by checking them out with your library card. For instance, if you use WordPerfect, you can begin with the basic WordPerfect video and move on to intermediate, advanced, windows, etc. These videos are wonderful references and you will gain an abundance of computer savvy from them.

There are also specialized videotapes on the market. These are a great resource for new WordPerfect users and others interested in learning WP tips and customized applications.

To get the most out of these videos, try to view them while actually sitting at your keyboard so you can practice the various techniques in the video demonstrations. If you do not understand something immediately, you can rewind the video and play it again. Through these various applications you will learn tips that will aid in cutting production time, improving transcription quality, and increasing profits.

You can easily bring yourself up to speed with self-paced audiocassettes. Put a tape in a Walkman™ or new transcribing machine, or slip a disk in your computer, and an instructor talks you through the program while you work directly on your computer. Two references for these self-paced audiocassettes are the following:

- **Personal Training Systems of San Jose**
  800-832-2499

- **Individual Software**
  800-822-3522

RECORDING YOUR COMPUTER AND SOFTWARE INFORMATION

It is a good idea to set up and maintain a file for detailed records of office equipment and computer hardware/software. It will be a valuable quick reference in case you experience office equipment problems. The file should include the following:

- Equipment model numbers

- Program names, dates of purchase, versions, serial and registration numbers

- Vendor names, telephone numbers

- Customer support phone numbers, software help line phone numbers

- Warranty information and expiration dates

BEWARE THE VIRUS

Software is subject to computer viruses that can contaminate data files and programs. To help prevent virus contamination, it is wise to invest in what the industry refers to as "virgin software programs" — software programs that are new and unused.

Invest in a virus check, too, even if you have purchased new software. Norton Disk Doctor, PC Tools and similar products are fine for this purpose. This is especially important if you plan to use a modem. It is truly sickening to see a software program self-destruct as a result of a virus.

As stated earlier, never borrow software because, according to the National Computer Security Association (NCSA), "borrowed" software could contain a virus that is put there by the manufacturer to deter copying. Viruses can also be introduced through other sources.

INCREASING TYPING SPEED WITH ABBREVIATION/EXPANSION SOFTWARE

I had seen demonstrations of abbreviation programs but was not enthusiastic about "retraining" in shorthand techniques . . . until I agreed to try PRD+ at the encouragement of a colleague. I was amazed at how quickly I adapted to it and was soon creating my own entries. Years later, I still feel that abbreviation software is the best invention since the agitating washing machine!

Even though abbreviation software can enhance efficient text production, it is not a substitute for in-depth knowledge of medical terminology and grammatical and transcription skills. Learning to spell and learning to type are two different things. An MT cannot be proficient in language skills without first having knowledge and understanding of the full word or combination of words that each character represents. Also, not all job settings will have abbreviation software available, nor will all those in charge understand and appreciate how they work.

A WORD OF CAUTION: Some home-based and classroom medical transcription training courses include instruction on abbreviation and word-expansion software programs, other time- and labor-saving devices, and information on how they can be obtained. However, we discourage taking courses that offer training in "shortcut" typing *in place of* learning the full meaning and spelling of the words and phrases being transcribed. Nothing can replace in-depth knowledge of medical language words.

KEYSTROKE/ABBREVIATION SOFTWARE

A keystroke/abbreviation software program can be a useful medical transcription tool, but it is most effective when used by a competent MT.

PROS

- **Reduces keystrokes** ... by compressing frequently repeated words, sentences and paragraphs into tailored abbreviations as short as two letters.

- **No stretching** ... to reach **ALT** or **CTRL** keys. With the stroke of a space bar or any "hot key," the abbreviation is expanded.

- **The savings** ... are in time and stress. Some transcriptionists report these programs save two or three hours in a 12-hour day.

- **Compatibility** ... with most word processing packages. You can easily customize your own abbreviations, phrases and formats.

I save approximately 45-60 minutes of keyboarding time in an eight-hour day with the WordPerfect macros and standard boiler plate documents I incorporated into my programs.

CONS

- Abbreviations can be mistakenly activated, so transcriptionists must edit documents with extreme care.

- Large abbreviations may sometimes be the same or similar (**ASHD** — arteriosclerotic heart disease and **AHHD** — atherosclerotic heart disease). Transcriptionists must be cautious when creating abbreviation menus. There is a toggle "on-off" switch that can be activated if you do not want phrase expansion, which would be helpful if you are typing a letter where a name like PAT might otherwise expand to a complex medical term.

PERSONALIZING AN ABBREVIATION SOFTWARE PROGRAM

Here are some of my favorite personalized abbreviation features:

- I enjoy the ease with which I can take the periods out of abbreviations like b.i.d. With abbreviation software, I type "bid" and it automatically expands to b.i.d. and includes the periods.

- Hyphenated terms are a snap because I've shortened words like "cul-de-sac." Now I just type "cds," hit the space bar, and "cul-de-sac" appears.

219

- I use shortened forms for words my brain has difficulty transmitting correctly to my fingertips — words like "epididymis" and "sternocleidomastoid." Now I just type "epd" and "scm."

- Other words I've included are those I tend to transpose — such as and (adn), with (wiht) and the (teh). Even if a word has been transposed when I type it, at the tap of the space bar it is automatically corrected.

Prices for these software programs range from a few dollars for shareware to over $400. We recommend you learn more about following abbreviation programs:

- **PRD+ MedEasy** — around $400 (Productivity Software Int'l, New York) 212-818-1144 or fax 212-818-1197

- **Shortcut** (Healthcare Technologies)
  800-648-0665
  www.hti2000.com/shortcut.asp

- **Smartype**
  617-566-1066
  www.narratek.com

- **Instant Text**
  800-355-5251
  www.twsolutions.com

- **WP Expand for WP** (Productive Performance)
  425-788-8300
  www.foxcomm.net/productive/WPEXPAND.htm

WHAT TO DO WITH THAT OLD COMPUTER

Well, suppose you have been in business for a few years, and during the past year you have made an excellent income. So, you decide to take the plunge and exchange your 386 for a 486 or pentium super turbo charged computer. What do you do with that old computer? Don't let it stand in a corner collecting dust; give it a new lease on life.

- **Pass it on.** Do you know a child or, better yet, have a child of your own, who would love to have his or her very own computer?

- **Sell it** . . . and brace yourself for rock-bottom pricing. If you thought your car depreciated fast, you're in for a real shock. Old computers depreciate faster! Don't ask a high price and expect to have people banging at your door. Be realistic.

- **Donate it.** Many schools, churches and charitable organizations desperately need computers. You might even be able to count your computer contribution as a tax deduction unless you have already written it off as a business tax deduction.

- **Dedicate it to a specific task.** Save memory on your primary computer by installing your database on the old one. You can even turn your old standby system into a useful telecommunications tool by installing a voice/fax/modem board.

MACROS

Macros are subprograms that assign a complete sentence, paragraph, page or document to simple keystrokes. For example, if a doctor dictates that a pelvic examination is negative, the typist, with a single keystroke, can initiate a macro that prints out the doctor's standard description of a negative pelvic exam.

If you have not yet learned to create macros, I suggest you take the time to do so. The keystrokes saved will result in valuable time saved.

If you use WordPerfect, you'll find several easy macros already built into the program, and each upgrade you receive will give you even greater flexibility. Try attending a WordPerfect workshop and learn even more about macros and other great techniques.

> *"I save approximately 45-60 minutes of keyboarding time in an eight-hour day with the WordPerfect macros and standard boiler plate documents I incorporated into my programs."*

COMPUTER REFERENCES AND RESOURCES

Generally speaking, there are two types of computer users: 1) users who want to know how their computer works, and 2) users who simply want the computer to work. When it comes to computer operating functions, I am no techie. I have learned about my computer through trial and error, and the more I learn, the more fascinated I become.

Through the years I have discovered a number of excellent computer references that have worked well for me. As many of you know, trying to decipher computer manuals that come with hardware and software can be like trying to learn a foreign language. Well, the light bulb finally went on and some enlightened soul came to the conclusion that all users aren't techies. Here are some very readable computer references.

- *DOS for Dummies.* This is a lighthearted reference that takes you through the operating system, provides the essentials and leaves out the heavy technical stuff you don't need to deal with. Helpful little hints and warnings are sprinkled throughout the text — a feature I especially enjoy. You will become computer literate after reading this, and the best part is, you will realize you are not a dummy after all!

There are many *"Dummies"* books including the following:

- *DOS for Dummies*
- *Dummies 101: Word for Windows ; WordPerfect for Windows*
- *Dummies 101: The Internet*
- *WP for Dummies: Windows*
- *PCs for Dummies*
- *AmiPro for Dummies*
- *UNIX for Dummies*
- *Word for Dummies*
- *QuickBooks for Dummies*
- *Quicken for Windows for Dummies*
- *1- 2- 3 for Dummies* ... and more.

- *OOPS! What To Do When Things Go Wrong*, Que.
  This reference offers computer basics for the technically timid. It lists the ten most common computer problems and offers advice on trouble shooting and problem solving. This is a very readable, fun, and easy-to-follow book.

- *Modems Made Easy*, McGraw-Hill.
  This is a great reference for telecommuters. It defines all basic aspects of communication, what is needed to set up, how it integrates with your other computer systems, different types of data and modem software, etc.

- *Voodoo Windows, Tips and Tricks with an Attitude*, Ventana Press.
  This is a well written, creative reference for learning Windows. The book is very understandable and eliminates much of the fear involved in working with windows. Technical details are simplified, which creates a comfortable atmosphere for learning.

RX FOR PC HEALTH

> ### WARNING
>
> Using a PC may be hazardous to your health.

Prolonged sitting at a PC can result in physical disorders. Herb Brody, writing in "The Body In Question," which appeared in *PC Computing Magazine* (March 1989) points out that, ironically, PCs produce discomfort, in large part, because the machines are just too good. Never before has it been possible to accomplish so much while using so few muscles.

The PC has given new meaning to the word "sedentary." Unlike typewriters, which force us to use some muscle mass loading and unloading paper, computers allow us to sit for hours in front of our machines, absolutely immobile, with eyes fixed on the screen.

Serious computer users are reporting a bevy of symptoms such as headaches, dizziness and blurred vision that are known collectively as repetitive strain injuries or RSIs. RSIs result from the constrained posture or repetitive motion involved in most computer work.

> *"Prolonged sitting at a personal computer can result in physical disorders."*

MOVE IT OR LOSE IT

There is no getting around the fact that you must exercise in order to keep your muscles functioning properly. The next time you sit at your computer for six hours without a break, evaluate how you feel. Not great, right? It's important to get out of your chair regularly and take breaks. If you do, you'll feel better and your productivity will increase.

You can work out with old exercise programs or try something more modern. A software program, *ComputerHealth Break,* is designed to help you exercise at the computer screen. Compatible with IBM PCs and DOS 2.1 or higher, the program pops up on your screen at scientifically defined intervals based on your workload. Exercises are different from day to day, so boredom is never a problem. Remember, the more work you do, the more exercise you need. Studies show frequent but short exercise breaks are very effective in preventing computer related injuries. Your total exercise time need be only 10-15 minutes a day — the equivalent of one coffee break.

Most of us who use computers have a love/hate relationship with them. When they are working, they are marvelous inventions. When they are down, we feel like throwing them out the window. Nevertheless, transcription life is better with them than without, and this new technology has resulted in some exciting additional comfort benefits.

> *"Sit loosely in the saddle of life."*
> —Robert Louis Stevenson

ERGONOMICS

Collectively, the authors of this book have worked as MTs for more than 65 years. Until the advent of the computer, medical transcriptionists had to suffer with the Chair from Hell (referred to in an earlier chapter), desks that were too high, bad lighting, and noise pollution from the constant drone of typewriters. Computer technology added a new word to the English language, *Ergonomics*.

Ergonomics! Almost overnight we were introduced to adjustable chairs that wrapped lovingly around our bodies, desks of varying heights, appropriate office lighting, quieter equipment, and reams of health and fitness information relevant to computer users.

We would like to think that all this innovative office comfort came about because someone was overcome with guilt about our Neanderthal-like office working conditions and was subsequently moved to improve our lot in business life. In reality, however, innovation probably occurred because individual and organizational office workers became a more significant market segment or because these improvements would result in fewer medical bills, physical and mental disability claims, and lawsuits. Whatever, we're delighted about the innovations.

We recommend that you take good care of your body. If you do, maybe you won't end up in a retirement home for medical transcriptionists, sitting on a porch with your right leg locked into an extended position, suffering from severe kyphoscoliosis, and wearing double hearing aids that get tangled in your cervical collar!

THE EYES HAVE IT — COMPUTER VISION SYNDROME

Chances are, if you use a PC every day, you suffer from Computer Vision Syndrome (CVS), which includes an assortment of eye and vision problems associated with computer use. The most common symptoms include eyestrain or eye fatigue, dry eyes, burning eyes, light sensitivity, blurred vision, headaches, and pain in the shoulders, neck or back. About three-quarters of all computer users suffer from CVS, and if you are among that number, you should visit your eye specialist.

Did you know that personal computer users blink less than normal people? We become so transfixed by the screen that we forget to blink, causing dry, itching eyes. Blinking, which normally occurs about every five seconds, is important because it lubricates the surface of the eye. Studies have shown that medical transcriptionists sometimes work for an entire minute without blinking. Contact lens wearers are at even greater peril since their lenses require additional eye fluids.

Don't get smug, you bifocal wearers. You are particularly vulnerable to VDT-induced eyestrain. The near-focus lens in bifocals provides correct vision at a distance of about 12 inches, the distance at which you normally hold printed material. However, your PC screen is typically situated 18 to 24 inches away. Moreover, opticians usually place the near-vision lens below the long-vision lens. This design forces you to tip your head back uncomfortably to view the screen, causing strain to your neck and back. The truth is, single vision computer reading glasses are less likely to give you a "crick" in the neck.

Whether you wear single vision or bifocal glasses for computer use, be sure your eye doctor adjusts your reading glass power for the average 19" to 28" computer distance instead of the usual 16" distance generally used for reading hand-held materials. Measure the distance from your eyes to your computer screen. How many inches is it?

Do you know that you can actually buy "computer glasses" to alleviate the symptoms of CVS? These glasses are designed specifically to provide sharp focus at the distance you sit from the screen. There are several different types of lenses from which to choose, and computer prescriptions are also available in clip-ons that attach to regular eyeglasses. Check out your options. The right computer glasses can make a tremendous difference in your comfort level both during and after computer use. Some of the more popular types include the following:

- **Occupational Progressive Lens**
  This is a no-line multifocal lens that corrects near, intermediate and, up to a point, distance vision. It has a larger intermediate zone than regular progressive lenses, leaving less space for distance. It is very effective in the office, allowing you to see clearly across the length of a standard room, but the lens is not well-suited for daily use outside the office where greater distance viewing is necessary.

- **Lined Trifocal Lens**
  The lined trifocal has a larger intermediate zone than regular trifocals, but, like the lens above, it is most effective when the wearer is using a computer and not for other daily activities.

- **Bifocal**
  Some people need only a bifocal, either with intermediate and near correction, or intermediate and far. Wearing bifocals for intermediate-to-far vision has a significant disadvantage for the transcriptionist, however. He or she has to switch to regular bifocals to read printouts or other documents.

Regardless of technological advances in computer glasses, some people still prefer the classic single-vision lens with an intermediate power, which they use for computer work only.

Make an appointment with your ophthalmologist or optometrist to determine which lens design best suits your needs. Compare local and online lens and frame prices, which can vary considerably.

You can also research the latest technological advances on the Internet by typing in the keyword "computer eyeglasses" or visit the following websites.

- **www.allaboutvision.com**

- **www.PRIO.com**

LIGHTS OUT

Some MTs like to work in a light room while others prefer working in a darkened room. The facts in the following paragraph build a solid case for the latter.

The computer monitor produces its owns light and readability requires contrast. In other words, the darker you keep the screen, the better. Dim the lights, kill the overheads, and close the window blinds. (So much for a room with a view!) Illuminate your work area with a desk lamp and keep the light off your computer screen.

Working in the dark is generally easier on your eyes. Every time you look away from the screen, your pupils must adjust to the different levels of brightness in the room. In dim light, pupils relax and expand to let in more light, while they constrict in a bright room to diminish the amount of light. Reducing the amount of light in the room decreases the dark/light contrast so your eyes have less adjusting to do.

Two of the most common office complaints are irritated eyes and headaches. One major cause of these problems is glare from the computer monitor. Direct glare can be created by the monitor itself so turn down the screen's brightness and turn up the contrast. Also, make sure your screen is clean. Dust builds up quickly, making your screen hard to read.

Positioning the computer screen properly helps reduce optical insult. Indirect glare arises when the monitor screen reflects surrounding lights or windows. If you tilt your screen up, it mirrors ceiling lights. Turn the screen away from windows to reduce glare and avoid tilting it up to prevent ceiling light reflection.

If your monitor does not move, consider purchasing a tilt stand, which is fairly inexpensive and allows you to move your computer screen into a position that is just right for you.

In addition to the above techniques, consider buying a glare screen. These mesh glass sheets fit over your computer and reduce reflection. Be sure the glare screen you buy fits your monitor, and check to make certain it does not degrade the image of the screen.

KEYBOARD TO SUCCESS

Workers who spend long hours at keyboards sometime develop wrist and hand pain, and many medical transcriptionists develop carpal tunnel syndrome. The fault, dear readers, lies not in our keyboards but in ourselves — at least that's what some experts say.

How we use the keyboard may hold the key to avoiding discomfort and pain, carpal tunnel syndrome, and other cumulative trauma disorders (CTDs). Factors such as typing, posture, working without breaks, stress, and even certain hobbies can contribute to the development of CTDs. Reforming your keyboard habits can often solve wrist problems.

The most common CTD is CTS (carpal tunnel syndrome), a form of compression neuropathy. The QWERTY keyboard (the one you see before you each time you put your fingers to the keyboard) was developed in the 1860s. It actually was designed to slow down typing on keys that tended to clump together in the original manual typewriters.

Development of computers and laser printers alleviated the key-clumping problem, but the keyboard remained the same. No one seriously considered changing the keyboard format because, although it was admittedly inconvenient and inefficient, typists were accustomed to it, and they could type faster because the keys no longer clumped. In addition, typing speed was further enhanced because it was no longer necessary to remove one's hands from the keyboard to change typing paper, move the carriage return, change typewriter ribbons, clean typewriter keys, or make manual corrections to originals and carbon copies. Such efficiency . . . without a second's break! It is easy to understand how such unrelenting pounding on a hard keyboard can destroy wrists.

CUMULATIVE TRAUMA DISORDERS

Simple stretching and relaxation exercises can help prevent CTDs. Try each of these for ten seconds every hour:

- Gently massage the palms.

- Press the palm down to stretch top side of forearm.

- Press the palm up to stretch the underside of forearm.

- Rotate the neck from side to side.

- Wear wrist splints to avoid supination of hands.

One product that is currently getting a good deal of attention is the Handeze Glove. This type glove is made of special material called Med-A-Likra. This material reacts to each movement, producing an automatic massaging and energizing effect. The more you work, the more you massage. At first the gloves feel like support hose or Isotoner™ gloves, but after keyboarding for awhile, the gloves make your hands feel great — as if they had been massaged thoroughly. There is no restriction in keyboarding ability because the gloves are fingerless. These gloves retail for around $20.

- **Therapeutic Appliance Group**
  Box 339
  Woonsocket, RI 02895
  800-457-5535

NEW TOOLS TO RELIEVE REPETITIVE STRAIN INJURIES

For many decades, medical transcriptionists worked in unbelievably difficult situations with unworkable equipment. We used desks that were too high, typewriters (many of us started on manual machines), and chairs that fell apart at the slightest attempt to make ourselves more comfortable. Since the advent of ergonomics in the 1980s, there have been many advances to alleviate and prevent CTDs (cumulative trauma disorders) — work-related injuries that result from many hours of repetitive tasks, which places great stress on the nerves and muscles of the hands.

Some of the newer product lines designed specifically to prevent CTDs include alternative keyboards. According to the March 22, 1993 issue of *Advance*, these keyboards are radically different, ranging from keyboards that bend at 90 degree angles or in three parts, or use the Dvorak configuration rather than QWERTY. The strangest looking ones don't even use keys, but are "chordic." Like a court stenographer's dictation machine, certain keys stand for combinations of letters or functions. Some designs even place fingers in "wells," rather than on keys, to select letters by back-and-forth movements.

DataHand offers padded handrests with individual finger wells that operate switches.

- **DataHand**
  Scottsdale, AZ
  602-860-8584

MIKey is a fixed keyboard with 12 function keys arranged in clock-face pattern.

- **Dr. Alan Grant**
  Chevy Chase, MD
  301-933-1111

The **Comfort Keyboard** is broken into three pieces, which can be rotated in any direction. It incorporates familiar key arrangements.

- **Health Care Keyboard Co., Inc.**
  Menomonee Falls, WI
  414-703-0170

THE EMF FLAP

Some health concerns have to do less with pain today than with illness tomorrow. One potential problem in particular stands out -— electromagnetic fields (EMFs). EMFs are a form of radiation emitted by computer monitors and many other electrical devices in our homes and offices. Some researchers argue that repeated exposure to EMFs can cause cancer, birth defects, and other health problems. The idea isn't without controversy, however, and all scientific facts aren't in yet. If you remain worried, however, about potential hazards of EMFs, you can take several precautions:

- Try to stay at least an arm's length from your monitor. EMFs decrease rapidly with increased distance.

- Avoid sitting near the sides or rear of computer monitors. Most units emit higher levels of EMFs in these areas than from the front.

- Use monitors designed to emit low EMFs. This isn't an option for most people. To find these monitors, check with computer dealers or look through manufacturers' product literature. Also, watch for reviews of monitors in computer magazines.

FIVE EXERCISES TO PREVENT INJURY

- **Neck glide**: Glide your head back as far as it will go, keeping your head and ears level. Doing it correctly creates a double chin. Now glide your head forward and repeat three times.

- **Wrist flex**: Hold your right arm out, fingers pointed up. Take your left hand and gently bend your right hand back towards your forearm. Hold five seconds. Repeat on the other side.

- **Finger fan**: Hold your hands out in front of you, palms down. Spread your fingers apart as far as you can. Hold for five seconds, then make a tight fist. Repeat three times.

- **Upper/lower back stretches**: *Upper stretch* — raise your hands to your shoulders. Then, using your arms, push your shoulders back. Keep your elbows down. Hold for 15 seconds. Repeat three times. *Lower stretch* — lower your head and slowly roll your body as far as you can toward your knees. Hold for ten seconds. Push yourself up with your leg muscles and repeat three times.

North Coast Medical, Incorporated sells everything a medical transcriptionist needs to ensure a safe and comfortable working environment. You can get a variety of wrist rests for keyboards, mouse pads, lighting, chairs, foot rests, lumbar supports, protective and strengthening products for your hands. They also carry an interesting product called *TheraPutty*™, a silicon rubber compound that promotes increasing range of motion, hand closure, tendon gliding, and hand strength. *TheraPutty* comes in different consistencies and costs around $4.

You can order a sample kit of all eight putty resistances for $24.95. Contact North Coast for a catalog.

- **North Coast Health and Safety Products**
  800-821-9319

MASSAGE THOSE MUSCLES

Medical transcriptionists spend many hours in front of computers. As a consequence, our muscles frequently get very tense and remain that way for painfully long periods because, unfortunately, we usually cannot run to our local massage therapist to work out the kinks. Recently, an OR nurse and friend shared a self-help therapy workbook she thought was wonderful. She was right! I found the guide very helpful in locating my myofascial trigger points and working out the kinks. The book, which gives basic, crystal-clear instructions for self-massage, is *The Trigger Point Therapy Workbook Your Self-Treatment Guide for Pain Relief* by Clair Davies, N.C.T.M.B. U.S. ($19.95, New Harbinger Publications, Inc., www.newharbinger.com)

REFERENCE BOOKS

Every medical transcriptionist's office should contain copies of references . . . and more references. They are essential and well worth the investment. There are numerous medical reference books on the market today, available through a variety of publishers. Gone are the days when the only reference book for MTs was *Taber's Dictionary*. Do not, we repeat do not, scrimp on these. Lippincott, Williams & Wilkins and W. B. Saunders Co. have entire libraries of medical reference books as well as electronic reference resources.

My reference library contains more than 100 books, many of which are medical references by specialty. All are essential for my work as a home-based medical transcriptionist. I update these reference frequently — some each year; the others, never later than three years or whenever updates are available.

Other essential references for the medical transcription library include grammar and punctuation references, a good collegiate dictionary, medical dictionary, anatomy book, and abbreviations, acronyms and symbols book. You'll also discover many other books that will prove helpful in your specific work.

Be sure to attend seminars, conventions and trade shows and visit the book vendors in attendance. You will see more books than you know what to do with. Once upon a time there were so few books it was easy to choose; you just bought one of each. Today there are hundreds of good references, and it will make your choice much more difficult. Purchase those that will meet your specific needs and keep them conveniently at hand.

For a list of some of our favorite reference books, check the reference books section at the back of this book. In addition, to obtain an excellent and comprehensive medical transcription reference list, contact the American Association for Medical Transcription, 800-982-2182.

Several publishing houses also specialize in books for the health care field. To obtain a list of titles available, contact our recommended book publishers listed in the reference section at the back of this book.

UTILIZING CONSULTANTS

Like all professionals, transcriptionists sometimes need the help of experts outside their field. These may include a lawyer to review contracts, an accountant/tax consultant, computer specialist, insurance agent, graphic designer, etc.

When possible, obtain personal recommendations for consultants from business associates. You may also call specific professional associations for referrals or find consultants listed in the yellow pages of the telephone directory. Contact potential consultants regarding their consulting procedures and fees. You may want to interview them. If you do not feel comfortable with a consultant, do not hesitate to seek another.

When consulting with specialists, do not expect them to make your decisions for you. They will make intelligent recommendations based on their knowledge and experience, but decision making related to your business is ultimately your responsibility.

When working with consultants, be open about your knowledge level of the subject and insist that explanations be in language you understand. If you do not understand something, ask for clarification. Remember, it is no disgrace to acknowledge that you are uninformed in this particular subject. That's why we hire consultants.

233

We suggest that you attend seminars, which are educational and also give you access to experienced professionals with whom you can speak — a type of informal consultation. Also, subscribe to publications that have Question-and-Answer columns that offer advice on issues and problems related to your business.

WORKSHOPS AND SEMINARS

Workshops and seminars are some of the most powerful self-improvement and professional development tools available today. They offer a refreshing change of pace from routine work — even if for only a few hours — and spending time in a stimulating, idea-filled environment is a motivating experience. It is also a great place to network.

Hundreds of millions of dollars are spent each year on professional training conferences. These events are excellent professional opportunities, especially when you plan ahead:

- **Write out your expectations before the event**. Think about conditions that currently affect your work environment. What skills you would like to learn? Make up a list of ways you would like the conference to help you and keep the list in front of you during the meeting.

- **Obtain information and plan conference activities ahead of time**. If you have decision-making authority over your attendance, or if you haven't yet committed to attending, ask the seminar sponsor to give you a detailed outline of seminar presentation materials, presenters' names and information about their experience and expertise. Study the outline and speak with past attendees. If one conference isn't right for you, chances are another will be.

- **Aim for comfort**. Dress flexibly and comfortably. Wear light, loose-fitting clothes and carry a sweater or jacket. Layering is wise because air-conditioning in some facilities is uncomfortably cool or downright cold; other times, it's stifling.

- **Make action notes during the conference**. As you listen to the speakers, divide your note pad into two columns. In the left-hand column make notes about the speakers' comments; in the right hand column, jot down "to-dos" and ways you can apply the information and ideas presented. These notes will be valuable to you later on.

- **Get to know other conference participants**. Every conference you attend provides great opportunities to meet your colleagues, learn about their businesses and accomplishments, and share mutual concerns. Share with others your expectations as well as your successes. Be prepared to LISTEN. Meet as many people as possible, exchange business cards, and establish a personal network that you will be able to use in the future. It will prove invaluable.

- **Get to know the conference leader**. While you may not be able to spend a great deal of time with conference speakers, they probably have some free time before and after conference sessions. Leaders expect participants to talk with them informally during these periods. Don't hesitate to explore a topic in more depth with the speaker or ask to discuss it during a break. Conference speakers have a wealth of information about topics they present.

- **Discuss the conference with others when you return and offer your impressions**. They will appreciate your sharing your time and valuable information.

- **Be prepared to implement what you have learned**. Start an idea file, keep one or two ideas in front of you at all times, and take the steps necessary to put these to work. The knowledge and ideas you bring back from each conference will help develop your skills. Exercise these skills and your seminar experience will pay big dividends to you in the months and years to come.

BEWARE OF EXPERTS WHO AREN'T

When I started as an IMT, there were no experts to whom I could turn. As with everything else I have done in my life, my experience came from "The School of Hard Knocks" (i.e., if Plan A fails, go on to Plan B. I spent hours in the library trying to gain insight into the steps I needed to take to achieve my goals). At that time, most of the books available were published in the 1970s when the typewriter was king.

Then there was the government bureaucracy to deal with. Those of you who have navigated this territory probably understand the depths of frustration I experienced trying to get information about zoning laws and tax regulations. Translated in typical government double-speak, public information was generally oppressive.

The end of the 1980s was a time of self-discovery and an "I want it now" mentality. Schools sprang up promising would-be medical transcriptionists a full-fledged medical transcription training program in an unrealistically brief period of 3-6 months and a job at the end of the program paying a grandiose $35,000-a-year medical transcription salary.

Currently there is a proliferation of books and seminars on how to start home-based businesses. Working at home is a viable business option in the 1990s and it seems everyone wants a piece of the action. Be forewarned: not all how-to books and seminars are equal.

Before you buy how-to books or attend how-to seminars, check promoters'/ authors' credentials. Is the "ultimate book on Victorian home restoration" written by someone experienced in Victorian construction, or is his expertise limited to wallpapering a bathroom? Did the author of *You Too Can Work at Home and Become a Bazillionaire MT?* ever actually own and operate a home-based medical transcription business? Has that seminar coordinator on starting a home-based medical transcription service ever typed a medical record report or owned a successful medical transcription home-based service, or was she only employed as a marketing rep for a computer company? Did that educator for the *Get-Rich-Quick School for Medical Transcription* ever work as a medical transcriptionist and become certified, or was her experience limited to legal secretarial work for a medical malpractice attorney?

Much misinformation is disseminated by so-called "experts." These people purport to know what is best for **us** and our profession even though they have no firsthand experience in actually running a successful home-based medical transcription service. Our profession is very specialized — unlike any other in the world. What works in our businesses doesn't necessarily hold true for other businesses.

ACCOUNTS AND SUPPLIES

When you acquire accounts, you will find that there are a variety of forms and formats you can work with. Individual accounts frequently have specific formats and sometimes their own paper supplies.

You can also use desktop publishing techniques, which are available in programs like WordPerfect, to create letterhead if there is an issue with your client supplying paper, which might jeopardize your independent contractor status as defined by the IRS. If the client does supply you with letterhead, be sure to return it if the business relationship is terminated.

If you are self-employed but your clients provide the paper, consider purchasing your own. In addition to denoting your independent transcriptionist status, you will also have another business expense to write off at tax time. Explain the rationale to your client. You may have to factor this expense into the rate you are charging for your services.

Hospitals often use tractor-fed, continuous feed paper preprinted with their name and logo, but many are now switching to plain paper documents generated through laser printers. Some clients have the transcriptionist modem files to their transcription department so they can be printed on their laserjet printer. Others may ask that you print the documents at your worksite on plain paper with their hospital format and deliver the documents. They may also request the documents on disk along with the hard copies. Doctors' offices usually provide letterhead for letters of consultation.

Paper for chart notes varies. Some transcriptionists prefer continuous feed, peel-off, or "sticky-back" paper for chart notes. Chart notes can be set up easily with the patient's name and date, body of report, and physician's signature line. They can be cut with a paper cutter and returned to the doctor/clinic office, peeled off, and placed in the patient chart. This eliminates handling charts and removing and replacing chart note sheets.

This paper can be purchased by the roll or sheet, for tractor-fed or laser printers. It is available with or without perforations. That without perforations offers somewhat more flexibility, allowing the transcriptionist to cut it wherever the chart note ends. Companies that sell this type paper — in continuous rolls and laser sheets — are listed below.

- **Script-Ese**
  800-553-7711

- **Briggs**
  800-247-2343

- **Pat Systems**
  800-543-1911

- **RayPress Corp.**
  205-254-3731

- **Professional Health Care Systems**
  800-445-5875

Radiology departments have special forms and formats, but many are converting to laser printed forms that are easier to use. Many radiology departments have their own dedicated *radiology information systems (RIS)* which incorporate all patient demographics. The transcriptionist only has to type the body of the report, which is printed out in the department or wherever routed. In RIS systems such as these, patient demographics are entered into a computer when the patient registers for the procedure. Physicians love this because they no longer have to dictate all the patient ID information, requesting physician, x-ray report, etc.

With the RIS system, transcription is done online and can be completed on site or through remote transcription connected by modem to the RIS. Transcribing is in real-time over the phone line. As the transcriptionist types, the information systems department in the hospital can monitor the document on the screen as the transcriptionist actually inputs information. This type technology brings us closer and closer to real-time transcription, which offers an almost instantaneous turnaround time.

Pathology departments also have individualized formats and these formats may vary from client to client.

If the client has no preference regarding format, prepare a generic format (e.g., block letter style, standard H&P, discharge, operation, consultation, etc.) for their consideration.

When establishing a working relationship with a new account, come to an agreement regarding format to be used. This helps prevent misunderstandings. If the account staff prefer a specific format that is currently in use, they may make copies of chart notes and letters for you to use as references. However, they may decide to take this opportunity to update or make revisions to existing formats. They may even ask your opinion regarding formats.

If you are picking up tapes of dictation from a doctor's office or a clinic, check to see if the tapes have been scanned. If not, request a list of names on which the doctor has dictated.

Unscanned dictation tapes are a risk to transcriptionists. If a doctor claims to have dictated a report on a patient but no transcribed report is available, the transcriptionist may be accused of losing the dictation. Generally, when a patient is seen in a doctor's office, the receptionist will check off or line out the patient's name after the appointment. The appointment book page can easily be photocopied for you.

> If a doctor claims to have dictated a report on a patient but no transcribed report is available, the transcriptionist may be accused of losing the dictation.

You can check patient names off as you transcribe and return the list to the office with the transcribed reports. If there are names not checked, the doctor's office staff can easily see that he or she still needs to dictate on those patients. If a log is not provided, I suggest you create your own log for reference and billing. List the subjects/names that were on the tape that you transcribed. (For more information, see section on medical transcription logs.)

In many offices, appointments are logged on computers, making it easy for staff to provide you with a printout of the day's patient register. This list will also assist you with correct spelling of patient names. Doctors are notorious for not spelling names and sometimes they even forget to give them! In those situations, note any discrepancies. Leave a blank for the patient's name with a note ("name not given"). Office staff will solve the mystery by locating the patient's chart. After picking up dictation tapes, be sure to confirm your turnaround or delivery time and dates, as well as the name of the office contact person who assists you with confirmations and details. Request a list of medical staff physicians (physicians list) to assure proper name spelling.

Hospital dictation should be handled the same way. A printout of patient name, medical record number, and physician name/identification number should be transmitted to you along with the dictated tapes. If computer printouts are not available, the hospital can provide you with the A&D (admission and discharge) sheets. These are generated daily on all patients admitted and discharged from the hospital.

You must have this information to transcribe the reports correctly. Hospital records require that the patient's name and medical record/identification number be present on each page of the record. Upon completion of transcription, these sheets can be returned with the transcribed tapes, or whatever you negotiate with your client.

ALERT! ALERT! ERASING TAPES

Erasing tapes after completing transcription can be risky. Some transcriptionists never erase tapes, even if asked to do so. They leave this responsibility to their clients. Other transcriptionists erase tapes upon request, following meticulous procedures to avoid potential problems. If you choose to erase tapes, the following guidelines will be helpful.

Never erase a tape of dictation until you have printed or transferred completed reports by modem. We all have horror stories to tell about the tape that got erased, the report the computer ate, etc. I keep a little colored basket/bin labeled "tapes to be transcribed" on the right of my desk and a different colored basket labeled "already transcribed" on the left side of my desk. When I have completed my work for that account, or that day, and the reports are printed out and secured in the delivery portfolio, I finally erase the tapes and include them in the envelope.

For accounts handled by modem, I first back up all reports onto floppy disks as my insurance; then I transmit the reports to the hospital, modem to modem. When my computer tells me the transfer is complete, I then erase all the tapes. If for some reason the transmittal did not go through and the hospital did not receive my reports, they are still on the floppy disk, and I can easily transmit again.

If you are downloading work off a digital system, you have completed the job and it is gone from your system, it can be recaptured. Usually the digital system will hold the signed-off jobs for 24-72 hours. If you find that you have accidentally deleted a report and you need to retranscribe it, you can call the client and ask to have that job reassigned to you if it is still in the holding/suspension mode. This happens!

Aren't computers wonderful! We have been transcriptionists long enough to remember when state-of-the-art electronic typewriters sometimes wiped out entire tapes of transcription, which then had to be typed again. That was extremely frustrating and an incredible waste of time! For the most part, computer technology has solved that problem.

Always check with your clients beforehand to determine if they prefer that you erase their tapes after completing the transcription, or simply return them rewound.

If working with digital systems through telecommunication, always identify the job number, which will be somewhere on your transcription log or somewhere on the report that you are transcribing, so the dictation can be recaptured by that job number if necessary.

Telecommunications

"Nothing, I am sure, calls forth the faculties so much as being
obliged to struggle with the world."

—Mary Wollstonecraft Shelley

Telecommuting is sending completed work to a client's computer via modem. Modems allow your computer to connect to telephone lines and transmit data to and from other computers or online services. Online services can range from a local bulletin-board service, or BBS, to a large international data center such as Prodigy and CompuServe.

Telecommuting eliminates pickup and delivery time and expense. You must have a modem and the client must have compatible software and a modem to receive the work.

REASONS TO TELECOMMUTE

Natural disasters: As a result of the 1994 earthquake in Southern California, commuter gridlock sometimes lasted for five hours. Employees for The City and County of Los Angeles were encouraged to work out of their homes two to three days a week by leasing equipment from the County.

During recent disastrous floods in the Midwest and hurricanes in Southern Florida, entire regions were able to communicate their needs immediately through telecommunication. It was their only link with the outside for long periods of time.

In Washington D.C., because of extreme weather conditions and hazardous commuting conditions, government employees were sent home to work. If they had not been able to telecommute, many employees would have missed work, forcing government agencies to shut down.

During all of the above natural disasters, the first computer information networks — online services like Prodigy, CompuServe and America OnLine — were heavily and beneficially used. At this point in history there is no question that whether we're faced with overwhelming natural disasters or balmy days of routine living, online services and telecommunication offer many positive benefits.

Environment: Telecommuting has a positive impact on the environment in terms of reducing air pollution by cutting back on commuter traffic. Many cities across the U.S. are imposing environmental ordinances that are mandating workers work from home at least two or three days per week in an effort to reduce air pollution.

Time, Productivity, Dollars: Tremendous amounts of time and energy are saved and employee productivity is greatly increased when workers telecommute. Consistently, employers report an increase in productivity of 12%-20% per employee, estimated to be a savings of $6,000-$8,000 per employee per year.

Office Space and Equipment: Telecommuting is kind to employers, too. With employees or independent contractors working at home, there is no need to invest company dollars in office expansion and added staff. In addition, smaller departments can be run more efficiently, making the company more competitive, and there is less managerial stress with fewer on-site employees and tasks to manage.

Flexibility: Businesses and individuals enjoy increased flexibility in performing their work.

Computers, fax machines and emerging telephone services are all developing in the same direction — to give us more control over where, when and how we conduct our work.

WHO ARE THE TELECOMMUTERS?

Telecommuting is best suited to people who like to work, who don't mind working alone, and who enjoy combining home and business activities. Those who have made the switch successfully praise the telecommuting lifestyle and its life-enhancing qualities.

The SOHO business market supported an estimated 6.6 million Internet-accessing telecommuters in 2000, roughly 28% of the segment's total workforce. The small business market was home to more than 5.3 million Internet-accessing at-home workers in 2000, making up 13% of the small business workforce.

TelNetwork, an Oakland-based association that researches the impact of telecommuting, recently estimated that at least 90,000 people in the San Francisco Bay Area alone now telecommute, and that another 700,000-1,000,000 commuters might be able to telecommute one to three days a week.

Air quality legislation, a more in-line work force, greater comfort with technology, and the dropping costs of high tech products are all fueling the growth of telecommuting.

> *"Even if you're on the right track, you will get run over if you are not moving fast enough."*
> —Will Rogers

TELECOMMUTER — THE PROFESSIONAL

Telecommuting is now established as a formal job description. More than ten million Americans are telecommuters.

Increasing numbers of health care facilities are negotiating off-site work arrangements to reduce overhead expenses, taking into consideration that telecommuting has proven to significantly increase quality and productivity. The same transcription services that once boasted they used only in-house transcriptionists are now aggressively recruiting skilled off-site MTs throughout the world.

Occasionally telecommuters do encounter resistance from those who aren't comfortable with such arrangements. But despite occasional skeptics, the trend toward telecommuting represents a large — and probably unstoppable — shift in workplace priorities.

As medical transcriptionists shift to telecommuting, we are more adaptable to industry shift because ours is a profession of individuals who can work on our own and require little face-to-face contact. There are prerequisites to successful telecommuting, however.

The downside to telecommuting can be loneliness and overwork. You may work extra hours to prove your dedication and the worth of your service. You may be tempted to stop working, wander from your desk and start doing something not related to your work. Keep focused. And if you find yourself cruising the refrigerator during working hours, take a brief walk elsewhere instead.

You must have an end-of-the-day routine or you may find yourself wandering back into your office and working again. Tell yourself, DON'T GO THERE!

TRANSCRIPTION ANYWHERE

More and more health care facilities and transcription services are utilizing skilled off-site transcriptionists at satellite locations to meet the ever increasing demand for transcription of dictation. The dictated data must be moved rapidly to resources that are the most available and cost-effective. The development of digital dictation has revolutionized the industry and, more recently, rerecord technology has been introduced. This allows transcriptionists to access dictation and download at a higher rate of speed than real time, thus cutting down on telephone rerecord costs.

There are now systems available, such as Dictaphone's STRAIGHT TALK system, that offer cost-effective solutions to high speed rerecording. This equipment can be programmed for the home-based MT to download dictation at any given time, and transcription can begin as soon as rerecording begins. This means no more waiting for cassettes to fill up or for the entire transmission to conclude.

> *"You must have an end-of-the-day routine or you may find yourself wandering back into your office and working again."*

INTERNET

The Internet is the mother of all computer networks. It is actually a collection of networks with shared software standards. The system allows millions of people in business and academia around the globe to communicate. More than 15 million users are currently on the Internet network and the number of users is increasing rapidly. Several hundred libraries worldwide have added their catalogs to the system. Full text data bases will likely evolve from this.

The beginning stages of a multibillion dollar user electronic highway are in place and it is anticipated that this highway will do for the flow of information what the first transcontinental railroad, and later the interstate highway system, did for the transportation of goods and people. Unlike those earlier communication networks, however, whose costs were supported by government, it appears that the costs of our multibillion dollar information highway will likely be borne by private enterprise.

From medical images and billings for physician services to movies and telecommunication, the Internet's electronic highway promises to transform the flow of information from a paper chase to almost instantaneous retrieval.

Internet services and data bases are so bewildering that software is being developed to specifically search for desired information. The overwhelming majority of revenues we get by the end of the decade will be from services and products that have not yet been invented.

To keep up with the digital revolution, there are many references we recommend reading. You may have heard of *Wired*. This is one of the first publications to actually capture the excitement of the merger of computing, communications and media that is changing every aspect of our lives from business to politics and education to entertainment. For more information or to subscribe, contact *Wired*.

- *Wired*
  P. O. Box 191826
  San Francisco
  14119-9866
  800-SO-WIRED

ONLINE GLOBAL COMMUNICATIONS

There are many resources available for learning to navigate the internet but one of our favorites is *NetPractice, A Beginner's Guide to Healthcare Networking on the Internet*. NetPractice is a self-instructional guide designed to give health care professionals a no-nonsense approach to navigating on the Internet. It doesn't try to overwhelm you with a conglomeration of Internet services but lays a foundation for the most common and practical uses of the Internet. Contact Opus Communications for more information.

- **Opus Communications**
  Fulfillment Center
  P.O. Box 9214
  Waltham, MA 02514-9214
  E-mail at customer_service@opuscomm.com.

THE SEVEN-SECOND COMMUTE

According to the report *Entering the Access Era: U.S. Telecommuter Demographics & the Impact of Fragmentation on IT Platforms*, new research on U.S. telecommuters indicates that employees have more freedom than ever to set up a home office, with roughly 24% of the U.S. workforce estimated to telecommute some time during the week in 2001. This works out to be more than 30 million at-home workers. *In-Stat* expects this percentage to increase to 28% in 2004, growing to nearly 40 million telecommuters. By the year 2010 a quarter of a billion people will be telecommuters, according to *Link Resources*.

Employers are finally realizing that where work is concerned, ***the important thing is the individual and the quality of the work he or she produces***, not the location where the work is produced.

For many years, large transcription services have boasted that their work is completed by only the most qualified transcriptionists. Some brag that they use only "in house" MTs. These individuals supposedly work in a controlled environment where confidentiality is a priority, use the best technology to produce excellent transcription in prompt turnaround time, etc. Some of the large services offer employee benefit packages and incentives. These perks used to be available only to those working in the office, but now these same services are promoting their employment packages to home-based MTs, to work as at-home employees with benefits or as independent MTs. This opens up great opportunities for home-based medical transcriptionists.

Large services have done an "about face" since our last edition of this book. They once suggested — either openly or indirectly — that independent transcriptionists were a threat to medical record confidentiality, but my experience has found that to be absolutely untrue. I have had the opportunity to transcribe reports in the acute-care hospital setting, as a transcription manager for a service, and as a home-based transcriptionist. Of these three environments, I found the home-office to be the most confidential.

Think about it. In the hospital setting the medical transcriptionist is the first one to see the patient's medical record, but she is certainly not the last! While the patient is in the hospital, that record passes through the hands of approximately 75 health care professionals — doctors, nurses, lab and medical imaging technicians, therapists, social workers, discharge planners, utilization reviewers and others. In medical records departments, the patient's record is seen by chart assemblers, coders/abstractors, and other medical personnel. And what about accounts receivable? In my experience, the transcriptionist is not a major risk factor in issues of patient confidentiality.

I live on a remote island in the Pacific Ocean, far away from the nearest transcription service. I'm a skilled, experienced, highly qualified transcriptionist. I, too, have a controlled office environment, confidentiality is a priority, my technology is up-to-date, and I provide great turnaround time.

This is the age of moving information through telecommuting and working where we choose. There is no reason why a person should have to sacrifice time and energy to commute hours on end just to get to a job, or get a job done! Transcription services that offer benefits can now have the best of both worlds. They can utilize qualified MTs who will gladly be a part of their team through telecommuting. With sophisticated technology at our fingertips, we can process data faster than Superman can fly to the top of a tall building, from anywhere in the world to anywhere else in the world — from where we are.

My work and lifestyle as a home-based transcriptionist suit my needs. I do commute thirty seconds every day to get to work, but I begin work when I like, and my schedule is flexible. In my Hawaiian office I enjoy warm tropical sunshine, cool breezes blowing through open plantation shutters, and a spectacular view of the ocean. In this setting, I am able to work longer and with less stress.

My work is done in a controlled office environment. My reference library is up to date, and my computer technology is state of the art. I have my own clients and service them through telecommuting. I also do work for a larger service when my own client load slows down. My professional life and my personal/family life are kept completely separate.

The work does have its ups and downs and many times it's feast or famine, but that's true in a large service as well. Ultimately, a career is what you make it. I choose this home-based independent working situation as do thousands of others. With modems and fax machines we are able to receive patient information, job numbers, and admission and discharge logs.

RIDING THE WAVE

With digital phone systems and rerecord devices now available, we can access dictating systems and offer incredible turnaround to our clients, just like the "big guys." And look what is coming now . . . the WAVE. Soon WAVE file technology will be an everyday medical transcription word . . . someone in New York will be reading what I am currently typing . . . that's what happens when we ride the WAVE!

You may need to purchase voice wave technology to access some of your clients. Bob's PCWerks has a VoiceWave transcriber for approximately $195 that is compatible with a number of products. The foot pedal connects directly to the PC.

- **Bob's PCWERKS**
  214-763-3768
  www.bobspcwerks.com

ASP/TASP - APPLICATION SERVICE PROVIDERS

Internet services continue to expand and enhance the support provided to transcriptionists. Transcription application service providers are fee-based upon use. The TASP provides end-to-end technology from the physician/client to the IMT or MTSO and back. With new regulations addressing the electronic delivery and storage of medical information, many old methods of file transfer are no longer acceptable. Documentation of security is a requirement in today's health care environment. This includes password protection, firewalls, and 128-bit encryption for all transcription file delivery. TASP utilizes these methods for high level security and work-flow automation that meets HIPAA security standards.

These providers also provide portable digital recording systems and upload of sound files and toll-free call-in to access their systems. Instead of chasing your tail trying to keep up with the latest technology, using an application service provider will allow you access to the type of technology you need for just a few dollars a day on a pay-as-you-need basis without the need for expensive equipment. There is no big up-front investment.

Some services require a sign-on fee similar to subscribing to a DSL or cable network. Service providers may charge you a "minute" plan based on your expected need, a fee of two cents per line, or fees based on minutes of dictation used. Clients can also utilize their telephone to access dictation via a toll-free number, and there are generally no geographical limitations within the US. Services are available 24/7, 365 days a year. Detailed usage reports are also available for billing purposes. Transcription can be done via any waveplayer that is compatible.

The ASP industry plans to conduct an international trend analysis study to measure change in both the demand for and supply of ASP services on an annual basis, over the next three years. The results should be available to the public in 2004-2005.

THE C-PHONE

The C-phone is still one of the most common and popular pieces of equipment for accessing dictation. It is a digital receiver/transcriber/phone that accesses digital dictation from another location via telephone lines.

PREPARING TO TELECOMMUTE

Whether you're planning to talk to multiple businesses across the nation or simply connect to local clinics, technical requirements are essentially the same: a personal computer at your end hooked to a modem attached to a phone line. Whomever you're telecommunicating to will need the same equipment. Each computer configuration is a little different, but here are some suggestions for an "ideal" setup and the reasons for each recommended component.

- **The most current PC you can reasonably afford.** A Pentium class PC with at least 64 megabytes of memory and Windows loaded would be a minimum desirable configuration. It's a fact that you can run WordPerfect for DOS on an old AT with 640K of memory, but the main advantage a Windowed-machine gives you is multi-tasking or background processing. This means you could be sending or receiving files or faxes in the background while processing documents, spreadsheets or other items at the same time. This may seem trivial, but if you're spending five to ten minutes sending or receiving, that can add up to over 300 hours a year!

- **An external, high speed, data/fax modem.** *External* because it frees you from being locked into a specific computer. *High speed* because it minimizes your line charges and increases efficiency. *Data/fax* because sooner or later someone will need to fax you a hard copy or you will need to fax a hard copy to them. (Remember, you'll need a fax software package to utilize the faxing capabilities of your fax/modem).

  A 33.6K bps modem costs around $99. You can get higher speed 56K bps external fax/modems for as little as $159! In addition, newer modems are more reliable and more compatible with other systems.

- **A *common* communications package. DON'T** use some hokey piece of software your brother or friend gave you for "free." Check the market you'll be talking with. What do they use — *PC Anywhere*? *Carbon Copy*? A combination? *PC Anywhere* and *Carbon Copy* (and *ProComm Plus*) have a distinct advantage over others in that they are easy to set up and can talk to most anything else. That means if you have PC Anywhere but the clinic has Carbon Copy, you can still communicate. If possible, stick with the commonly used products. Check the references and resources in the back of this book.

> NOTE: If a business **insists** on a specific software package you don't have, ask for a copy of their software and adequate licensing documentation. Often, the license they've purchased will allow for your use of the software, too. Conversely, your license will often allow you to load the product on both your home PC and that of another host computer.

- **If you have substantial online time, a separate phone line for your fax/ modem.** If your time online is usually short, a separate phone line for your fax may not be necessary, but if your phone has various options like call waiting, etc. you might experience connection interruptions. Check with the phone company to see what impact, if any, such services could have on your data transmissions.

Whenever possible, remain independent of the remote business. Sometimes, however, the business will require you to work online. In this situation you dial the business and do your work on *their* machine. Although your body is home, your transcription is in their office. There are two disadvantages to this scenario:

1) Most transcriptionists can out-type even the fastest phone line connection.

2) You are at the mercy of communications lines and hardware at the business site. If either fails, you're out of work until repairs are made.

Remember, too, that all communications packages provide dial-back capability. This means you can call a business that is long distance and the business's modem can dial your modem back to establish the connection. You benefit because that telephone call is on their dime (or dollar!), not yours. In addition, it gives them more security because they control outgoing calls from their modem.

Get to know your computer. Books like *DOS for Dummies* are a quick way to gain basic knowledge about your computer and telecommuting.

THE MODEM

To telecommunicate you must connect your computer to a phone line. For that capability, your system must incorporate a modem. In essence, a modem is a small electronic telephone. It can be installed either on a card inside your system unit (internal modem) or outside the unit, hooked up to a communications, or COM, port (external modem).

Your modem accepts data you input via your keyboard and translates that data into bits and bytes, which the modem then transmits across phone lines. After another computer or online system has received your telephoned transmission, its modem translates these bits and bytes back into readable form, and your telecommunicating begins.

Internal modems cost less than external modems, but whenever possible buy an external modem. External modems are easier to install than internal modems. You don't have to remove the cover from your PC and squeeze another circuit card into a tight-fitting slot. Most important, you will not have to reverse the process if the modem is set up wrong the first time you install it. If an external modem needs service you just unplug it! Removing an internal modem requires much greater effort.

Another advantage of external modems is their indicator lights, which are located on the front of the modem's case. These lights are computer status indicators and are great troubleshooting aids. After a short time, you will be able to tell which lights should be on, or blinking, during transmissions.

Internal modems are not helpful at all when something isn't working right, and some computer techs tell us they are discovering that internal modems are rough on the computer's hard drive and eventually cause failures more often than external modems.

The greater the baud rate, the faster information is sent over the phone line . . . and the higher the price of the modem. However, just because your modem may be a 33,300 baud, it doesn't guarantee that your data will **always** be transmitted at that speed. Data is transferred according to the availability of phone space through the lines, so during peak hours of the work day your modem may automatically bump down to whatever baud rate it needs to get the data through the line.

If you are anxious to try out your modem after installing it, and perhaps feeling a little insecure, contact a friend who has a modem and experiment. Connect with him/her and practice using the chat mode. Practice exchanging files, uploading and downloading. (Note: To send a file is to **upload**, to receive a file is to **download**.)

THE TELECOMMUNICATIONS PROGRAM

A telecommunications program is software that controls the connection between your computer and some other remote computer system or online service.

Some online services such as *Prodigy* or *America OnLine* provide special software.

To call another computer system you need to know the following about the other system:

- The phone number to call

- Any password or log-in procedure the other system requires

- The baud rate (for example, 9600 bps, 14,400 bps)
  (Most new computer software will search your system and set up parameters automatically.)

- Number of data bits (usually 7 or 8)

- Number of stop bits (usually 1)

- The parity (odd, even, or none)

Software programs for modeming vary in price but, generally, they perform the same functions. Do some comparison shopping before making your final decision. Pro-Comm Plus is one software program that does the job for about $80.

SERVICING CLIENTS THROUGH TELECOMMUNICATION

In the old days, hospitals mailed tape cassettes and waited several days for reports to be returned. Through telecommunication, digital dictation systems allow the transcriptionist or service to dial in and transcribe off the system, send files back via modem, at which point hard copies are printed at the facility. Turnaround is decreased to HOURS instead of days and weeks.

Telecommuting can be utilized to access dictation through the telephone system with digital dictation and using a modem to transfer or deliver transcription over the phone to another computer.

Computer bulletin boards (BBs) are also accessed through telecommunication. The Federal Drug Administration (FDA) has a computer bulletin board, as does the Small Business Administration (SBA). Both are very helpful resources for home-based businesses.

Servicing clients from the home office through telecommunication is now very popular and very cost-effective. It eliminates wasted time and travel expenses in pick up and delivery, and expensive courier fees required for rush jobs. With telecommunication, a two- or three-minute phone call transmits your transcription across the street or across the country. The cost for this type of service is a modem, software and a telephone call.

Currently, using modern technology and telecommunication, it takes me *three hours* to do what it took me eight hours to do ten years ago! My clients benefit from this improved service, and so do I — with less stress, increased productivity, and greater profits.

WHAT IS PRACTICAL FOR INDIVIDUAL CLIENTS

Telecommuting isn't always practical for physicians' offices, especially in remote areas. With health care policies and impending government reforms, many physicians are gearing up to implement a variety of cutbacks and reduce overhead expenses. We anticipate that one of the first cutbacks will be clerical and transcription services.

If you plan to market your services to physician accounts, be prepared to pick up and deliver cassettes, for this will probably be the most cost-effective plan for one- or two-client offices. Other doctors will prefer cassettes because, although a dial-and-dictate system might work well in their office, they do not have time to dictate in that setting. They are doctors who frequently use a hand-held recorder and dictate chart notes wherever they happen to be — in the examining room during or after a patient's exam; in their car on the way to the hospital or on their way home; in the recovery room after performing surgery; at home after dinner; or at the park while watching their kids or walking the dog. Their time is precious and they squeeze dictation duty into their busy schedules whenever and wherever possible. For these doctors, cassette tapes continue to be ideal.

Telecommuting and dial-and-dictate systems are very effective for hospitals and larger clinics where there is shared financial responsibility. These facilities are able to contract with remote services, use home-based medical transcriptionists who can connect directly to their dictation systems via modem, and even home-base their own employees.

TELEPHONE CHARGES

As a telecommuter you are responsible for telecommuting phone charges, and one of your biggest expenses will be long distance charges. If your potential clients are long distance, carefully weigh the cost of telephone charges against what you will earn. For current clients, consider rerecording or using your digital system during less costly off-peak telephone hours.

If you are interested in telecommuting with a service, look for a reputable service in your area that hires home-based telecommuting medical transcriptionists. If you are fortunate enough to find a good company locally, you will avoid the expense of long distance phone bills.

If you are hired by a service as a home-based employee, the service should provide you with tools to perform your duties for them. This should include their paying one-half of your social security payroll tax, covering costs for your computer, printer, toner, phone, paper, transcriber, and other necessary supplies.

If you contract with a service as an independent contractor, you should supply all of the equipment necessary to perform services for them — including the cost of accessing dictation.

RESEARCHING TELEPHONE SERVICES

If you are preparing to service long distance clients, you should definitely research long distance phone carriers. There are hundreds of long distance phone carriers (in California alone there are over 110 long distance carriers). Ask one or more long distance providers to do a traffic analysis of your phone calls. Check on special phone discounts, WATS lines, Circle Calling, etc.

Investigate telecommunication resource and management companies that specialize in recommending and implementing long distance, local data and other telecommunication services to customers. These companies research and find phone carriers for clients at a lower cost than companies can obtain on their own. With this service you benefit from cost savings, administrative benefits, and ongoing telephone line management and monitoring services. These companies also negotiate with many carriers in order to offer clients services that provide high quality service at the lowest rates.

You will find many resources for long-distance telephone carriers on the following website:

- **telecommunicationsinformation.com**

TELECOMMUTING FOR REMOTE SERVICES AND CLIENTS

To locate services that use medical transcription telecommuters, investigate ads in trade journals and publications. If you are interested in working for a remote service, you will be asked to submit a resume of experience. After reviewing your proposal, they may ask you to transcribe a tape so they can review your transcription quality. Often, they will simply have you modem the transcribed documents back to them. Other services will mail a tape to you and ask you to mail your transcribed documents back. If the company decides to use your services, they may require a trial period during which you will be given a limited amount of work. Some companies also require on-site training.

Many remote companies require that you dial into their dictation system and download onto tapes, then transcribe and modem the files back to them. (The service will provide you with instructions for setting modem parameters to send and receive files).

Technology now available to home-based medical transcriptionists is becoming much more sophisticated. For instance, systems such as PC Dart allow transcriptionists to download dictation into their computers, which eliminates tapes altogether. And, transcriptionists can begin transcribing during the downloading process.

Be forewarned: Remote service downloading of dictation onto cassette tapes can be very time-consuming. However, the alternative — transcribing over telephone lines — would be far too costly.

Utilize time wisely while you are rerecording by organizing the office as you monitor the rerecord process. Update reference materials and finish other clerical tasks that you generally don't have time to do when transcribing. If you are working full time at least 40 hours per week transcribing, you will probably appreciate this "extra" time.

Some rerecord units can be set to automatically dial into the service system and start the recording process (even while you sleep). Many systems now have technology designed to download at a higher rate of speed, thus reducing your rerecord time. Other rerecord networks require you to key in numbers to begin and end each dictation. Rerecording is time consuming and you may lose some dictation quality/clarity in the process.

A reputable service will have quality standards which you will be expected to meet. These standards are usually outlined in the contract you enter into with the service. Typically, if you do not meet their standards, for instance, if your error ratio is too high, it is acceptable procedure for them to impose a penalty or cut the rate of pay you agreed upon.

When working remotely for a service, remember to follow through on your commitments. Keep an open mind about upgrading systems and improving your efficiency. Be professional when accepting constructive criticism, and encourage feedback regarding your work.

If possible, before accepting work, try to visit the service in person to get a feel for their organization and the people you will be working for. Some services **require** that you arrange to visit their facility and participate in a training session before you begin working for them. Never hesitate to ask questions. Remember, you are an independent transcriptionist and are responsible for YOU, INCORPORATED.

GOING MOBILE

> *"Thanks to technology, taking your home office with you*
> *when you travel is a viable option."*

We know that the home office can at times be confining, so it does us all good to get out and about occasionally. We also know that as independent transcriptionists with major responsibilities to clients — sometimes 24/7! — it is difficult to schedule getaways, even for occasional professional conferences or for those much-needed family vacations.

There may be a number of reasons that you cannot take two weeks away from your business: 1) You cannot afford it; 2) You have no alternative coverage for your clients; 3) You have a stack of unfinished projects; 4) Your turnaround commitments do not allow it; 5) You're a workaholic; or 6) You just want to be adventurous and try something different.

Fortunately, technology has opened up some wonderful opportunities for busy IMTs who needs a break from life's workday routine. If you want to get away but can't leave your work behind ... GO MOBILE! Thanks to technology, taking your home office with you when you travel is a viable option.

One of our goals, which we look forward to enjoying very soon, is to pack up a motor home and travel extensively across the U.S.A. to see this great country. This won't be a totally new experience for us, because we have taken trips before to visit family members and friends in various parts of the country. On occasion, I have taken my clients with me, so to speak, fulfilling my transcription responsibilities along the way.

If you are motivated to pursue this option, then we recommend you learn everything you can about mobile computing. Regardless of whether you plan to work a little or a lot while traveling, you will need to think ahead and plan how you will manage hardware and software challenges, security, communications and various other business issues that may arise. In addition, you will need to maintain contact with your customers if "glitches" arise. Will your work and turnaround be reliable once you "hit the road" or will your clients lose faith in your ability to live up to your commitments?

If you want to schedule a working road trip, we suggest you "test the waters" with some short excursions before allowing your nomadic spirit to take over and launch you on an extended travel adventure. To ensure that you will have an enjoyable trip and avoid potential work problems, be sure your plans are well thought out and your mobile computing equipment needs will be met.

> *"The number of transcription services that utilize home-based transcriptionists has signifigantly increased in the past three years."*

SITE PLANNING

If you are contemplating including transcription work in your travel plans, you should take time to strategize before hitting the road. When planning a mobile "work vacation," there are a number of options you need to consider. If your office suite will be the family motorhome, you will want to determine which equipment you will need for the road — PC, laptop, printer/scanner/fax/copier, transcriber, good quality headset, etc. Consider investing in a combination printer/scanner/copier/fax machine. Hewlett Packard has a great one for about $150.

Whether you are on the road, at the beach, camping, renting, or visiting, select the computer that meets your needs . . . and price tag. The same with transcribing equipment. If you are online with an Internet Service Provider (ISP), you may utilize a PC-based pedal/player combo, or use a stand-alone transcriber. There are many moderately priced transcriber/recording units on the market that would work well. Panasonic has a great model that I use to download and transcribe from tapes, at a cost of around $225. With the PC-based pedal/player combo the foot pedal plugs into the computer's serial port and the player portion is a software component.

Consider how you will access your dictation. Make sure the motor home has the appropriate phone line setup. Will you utilize an Internet Service Provider, have access to 800 numbers and/or download onto tape cassettes? Look into a DC to AC inverter to convert the 12 volts DC vehicle battery to household 110 volts AC. An inverter producing 400 watts can power up both transcriber and laptop and could easily support a desktop PC and monitor. Costs can range from $59 and up, depending on where you purchase the inverter. Many motor homes are equipped with power generators that can accommodate computer equipment; so investigate this information and the motor home you are planning to travel in.

Before visiting friends or relatives, check to see if they have a computer available with Internet access, fax capabilities, phone lines, etc. If so, you may only need to take your c-phone, transcriber, and/or rerecord device and download your dictation onto tapes. If you bring tapes with you, will you be able to telecommunicate the reports back to your clients? Can you send via e-mail in zip files? Or, will you need to Express mail the reports back to them? These are things you will need to arrange prior to your departure. And, be sure to include that extra long phone line with your traveling equipment stash. You may need it if the location of phone jacks en route are some distance from your mobile workstation.

When packing for your much-needed stay at a vacation rental, you may want to include your laptop. Before traveling, get information on phone lines and Internet access in the unit you will be renting. You can telephone or investigate using one of the many ISPs — Internet Service Providers. If the right equipment is provided, you can avoid taking unnecessary dictation/transcription equipment along with you.

Is the rental furnished? If not, be sure you take along a portable desk setup. A portable sewing machine table works great, folds flat, and will fit in the trunk of your car or back of your SUV. Unless you plan to ship your entire computer, it may be wise, depending upon the distance of your destination from your home, to utilize a laptop, which will be less cumbersome. Also, laptops withstand the bumps and bruises of travel a little better than desktop PCs, but this difference is narrowing with each piece of new technology that hits the marketplace. Nevertheless, if your destination is within driving distance, by all means consider the PC setup. I have done this and it has worked very well. Put the tools of your trade in your travel trunk, along with other equipment you will need.

Foreign travel is sometimes a little more complicated. If you plan to go mobile and global to some international destination, research the types of plug adapters and voltage transformers that are standard in the country you plan to visit, and, if needed, acquire them.

Of course, in all the scenarios discussed above, a good desktop and comfortable chair are important. If you plan to bring your own desk, check out Home Depot, IKEA, WalMart and Kmart. They have some small, convenient computer desks that assemble and disassemble easily. Or, as mentioned earlier, use a portable sewing machine table, which folds flat and can be set up and stored easily. Consider getting a lightweight pad to put under your computer gear to avoid slipping and sliding.

You may also want to consider such items as a cordless mouse for easier maneuverability, and a high-quality headset, especially helpful if you will be working in areas near a lot of noise. Dictaphone and Lanier have some excellent lightweight headsets. I prefer the soft wire type that is very mobile as well as top quality. They cost about $75 and are well worth it.

A cellular phone can also increase your telecommuting efficiency. Some cellular phones are capable of receiving e-mail and supporting modem transmissions. Just be sure, when shopping for the perfect cellular phone system for your trip, that the phone setup you select includes all the essential accessories Also, it's a good idea to find out if your travel destination has adequate cellular coverage.

If your destination is very rustic or rural, your options may be limited to mail drops, or scouting out for cybercafes, libraries and truck stops that may have high-speed Internet connections. Hotels, even rustic ones, generally have Internet access available. Before or when checking in, request this service. If it's available, you will have access to connections and jacks for use with your laptop or PC.

MOBILE SECURITY

Remember that security is as important on the road as in your home office, so plan carefully and design your travel workspace so that it is secure and will remain secure throughout your journey. Office supplies will need to be safe and secure. Protect them in plastic containers, which come in all sizes and make great storage receptacles. Plastic containers work well for safeguarding computer equipment, too, from potential dangers, including the weather. Be ever aware that radical changes in temperature, which may occur unexpectedly while traveling, can be hard on computers.

Review your computer's maintenance manual and make provisions for protecting computer hardware and data, perhaps installing a personal firewall to protect your sensitive data. In addition, be sure the phone line you are using is a modem-safe line to prevent "frying" your modem. As you prepare to travel, plan to be as organized as possible from the beginning to the end of your trip. Personal and professional pursuits can easily spiral out of control if you lose control while traveling.

Make a list of items you will need in your mobile office, which might include the following:

- Surge protector
- Multi-phone jack adapter
- 25 foot cord
- Additional power cords
- Telephone (if needed)
- AC/DC adapter
- Transcriber/recorder
- High quality headset

- PC/Laptop
- Printer/scanner/copier/fax (optional)
- Portable file cabinets with latching tops to prevent spills
- Equipment covers
- Breakout work station (if needed)
- Other office supplies, as needed

And, last but not least, none of the above will result in success if you don't bring along the ever-needed REFERENCE BOOKS! Reference book essentials can include (Pocket size books are ideal for traveling.): Lippincott, Williams & Wilkins books, Dorland's books, *Nursing Drug Handbook* (latest edition), Mosby's pocket medical dictionary, Vera Pyle's *Current Medical Terminology*, laboratory/pathology book, radiology, surgical, and other . . . whatever specialties you service.

Going mobile is ideal for many telecommuters, but it is somewhat less than ideal for those who must print documents and mail or fax hard copies. Think carefully about the pros and cons before you decide to try mobile transcription. You will avoid many disappointments if you plan carefully and do your homework, investigating and analyzing your client base, the appropriate tools and technology needed, your estimated investment in the project, the uncertainties of locations you will travel to, your transcription skills, your ability to manage the challenges of mobile transcribing, anything else that may impact you personally and professionally.

Somewhere, in the South of France, there is a stone cottage with my name on it. Where do you dream of transcribing?

For more information on going mobile, check the resources in the back of this book.

TRANSCRIPTION SERVICES THAT USE HOME-BASED TRANSCRIPTIONISTS

The number of transcription services that utilize home-based transcriptionists has significantly increased in the past three years and is now too numerous to list here. However, there is a directory on the Internet where this information is available. Do a search using Google, GoTo, Yahoo, etc, typing in keywords "medical transcription." Another directory, *The Nationwide Medical*

Transcription Service Directory (latest edition, about $40) is available from publisher Rayve Productions, 1-800-852-4890.

DOs AND DON'Ts FOR ONLINE COMMUNICATION

Make sure that both your modem and telecommunications software are set up correctly for the BBS or online system you are calling.

- Never disconnect your modem from a BBS or online service without correctly exiting the system, unless you absolutely must do so. Such abrupt exiting can damage a system.

- Use the highest baud rate possible when downloading data to reduce your on-line charges; *however,*

- Don't use a high baud rate when talking to another user in real-time on an online service; often the higher speeds are billed at higher rates, and you almost certainly type more slowly than your modem can transmit anyway.

- Use an automated program to download message headers and messages from CompuServe and other services; reading such messages online can run up big phone bills.

- Don't download program files from bulletin boards with which you are not familiar; such files may hide computer viruses.

- Install a separate telephone line for your modem if you can afford it. It frees up your regular line so that you can talk and type at the same time.

- Don't configure your modem to use the same COM port as any other device in your computer system, such as a mouse.

- Make sure your modem is connected correctly to both your computer and your telephone line.

> *"Nobody can make you feel inferior without your permission."*
> —Eleanor Roosevelt

TELECOMMUTING LINGO

- **Messaging**: Talking to others through the use of electronic mail.

- **Conferencing**: Talking to another in real-time. Your words appear on another user's monitor as you type them on your keyboard.

- **Uploading**: You transmit a file from your machine to a client or BB.

- **Downloading**: You transmit a file from a client or BB to your machine.

EXPRESSING YOUR EMOTIONS VIA TELECOMMUTING

When you "message" or "conference" online with other computer users, you sometimes want to express an emotion or attitude that may be difficult to convey in words on a computer screen. That's why a special system of expressions has developed among online telecommuters. These "*emoticons*" (emotion icons) use standard characters in set patterns to express specific emotions. When you look at an emoticon sideways (with your head turned to the left), it looks like a face in a particular expression.

For example :-) is an emoticon for happy. (It looks like a smiling face, right?) And :-(is an emoticon for sad. There are many different emoticons, including some that are completely off the wall. Plain bracketed comments also serve as emoticons to some users: when you see a <g>, it is shorthand for "grin" and it means the user is just kidding. Pretty cool, eh? <g>

PROTECTING E-MAIL COMMUNICATION

If you are communicating with your clients or transmitting protected health information via e-mail, consider including the following disclaimer with your e-mail message:

Confidentiality Notice:
This e-mail message, including any attachments, is for the sole use of the intended recipient(s) and may contain confidential and privileged information. Any unauthorized review, use, disclosure, or distribution is prohibited. If you are not the intended recipient, please contact the sender by reply e-mail and destroy all copies of the original message.

Quality Improvement

QUALITY VERSUS QUANTITY

> *"In personal and professional pursuits,*
> *I demand of myself an ever higher*
> *standard of excellence."*
>
> —Beatrice Gage

Much has been written in the past several years about quality versus quantity. Should we sacrifice the quality of the report in order to produce more transcription in a given day? The consensus has been a definite "No."

This certainly holds true for the home-based medical transcriptionist. If the quality of your reports suffers, the patient may suffer, your client may suffer, and so may your income. It is impossible to maintain accounts or procure new ones if your product quality is poor. The world of medical transcription is a very small one, and word does travel about the quality of one's work.

This author has worked for two large transcription services, one that provided an in-house proofreader and one that did not. The service with the proofreading staff sent out A+ quality reports, while the latter did not. The latter was more interested in format than content, and the firm had difficulty retaining accounts for any length of time.

During my tenure with the first firm, I learned more than I ever had about medical words and usage. It held me in good stead when transferring to a second firm and eventually establishing my home-based business.

ERRORS IN THE MEDICAL RECORD

As professionals, we want our transcription of the medical record to be as accurate as possible for the sake of patients and our clients, but being human, we do make errors.

Sometimes a transcription error will occur through no fault of our own. Other times, it will be decidedly our mistake. No matter where the fault lies, it is important to learn from the mistake and find ways to prevent the same error in the future.

Most dedicated professionals strive for perfection in work as well as in personal life. In truth, we realize that perfection is unattainable except for small slices of life, but even small slices of perfection whet our appetite for more. As a group, we medical transcriptionists tend to be perfectionists by nature, workaholics who thrive on challenge and look forward to the day when innovation by man and/or technical beast solve the problem of errors. Until that time, we will continue to persevere.

As medical language specialists, we must keep in mind that the English language, as well as the language of medicine, is still evolving and new words are added every day. Discovering new words is an exciting and worthwhile experience. Skilled transcriptionists never stop learning.

Perfection may not be attainable, but transcriptionists must always strive for knowledge, understanding, innovation, and creative ways to improve our product while remaining adaptable to changes in our profession. We must be objective and able to accept criticism. We must learn to work with and through fellow transcriptionists and other health care professionals. After having sat through a grueling and tedious dictation, there is no greater satisfaction than to sign off a report with my initials, knowing that I have done my very best. It feels very much like perfection.

THE FINE ART OF EDITING

Unless the dictating physician was also an English major in his premed days, most medical reports you transcribe will require some form of editing. Editing can be as simple as changing plurals to singulars, correcting punctuation (semicolon instead of a period), or correcting a medical inconsistency (changing metatarsal to metacarpal).

A useful resource book for answering questions regarding editing is the *Style Guide for Medical Transcription* published by the American Association for Medical Transcription. In 1982, Vera Pyle, CMT, addressed the issue of how and when to edit in an article published in the *Journal of the American Association for Medical Transcription*. The article is reprinted in the *Style Guide*.

Vera Pyle is quoted as saying," In editing we do not go charging in, doctoring up reports in an aggressive way, in an intrusional way. It has to be done so subtly, so delicately, so carefully, that we get a favorable response from the author. We must be so involved with what we are transcribing that we know what is going on and can detect something that is dictated that does not make sense, that does not flow, that does not add up. We must listen with an educated ear, with an intelligent ear, so that we can produce an accurate, intelligent, clear document, always remembering the fine line between editing and tampering."

On the subject of when ***not*** to edit, Pyle asks," What about those who are inconsiderate of us? What about those who mumble? What about those whom we can't help because we don't know what they mean? If you know what they are trying to say, you can help clarify the dictation. If you don't know, that is the time to transcribe verbatim; it's our only recourse."

Editing has changed considerably during the past fifteen years. In the United States, many changes are a result of the influx of foreign-born physicians, who are popularly referred to as ESL or English-as-a-Second-Language physicians. Although most of these doctors are very conscious of their accents and do an exceptional job dictating, there are others who have not quite mastered the intricacies of English, especially in differentiating between past and present tenses and noun and verb usage.

As a medical transcriptionist, you must have a good grasp of the language, not only of English but of medicine, to equip you for some very complex editing challenges.

According to the *Style Guide*, it is important that you retain the dictating physician's style. We have no right to impose our style on the report. As a good rule of thumb, edit grammatical, punctuation, spelling and similar dictation errors as necessary to achieve clear communication. Edit slang words and phrases, incorrect or verbal inconsistencies and medical inconsistencies. Edit inaccurate phrasing of laboratory data.

Physicians also tend to talk with colleagues when dictating and sometimes make inadvertent, derogatory comments about the patient, which, of course, should not become part of the medical record! Never include informal, inappropriate statements in the transcribed medical report.

QUALITY IMPROVEMENT

Developing good quality in your medical transcription business is essential to your success and survival as an independent transcriptionist. Continuing quality improvement (CQI) should be an ongoing process in your business. Developing quality guidelines should be established at the onset of business. AAMT has established recommended guidelines for such quality control (see example).

KEEPING ONE STEP AHEAD OF THE HEADHUNTERS

Medical transcription companies merging is hot news on the Internet. Recently there was a post stating that this is good news for MTs working for services, home-based MTs and independent MTs.

I guess it's good news if you want to work for someone else. Personally, there are MTs who prefer to remain *"independent."* The latest merger means a work force of over 2000 MTs throughout the US. The merger will also mean better bargaining power with health care corporations in negotiating contracts for less. The bigger the bargaining power, the better the price.

This is just another example of why the IMT must keep pace with industry trends and technology, because when the dust settles, and work is being done for fewer dollars, in less time, with fewer people, only the *creme de la creme* will be skimmed from the top of the bucket. The most technically savvy and knowledgeable, not only in medical transcription but in all aspects of professional and business management, will survive.

As health care corporations continue to acquire physician practices, clinics and outpatient centers, they will incorporate and manage their cost centers as well. And, as managed care continues to negotiate capitated contracts with these health care organizations, physicians will be required to cut operating costs to maintain a place on the provider list. This means that medical transcriptionists servicing individual physician practices may lose clients because those clients can no longer afford their services, or because this expense has been absorbed by a larger cost center which is negotiating cheaper rates elsewhere. Health care headhunters are already including a "medical transcriptionist" category in their marketing material.

Independent medical transcriptionists should focus on real-time (meaning, "happening now") business management practices. The medical transcription industry and technology are evolving more rapidly than ever before and to keep pace, independent medical transcriptionists must look at 1) how we do business and how we can do it better, 2) increasing our knowledge and 3) promoting our professionalism.

TAKING A PROACTIVE APPROACH
WHEN RENEGOTIATING CONTRACTS

At the start of any professional relationship with a client, the parties involved commit themselves to certain promises. This is done through agreement and is documented in a contract. During contract negotiations it is important to discuss policies and procedures on all items that will be incorporated into the contract. Once a contract is signed, both parties are expected to live up to the terms of the contract.

Regularly review how you are doing business and servicing your clients. This is important so you thoroughly understand what does and does not work for you and your business. Frequently one party or the other wants to change one or more terms or conditions in the ironclad contract. What should you do when faced with the need to change a contract? Renegotiate . . . wisely.

A valid contract involves *mutual consideration*. A term used to explain consideration is "quid pro quo," meaning *"this for that."* When renegotiating a contract, the parties are required to come up with new consideration in order for the revised agreement to be equally binding. Here are some cues to aid in successful renegotiations.

- **Keep in touch with your client**. Frequently touch base with the client to review any problems that arise and keep notes in your contract file. Also document activities so that new policies can be written into the contract.

- **Offer something new.** Offer something of value to the client that is not already in the deal (e.g., your new technology and ability to provide more efficient "quality" service, discount for quick pay, rate break for volume of dictation, etc.).

- **Be creative and flexible**. When situations change and there is a need to renegotiate the deal, recognize that the other side's wants and needs may have changed from the time the contract was initially negotiated. Be sure to include these in your renegotiation considerations.

- **Use a cooperative approach.** Remember that cooperation, creativity and flexibility play an important part in your success with clients. Both sides need to realize that they are negotiating with feeling people. If you are initiating the renegotiation of your contract, your approach should convey a sense of cooperative teamwork so the client does not feel you are an adversary or merely trying to escape your commitments. Likewise, the facility needs to cooperatively reciprocate, maximizing goodwill and reputation to make you feel like a winner. Ultimately, of course, a truly successful relationship will depend on the cooperation of the facility staff. In renegotiation, both sides should feel they have received more than they gave up.

- **When terms are finalized, have legal counsel review the contract before signing.**

NOTE

It is important to remember that the Internal Revenue Service does not recognize a written agreement as verification of your status as an independent contractor. Contracts and agreements only provide details and terms of your services with the client. Even if your contract states that you are acting and operating as an independent contractor in providing your services to the client, this has no effect on IRS determining whether you are an independent contractor or an employee.

THE POWER OF SHARING EXPERIENCE

We are living and working in an ever-changing communication age. Old conventional ways of gaining knowledge about our profession and marketplace through professional organizations are not as effective as they once were. Many professional organizations are no longer able to hold the interest of members, for whom they were developed to serve.

Throughout history, there has been a tremendous amount of information to be gained from collective, tribal sharing of information and experience, and that continues to be true today. In modern times, many of us have grown up working within and serving relatively homogenous social, business and organizational groups with a fairly narrow, inward focus. For many decades, the knowledge and professional contacts gained in this manner were adequate for professional growth. However, in the past few years some organization members have discovered they are learning more from one another, as well as from many other sources, than from presenters at association meetings.

As independent transcriptionists and business owners, our professional needs have gone beyond what is offered by inbred, narrow-minded, myopic organizations that are not keeping pace with worldwide business trends. More often, the linkages we need to gain knowledge about professional practices, business management, and marketing are not with the people who are like us but with dissimilar stakeholders who complement us in unique value-adding ways.

Homogenous groups always risk becoming self-absorbed. It is critical to the success of our business, and as independent medical transcriptionists, to continuously address new issues and process diverse views. Today, we need to invest our valuable time in a network of resources. An internally focused association too often inhibits this process.

People need new ideas and new methods if they are to achieve their goals. In health care, with the physician shift from "boss" to "team member," there is greater involvement of nurses and other allied health professionals at medical conferences. In fact, most conference audiences are composed of mixed groups of health care professionals.

The world of the CME (continuing medical education), CEU (continuing education units) is rapidly becoming the CPE (continuing professional education). As an independent medical transcriptionist, the more diverse your communication experience, the more positive the effect on your business. As a solo business owner, you should seek out new, updated, comprehensive information and resources on managing your business, accessing and marketing on the Internet, dealing with difficult personalities, quality and productivity enhancements/ standards, risk management, negotiating skills, self-improvement, finances and record keeping, long-range planning, and other relevant topics. Search for and interact with specialized groups that provide seminars on many subjects that will enhance the operation of your business, and for which you can receive CPE (CEU).

THE "NET SET"

Although the World Wide Web cannot yet substitute for good old face-to-face networking, the base of online medical transcriptionists is steadily growing throughout the world. The Net was not meant to be monitored or moderated by one personality over the other, and merely because one is found online does not necessarily make him or her an expert. Rather, the net should be utilized as a resource to communicate with other professionals, provide support for newcomers in the field and to share knowledge, experiences, bits and pieces of miscellaneous information and opinions, agreeable or not. What works for one may not work for another, for our careers are shaped by many factors — education, training, experience, attitude, personal preference, technology, work environment, social arena, etc.

A recent Internet trend is for individual MTs and organizations to set up their own online websites. You will find websites for Health Professions Institute, AAMT, MTIA, AHIMA and many other health care and business networks. Associations are beginning to take advantage of the Internet to promote conference programs, which will save organizations a tremendous amount normally spent on marketing and reaching a greater target market. At the same time it will provide the Internet visitor with additional educational opportunities they probably would not have been aware of otherwise.

Even more important is the immediacy of the Web. For educational programs, registration can be completely automated, the program schedule detailed before your eyes, and information provided about CEU available, product exhibitors, host city amenities, hotel reservations, airline schedules and prices, and more. For information on other conferences just do a search for "conferences." Log on and take a look!

CREATING YOUR OWN WEBSITE

Perhaps you are interested in creating your own website. If so, create a site that will compel visitors to return again and again.

- **Make it interactive.**

- **Promote participation from "visitors."**

- **Keep it simple.** Visitors prefer to read through information quickly. Don't make them wade through large blocks of text or wait for large amounts of information to be downloaded onto the screen. This frustrates your audience and they may not return. Having a "tool bar" on every screen helps ensure easy navigation around the site.

- **Target your information.** Offer a menu of information by subject matter so visitors do not have to spend time scrolling through all your data. A well-designed site will lead them to the specific information they are seeking.

- **Keep the page current.** Update information continually. Fresh information encourages repeat visits.

- **Strive for consistency.** The "look" of a website makes a statement about the sponsor. Develop site architecture that makes the visitor's experience seamless, intuitive and effortless. Be creative but make sure your resources are accurate. Consider offering "sneak previews" of information, products and trends. Make your website a place where visitors will enjoy a unique experience. Since it is easy to put up-to-the minute information on the Internet, make your site "the place" for the latest-breaking industry news.

- **Respond to website visitors.** Offer an e-mail component to your site to help visitors get answers to questions they may have.

- **List your site in appropriate online directories and search engines.** Remember to include website promotion in your printed material. Add it to your letterhead. Mention it when networking with colleagues and other contacts.

- **Track website hits.** Establish a method of tracking "hits" to see how many visitors your site is getting.

The cost of a website varies depending on the complexity of the architecture. Paying for a website is much like building a home. There is a one-time cost to lay the foundation and put up the frame. Additional improvements increase costs. You can change the content of a site whenever you need to. Updates may be at half the initial cost. Some changes and updates will be essential to keep your site current, others optional.

Internet advances and worldwide business trends will seriously impact all professionals in the years ahead. These authors have been working independently since before "home-based," "solo," "SOHO" or even IMT or the Internet were recognized. We have seen and continue to see tremendous change in this industry. We have worked in the acute-care setting, in the service setting and independently. We choose to remain independent.

What does the future hold for IMTs? Will our independence be threatened? Will organizations attempt to employ or contract only with companies that have multiple transcriptionist employees? Will independents be faced with legislative changes and legal battles over restraint of trade? One thing is certain, if and when that time comes, we will fight for our right to work independently; we hope we will not be fighting alone. Both now and in the future, we pray for a strong professional organization supporting our cause.

AAMT QUALITY CONTROL FOR MEDICAL TRANSCRIPTION

- Medical transcription services within (or for) the health care organization are performed and supervised by qualified medical transcriptionists.

- Designated equipment is utilized effectively, skillfully, and efficiently.

- Patient identification and demographics are verified.

- Dictator identification is verified.

- Appropriate format is followed.

- Appropriate medical terminology is used, and English language rules are applied.

- Current reference materials are used appropriately and efficiently to facilitate accuracy, clarity, and completeness.

- Visual proofreading and spellchecking (and electronic spellchecking, if appropriate) are performed.

- Inconsistencies, discrepancies, and inaccuracies are recognized and appropriately revised, edited, or clarified, without altering the meaning of dictation or changing the dictator's style. All remaining inconsistencies, discrepancies, and inaccuracies are flagged for dictator review or brought to the attention of supervisory personnel for appropriate action to assure accurate completion of the document.

- Appropriate personnel are consulted regarding dictation that may be considered unprofessional, frivolous, insulting, inflammatory, or inappropriate.

- Appropriate risk management personnel are consulted regarding unusual circumstances and/or information with possible risk factors.

- Quality and productivity standards and deadlines are met.

- Appropriate measures are taken to protect the confidentiality and security of the record.

- Administrative procedures are followed (e.g., copy distribution).

- If amendment or revision of the record is required, appropriate policies and procedures are followed, with corrections or revisions made according to established medicolegal guidelines.

- Document storage, security, and retrieval guidelines are followed.

- Random quality control review is performed by a qualified medical transcriptionist.

Quality improvement standards require that documents produced must demonstrate continuing efforts to improve the process and content of patient-care documentation. The quality issue means that documents must be accurate in content and presentation, ensuring that patient confidentiality and privacy are protected throughout the documentation process, dictation, transcription and storage. Documents should be well organized and succinct, and reflect a commitment to professionalism and quality.

Monitoring quality should be done by independent medical transcriptionists as well as in-house transcriptionists. Quality checks should include correctness of grammar, patient identification and errors. Develop a quality audit program for your business. During times of low volume, randomly select twenty-five reports for review. Your CQI program could contain some of the items listed below.

- Enhancement with productivity software

- Turnaround time

- Quality management procedures

- Continuing education

- Technology and computer security

INCENTIVE PROGRAMS

A well-written incentive plan covers quality and quantity while monitoring results. Before incentive plans, quality of work was frequently poor. Incentive plans motivate employees and encourage top-quality work. If the quality is not there you will not be in business long, and if you work for a service as an independent, you may suffer a reduction in your rate of pay if your error rate is substantial.

PRODUCTIVITY AND TURNAROUND

Productivity software is computer software enhancements such as keyboard shorthand programs or basic macro commands. There are several programs like this currently available, and they make it easy to quantify improvement and reduce labor and keystrokes. Also, they create an atmosphere of excitement and have the added benefit of improving quality while decreasing transcriptionist fatigue.

The choice of productivity software should be made after surveying what is available, talking to users, and comparing prices and customer support. Adapting to this software takes time — usually about two weeks — so be sure to allow extra time for that in your schedule. You may want to modify your workload during this learning period, taking less work than usual.

Evaluate your productivity figures after two weeks and periodically thereafter, weekly or biweekly, to see how the program has benefitted your productivity in dollars and time. A logical time to do this is at the end of a billing period.

With productivity software you must also monitor your documents by proofreading on a regular basis. A spellchecker will not pick up expanded short-forms that are incorrect. For example, if the patient's name is Pat, she may end up as "paroxysmal atrial tachycardia" if "pat" happens to be your short-form for that term.

CONTINUING QUALITY IMPROVEMENT MANAGEMENT

Consider updating reference materials, macros, and updating and/or changing formats regularly. Perform quality audits of your reports and look into upgrading your computer technology.

Perform ongoing audits on your documents and consider developing a formal report of your audit procedure. This is essential if you are to provide ongoing improvement and enhancements to adequately meet the needs of your clients.

Medical record entries are only as accurate as the people who write, dictate and transcribe them. As businesses and service providers learn about continuing quality improvement procedures (CQI), they will expect them to be implemented in daily activities. We must always try to do the job right the first time, focusing on the benefits of timely, accurate and complete documentation and the effect it has on patient care and our professional lives. Errors, of course, will occur from time to time for a variety of reasons, including doctors who mumble crucial words that transcriptionists hear incorrectly or not at all. When errors are found, the recorded entry should be corrected as soon as possible.

> *"Perform ongoing audits on your documents and consider developing a formal report of your audit procedure."*

AUDIT LOG SHEET

Month Audited: _____

DATE	MT ID	DOCUMENT TYPE	NO. PAGES	POINTS	TYPE ERROR
					Rev: 7/02

TIME MANAGEMENT

Here are some tips for managing your time and productivity.

- **Organize and prioritize your responsibilities**. Use a notebook, calendar or a "to do" list. At the end of each day write down the next day's activities.

- **Give yourself deadlines**. If you estimate how much time you need to complete a task, you are more likely to finish it on time. Block out time on your calendar.

- **Determine your peak productivity period**. Try keeping an hour-by-hour log of activities for a few days. You may discover you are particularly productive during certain times of the day.

- **Make beneficial use of commuting and waiting time**. Carry a cassette recorder or note pad with you to record ideas and thoughts that pop into your head when you have unexpected spare minutes.

- **Take some daily quiet time**. Set aside a period of each day for uninterrupted concentration, planning and thinking.

- **Don't procrastinate**.

- **Combat clutter**.

- **Make efficient use of your telephone time**.

By using your time more efficiently, you may improve your productivity. It's definitely worth the effort.

FLAGGING AND LEAVING BLANKS IN A REPORT

*"Keep in mind that your goal is to type
the most accurate medical report possible."*

To safeguard the integrity of the reports you transcribe, never second-guess what a physician means. If something is unclear, don't hesitate to flag a report and ask for clarification. If in doubt, leave it out.

Be sure to leave enough blank space for the word or phrase to be inserted later. Make a copy of your "flags" for your records.

If you are working for a hospital account, ask for their quality assurance standards. If they have none, explain your standard editing procedure and use your best judgment on individual cases, always keeping in mind that your goal is to type the most accurate medical report possible.

You will occasionally encounter words that you have never heard before. Even the best transcriptionist has this problem, so don't feel bad. If you cannot find the term in your reference materials, flag the report.

Physicians sometimes get right and left mixed up. One minute they may be dictating an operative report on the right femur, only to switch to the left femur later in the report. Clearly, such a report should be flagged.

There are times when physicians are interrupted during their dictation and do not complete the report. Always be sure to flag that report as incomplete and keep a record of it on your transmit log sheet.

Avoiding second-guessing is especially important for laboratory data. Medical transcriptionists must understand the normal ranges for all laboratory work, so they can detect inconsistencies when they appear.

Sticky-notes are a blessing. Simply flag questionable reports where a word, phrase or number would have been typed and make a notation of what you heard so that the word, phrase or number is brought to the attention of the dictating physician. Some software systems also have flagging capabilities.

If you have consistent difficulty with a certain dictating physician because of accent, poor tape quality, or poor dictating habits — dictating while eating, dictating from an erratic car phone, etc. — talk with the transcription supervisor or medical records director. Most accounts are willing to work with the outside service to ensure integrity of the medical record and a satisfactory working situation for the transcriptionist.

Don't leave too many blank spaces, however. This will suggest a deficiency on your part. If you find yourself in this position, you should reconsider whether you have the background experience or are adequately qualified to take work at this level of technical difficulty.

ONCE UPON A TIME BEFORE COMPUTERS

Before the computer, reports were transcribed with pen and ink. Multiple copies were duplicated by hand. Next came the manual typewriter, followed by the electric typewriter, typing first and second drafts, multiple carbon copies, ink erasers, and that wonderful invention, "whiteout."

The computer has certainly changed our way of doing things, and editing is now as easy as hitting a few command keys. The computer industry has responded to our needs by giving us abbreviation, spellchecking and dictionary software. These are wonderful tools to aid us in quality control.

Remember, though, that your spellchecker is only as good as your computer dictionary, which should be updated on a daily basis. Also be certain that new words added to the dictionary are spelled correctly. The same applies to macros and abbreviations. And, most important, proofread your documents. Remember that a spellchecker cannot proofread your document for inconsistencies or omitted words.

When working for hospitals, it sometimes seems that medical records personnel are more concerned with format than content. Be sure to spend time with your hospital account contacts, and don't be afraid to ask questions. Discuss and come to agreements on quality assurance guidelines and formatting details.

We recommend that transcriptionists just learning to use computers find a programmer who understands the work of a medical transcriptionist, or ask a medical transcriptionist who is familiar with formatting to program the formats into your software. This will save you much time and aggravation and prevent your having to constantly experiment with formatting.

When working for individual physicians, their formats may not be a "statement of professionalism." Do not hesitate to point out that a different format may indeed be more representative of their professional image. It may also save them unnecessary expenses and win you a client for life.

Each physician has his or her own style of dictating and may use pet phrases or terms that cannot be found in any medical or English language dictionary. Keep the lines of communication open with those clients. If they consistently misspell a medical or English term which you know to be incorrect, don't hesitate to communicate that to them.

If a client continues to doubt your information, a good way to handle the situation is to take your reference material to the office for review. More often than not, your candor will be appreciated. On the other hand, the client may continue to insist that you type it "their way," in which case you have two options. You can do what the client demands or you can simply walk away from the account. The choice is yours, a decision not easily made nor to be taken lightly.

Risk Management and Insurance Protection

*"The Lord gave us two ends — one to sit on and
the other to think with. Success depends on
which one we use the most."*

—Ann Landers

In every business there are risks that must be managed, and the medical transcription industry is no exception to this rule. There are risks for every small business. Just think a minute about the hundreds of things that most business owners must worry about. Some concerns are predictable and can be eliminated or controlled to some extent:

- Volume

- Salary costs

- Taxes

- Overhead

- Equipment and supply costs

- The price you charge for services offered clients

Other risks are unpredictable and largely beyond your control:

- Competitors' actions

- Changing technology and trends

- Effects the above actions and changes have on your market and your clients

- The economy and its impact on your client base

Other events can also directly affect your day-to-day operations, reduce profits and result in unexpected financial losses serious enough to cripple or even bankrupt your business. You have probably already considered the most obvious risks, such as fire or injury, and have bought insurance to protect against them. But there are hundreds of other losses and liabilities that every small business faces, many of which are overlooked or ignored.

Large corporations often employ full-time risk managers to identify and analyze possible exposure to loss or liability. The risk manager takes steps to protect the firm against accidental and preventable loss and to minimize the financial consequences of unpreventable or unavoidable losses. As an independent business owner, you can't afford the services of a risk manager, even part-time, so you must take on that responsibility.

WHAT IS RISK MANAGEMENT?

Risk management consists of the following:

- Identifying and analyzing events that may result in loss

- Choosing the best way to deal with each potential loss

Let's discuss ways to help you identify, minimize and, in some instances, eliminate business risks.

Identifying exposure is a vital step to risk management. Until you know the scope of possible losses, you won't be able to develop a realistic strategy for dealing with them. Unless you've experienced a fire, you may not realize how extensive fire losses can be. For example, you may experience the following:

- Smoke and water damage

- Damage to your personal property and to the property of others that is left on your premises (e.g., data processing equipment you lease or client's property left with you)

- Business lost during the time it takes to return your business to normal

- The potential permanent loss of clients to competitors

Take a close look at each of your business operations and evaluate where losses might occur. For each exposure identified, determine how serious the loss might be and what that loss might cost.

Many business owners use a risk analysis questionnaire or survey, available from most insurance agents, as a checklist. In general, most questionnaires and surveys address the potential for these losses:

- Property losses

- Physical damage to property

- Loss of use of property

- Criminal activity

- Business interruption losses

- Indirect losses — Although insurance provides money for repairing or rebuilding property damaged, most policies do not cover indirect losses, such as income that is lost while the business is interrupted for repairs.

Business Interruption Insurance reimburses policyholders for the difference between normal income and the income earned during the shutdown period. During this period not only is income reduced or cut off, but business expenses such as taxes and loan payments continue. Frequently, interruptions in business also trigger extra expenses such as those incurred when subcontractors must be used to complete previously contracted work for clients. These expenses put an added strain on finances at a time when little if any income is being produced. Don't forget to protect your business against loss of income and unusual expenses that may result if indirect loss forces you to close temporarily.

- Liability losses

- Court decision (lawsuit charging negligence)

- Violation of contract provisions (a contract that makes one party responsible for certain kinds of losses)

- Public liability (injuries or loss to others)

- Key person losses — What would happen to your business if an accident or illness made it impossible for you to work? It is important for you to prepare your business for survival before you become disabled. Carefully evaluate the following questions:

  1) What impact would your absence have on your business such as volume, productivity, costs, etc.?

  2) How will you reassign duties to cover this period?

  3) What extra costs will you have to incur for a replacement to cover the operation of the business?

  4) How long will it take before the replacement is trained and productive?

  5) What would your source of income be?

  6) Who will continue your business? What if the person is not qualified or is a minor?

  7) If a will is not in place before your death, will the business close, or will someone inherit it?

  8) If your life-savings are invested will the family be able to use it wisely?

  9) What will the surviving family's source of income be?

The answers to the previous questions can be determined with the help of your business planner, attorney, accountant and insurance agent. Let them help you develop a risk management plan for your business.

As you can see, a business may face several types of risks and exposure. You must decide upon the risk management measures that will best protect your business.

- What can be done to prevent or limit exposure to risk?

- What techniques can be used to ensure that funds will be available for unavoidable losses?

LIMITING EXPOSURE TO LOSS — AVOIDING RISKS

One principle of loss prevention and control is to avoid activities that are too hazardous. For example, although exposure to loss from fire can seldom be eliminated completely, the risk can be reduced by installing smoke detectors and fire alarms and by having fire extinguishers readily available on the premises.

Insure business vehicles rather than take the risk of canceling collision coverage; or hire a delivery company, thus transferring the risk to the local delivery service.

TRANSFERRING RISK

The most common method of transferring risk is insurance. By insuring your home and car you transfer much of the risk of loss to the company that issued the policy. You pay a relatively small insurance premium compared to the risk of not protecting yourself against the possibility of a much larger financial loss.

With business insurance as with personal insurance, only you can decide which exposures you absolutely must insure against. Some decisions, however, are already made for you:

- Those required by law

- Those that others require, such as operating an insured business vehicle (required in some areas)

- Few lenders will finance property acquisition or construction unless it is adequately insured and the lender named on the policy as having an insurable interest.

ESSENTIAL COVERAGES

Four kinds of insurance are essential:

- Fire

- Liability

- Automobile and workers compensation. In some areas and in some types of business, crime insurance is also essential.

THE ROLE OF THE INSURANCE PROFESSIONAL

The professional independent insurance agent has been trained in risk analysis. He or she is familiar with insurance coverages and financial strategies available in your state and with regulations that govern them. With this expertise agents are able to point out risk exposures you may overlook. The agent can suggest a menu of risk-management strategies and amend a basic policy to suit your needs by adding special coverages and endorsements. The resulting policy will be custom tailored to your business's unique protection needs.

You may not be aware of other services that insurance companies provide to their policyholders:

- Legal defense — liability insurance usually includes legal defense

- Rehabilitation — Workers' compensation/disability policies may offer rehabilitation services and in some cases, retraining

- Claim management services for loss analysis

> *"The well-trained insurance agent is able to point out risk exposures you may overlook."*

INSURANCE PROTECTION

Safeguard your business with insurance. A home-based business is a significant investment. To be adequately covered for potential losses, you will probably need increased insurance coverage.

To protect business equipment in your home, you may need a special rider on your homeowner's policy. Even this, however, will generally not provide full replacement cost reimbursement, but only for the depreciated value of equipment at time of loss. Therefore, some home-based professionals invest in a personal property policy, which may require a hefty deductible but does reimburse at replacement cost values.

Don't depend on your homeowner's policy to meet all your personal needs in a crisis. You will also need some type of disability insurance. After all, your fingers are your life. How will you survive if you are suddenly unable to use them?

In the past, it was difficult to find a disability insurance carrier who would provide a policy for home-based workers, but fortunately, this is changing. There are now insurance companies that recognize home-based transcriptionists and are meeting our needs.

Contact your insurance agent to discuss your present business coverage, if any, and evaluate possible additional coverage. Your insurance carrier will probably need a written description of your business so be prepared to provide it to him or her.

Your insurance agent will assist you in obtaining appropriate protection from potential hazards resulting from your business operations.

STANDARD INSURANCE COVERAGE FOR
SELF-EMPLOYED BUSINESSES

- Fire, theft, and casualty damage to inventories and equipment

- Business interruption coverage

- Fidelity bonds for employees (if applicable)

- Liability for customers, vendors and others visiting the business

- Worker's compensation and worker's disability insurance

- Group health and life insurance

- Business use of vehicle coverage

- Business life insurance

- Disability insurance

- PC and software insurance

    . . . and also consider . . .

- Errors and Omissions

CREATING AN INVENTORY LIST

It is a good idea to make an inventory list of all home furnishings, business furniture and appliances, including model numbers, prices and purchase dates.

Photograph or videotape each room including interiors of cabinets and closets. Keep the inventory list, photographs and/or videotape in a safe-deposit box (tax-deductible) or some safe place outside your home. This will speed up the collection process should you ever need to file an insurance claim.

GROUP INSURANCE POLICIES

Health insurance is very expensive and individual policies tend to run higher than group rates. You may find a bargain in a group policy through a professional organization. As an organization member, you may obtain the coverage you need at attractive group rates.

> *"If you were caught in a natural disaster,*
> *would you have the means to rebuild your business?"*

INSURING AGAINST CATASTROPHE

As micro-businesses, MTs take pride in possessing the newest in technology, not only to be competitive but to make our working hours less stressful and our transcription output of the highest quality. Most of us have the latest turbo computer, software and peripheral programs; laser printers, fax machines, and digital dictation equipment; standard, micro- and mini-transcribing machines. Never forget, in just a matter of minutes, all this sophisticated equipment could go up in smoke, quite literally. It is reported that the two disasters most responsible for the demise of a home-based business are fire and water damage. However, most of us live with the added threat of earthquakes, tornadoes and hurricanes.

If you were caught in such a natural disaster, would you have the means to rebuild your business? The National Fire Protection Association states that 30% of all businesses that experience a major fire go out of business within a year; and 70% fail within five years. Those are frightening statistics.

Now is the time to evaluate your business and take steps to ensure that you would be capable of rebounding after a catastrophic loss.

- **Insure your business equipment and records adequately.** Take out a separate business policy that covers general liability and the **full** replacement cost of equipment and furnishings, including computer hardware and loss of your home office. Verify that insurance coverage that specifies "replacement" means "**full replacement value**." Also make sure operating a business out of your home does not invalidate insurance coverage.

- **Document valuables adequately and safeguard records.** Document your possessions including serial numbers, purchase dates, and prices, keep receipts and detailed descriptions as proof. Periodically send an updated copy of this information to your attorney or a relative in another state, or store it in a safe-deposit box.

- **Back up computer data and safeguard files.** Back up computer data regularly and store copies of data files in an alternate site or in a safe-deposit box. This is cheaper and more efficient than special data-loss insurance, and you won't lose valuable information.

- **Use UL certified transient voltage suppressors on your computer and other business equipment.**

- **Safeguard office equipment and records on-site.** Arrange furniture and equipment to guard critical items and records against leaks, floods, crashed windows, heavy vibrations or earth tremors.

- **Clean, organize and maintain your office.** Regularly pick up and toss those mounds of paper, the ones you think you can't possibly throw away because you might need them someday; or keep them and just call it "kindling."

GET WITH THE PROGRAM

Good risk management and good insurance management are achieved through good planning. A lifetime of work and dreams can be lost in a few minutes if your insurance program does not include certain elements. To ensure that you are adequately covered, take these steps:

- Recognize the ways you can suffer loss.

- Follow the guides for buying insurance economically.

- Organize your insurance management program.

- Get professional advice.

RECOGNIZE THE RISKS

The first step toward good protection is to recognize the risks. If you have costly equipment in your business, obtain special insurance covering loss, damage, or business interruption resulting from not being able to use the equipment.

HAVE A RISK MANAGEMENT PLAN

Have a definite plan that defines the objective of your business.

- Write down a clear statement of what you expect insurance to do for your firm.

- Select an agent to handle your insurance.

- Do everything possible to prevent loss.

- Don't withhold information about your business and its exposure to loss from your insurance agent.

- Don't try to save money by underinsuring.

- Keep complete records of your insurance policies, premiums paid, losses and recoveries.

- Have your property appraised periodically by independent appraisers. This informs you of your exposures and allows you to prove what your actual losses are if any occur.

GET PROFESSIONAL ADVICE

"Good risk management and good insurance management
are achieved through good planning."

Insurance is a complex and detailed subject. A qualified agent, broker or consultant can explain the options, recommend the right coverage and help you avoid financial loss.

Some small-business owners look upon insurance as a sort of tax. They recognize it as necessary but consider it a burdensome expense that should be kept to a minimum. But used correctly, the potential benefits of good insurance management make it well worth your study and attention.

THE ERRORS AND OMISSIONS CONTROVERSY

In the first edition of *The Independent Medical Transcriptionist*, we urged you to consider investing in an errors and omissions liability policy. However, after lengthy discussions with medical transcriptionists, attorneys and other business professionals, we have re-evaluated the fact and now believe this coverage is not a necessity. If you are just starting your business, the last thing you need is to spend $600 to $2000 per year on a policy that does nothing but cover the attorney fees should you be sued. In addition, most policies have caps of one to two million dollars.

While there have been a few cases in which medical transcriptionists have been sued, such cases are rare. If you contract with a physician who does not carry his own malpractice insurance, your risk for a lawsuit is increased; however, according to legal consultants, lawsuits are often initiated and targeted toward parties who have large assets (that translates "lots of money") such as the doctor, hospital, etc. Logically speaking, a larger medical transcription service would more likely be named in a lawsuit. For a single independent transcriptionist, it's unlikely.

In investigating the errors-and-omissions issue further, the authors sought advice from insurance brokers, underwriters, and lawyers, who advised against this particular type of insurance coverage at the present time. In most cases, insurance brokers weren't even sure what it was, why we would need it, or where we could get it! The feeling of these professionals was that with insurance being as costly as it is today, one is wise to spend money on insurance that is really needed and required by law — not on something you will probably never need.

In the process of consulting with an attorney for some business advice, the authors were presented with a six-page contract from the attorney that included his fee schedule. At the top of one page was a disclaimer:

"I DO NOT CARRY ERRORS AND OMISSIONS INSURANCE."

If an attorney does not feel the need to carry this coverage, why should we buy it? In the opinion of many experienced transcriptionists, this type of liability insurance is not necessary. Perhaps those who promoted errors and omissions insurance overreacted to unsubstantiated fears; perhaps they were ultra conservative; or perhaps they were simply greedy for the revenues that increased insurance premiums would produce. In any case, most medical transcriptionists feel that if the physician's signature is on the bottom line as required, it is the doctor's responsibility to read the transcription for accuracy and completeness. This is the position of health care regulators as well.

In talking with insurance underwriters, an errors and omissions policy basically provides coverage for attorney fees. IT DOES NOT PREVENT YOU FROM BEING SUED BY SOMEONE.

Instead of errors and omissions insurance, we suggest that all independent medical transcriptionists take measures to safeguard themselves against the trickle-down effects of lawsuits that could result from errors in dictation. When negotiating a contract with a new client, include a WAIVER OF LIABILITY clause (see two examples below). A waiver is the surrender either expressed or implied of a right to which one is entitled by law.

Ask your legal adviser to review the contract. By addressing this issue, your clients will appreciate your professionalism. If they do not, reconsider whether you want them as clients.

Within our industry, there is a definite need for discussion, clarification and definition of errors and omissions liability and other contract issues. It is the responsibility of every medical transcriptionist to help develop clearly defined and acceptable professional practice standards.

EXAMPLES OF LIABILITY WAIVERS

All technical terms and words shall be proofread and spellchecked. However, the parties agree that final responsibility for proofreading the transcript lies with the above named client. Client, therefore, agrees to waive any liability which might otherwise be asserted against (your business name) excepting breach of this contract. In addition, client agrees to indemnify and hold (your business name) harmless against any claims which might be asserted by third parties arising out of the performance of this contract.

. . . or . . .

It is my policy that computer-authenticated or artificial signatures generated by means other than actual dictating physician's signature are not endorsed by me. Therefore, the doctors should proofread the transcription for document content, accuracy and quality control. This means that they will accept the liability of the transcription and I will not purchase errors and omissions liability insurance.

In your contract with clients, also consider stating the following:

I DO NOT CARRY ERRORS AND OMISSIONS INSURANCE.

NOTE

Laws and procedures change frequently and are subject to different interpretations. Always contact a lawyer for specific legal advice. We have researched legal issues to the best of our ability, but it is your responsibility to make certain that facts and general information contained in this book are applicable to your situation.

PREVENTING D.P.S. (Deep Pocket Syndrome)

Because of the important services they provide, MTs, IMTs, MTSOs and the medical transcription profession are vital components of specific health care provider systems and of the general health care culture as well. As health care systems change so, too, will the role of medical transcription professionals.

The health care system continues to decentralize many services, including technology, support staff and programs, by outsourcing to contract services. The integrated local health care system is very patient-focused, sensitive to patient concerns, patient perspective, patient wellness, patient education and patient satisfaction. To meet patient needs and control costs, critical health care pathways and systems are being established to monitor appropriate use of resources and selection of technologies that provide information and service in the fastest, safest manner at the least cost.

Outsourcing of some medical transcription services has been occurring for years, but today's explosive outsourcing levels, which have surprised many health care professionals, is good news for independent medical transcriptionists. In a survey published in *Medical Records Briefing—Special Report* (January 1996) almost 66% of hospitals surveyed contract out transcription to independent contractors, transcription services, OR BOTH. This information continues to confirm what we have long been aware of: Independent medical transcriptionists are in demand, and those who maintain competency and professionalism will have successful careers.

There are many ways to determine competency. In the medical transcription field, a number of specific quality assessment mechanisms are used to measure competency: certification, documented ongoing continuing education, and quality improvement. For the medical transcriptionist, competency is vital because it leads to success and survival in a very competitive marketplace. If you are not competent, you won't keep old clients or get new ones. It is just that simple.

Maintaining competency will depend upon many factors besides just your education, training and fund of knowledge. Staying competent means addressing problematic areas within your business and reducing your professional liability through good day-to-day management. Begin by developing quality and productivity standards for your business based on your professional qualifications. For example, if your skill and experience are limited, your transcription output will also be limited. Therefore, you should set your quality and productivity standards at realistic levels and seek out clients whose needs will match your current potential production level. Given your level of expertise, it would be a mistake to set standards too high or market your services to hospitals or other highly sophisticated and demanding areas of medicine.

Develop a plan to evaluate and improve performance. Monitor quality comprehensively and continually within every aspect of your business: transcribed documents, service to clients, confidentiality, technology security and turnaround. Once problems areas are identified, implement methods to solve the problems, monitor them for effectiveness, and make adjustments as necessary.

If you discover weak or potential high-risk areas within your business, utilize the services of an appropriate consultant — accountant, lawyer, insurance agent, or experienced IMT. Dedicate yourself to being the best transcriptionist ever with the best service anywhere. Never forget that your competency is your best protection against liability.

LIABILITY INSURANCE

Liability is an issue in health care as in all professions, but is liability insurance really necessary for the medical transcriptionist? We believe it is not.

We recommend that you carefully evaluate any source that promotes liability coverage for medical transcriptionists. In our decades of experience as medical transcriptionists, we have never known nor heard of one incident in which a medical transcriptionist has been sued. We have heard *rumors* about such lawsuits, but no one has ever validated these rumors by presenting documentation of specific lawsuits or industry case rulings. Facts and facts alone are what we need. We cannot make wise decisions without evaluating the facts.

Rumor does not justify running out and purchasing a million dollar liability insurance policy. Of course, if we all purchase liability insurance there will be an enormous bank of funds which will surely encourage somebody to initiate a lawsuit, because there is insurance to pay for it! In such a scenario, who would get the lion's share from this new deep pocket? Insurance companies and lawyers.

Information from legal consultants indicates that lawsuits are often targeted toward individuals, groups, or facilities that have substantial assets, great sums of money or hefty insurance coverage. In investigating this issue further, the authors sought advice from insurance brokers, underwriters and lawyers, who recommended that we medical transcriptionists spend our money on insurance that is necessary or is mandated by law.

Currently, independent medical transcriptionists carry a variety of insurance coverages; some are essential; others, practical but optional: auto insurance (mandatory in most states), health insurance, life insurance, homeowners/renters insurance, personal liability insurance, business insurance. Depending on coverage, total insurance premiums can add up to thousands of dollars per year. To add professional liability insurance would cost an additional $250 to $2000 per year. Budgetary considerations cannot be ignored.

Then, too, if medical transcriptionists were to purchase professional liability insurance, we would also need to purchase errors and omissions coverage, which, if our sources are correct, is basically enough insurance to pay your lawyer's fees in the event of a lawsuit. To afford this type of coverage, we estimate an IMT would have to earn $100,000+ a year! Medical transcriptionists don't make that kind of money.

One professional liability policy currently being promoted has "limits of liability" of $1,000,000 each incident and $3,000,000 aggregate. These limits of liability are one-third that expected of the MD, DPM, DDS, and all other licensed allied health professionals.

It is important to differentiate between medical transcriptionists and the above licensed professionals, which are 1) ACCREDITED HEALTH CARE PROVIDERS, 2) LICENSED through state medical boards, and 3)

CREDENTIALED to practice. They have direct patient-care contact as well as health-record documentation responsibilities.

1. **Accredited Health Care Provider.** This category includes health care professionals such as the physical therapist (PT), occupational therapist (OT), registered nurse (RN), certified registered nurse anesthetist (CRNA), medical doctor (MD), doctor of osteopathy (DO), doctor of dental surgery (DDS), doctor of podiatric medicine (DPM), and many others. All are professions that have been accredited by their state medical associations and the American Medical Association through application and/or approval of education and training programs and have been given the official status of allied health care provider.

2. **Licensing.** The recognized health care professionals we have mentioned above and other recognized allied health professionals are, for a fee, licensed to practice in their profession through their state licensing boards (in California, the Board of Consumer Affairs; in New York, the New York Board of Medical Licensing, etc.) The license is generally for two years. Along with this license, they must document their continuing medical education units with their State licensing board. There is a reporting mechanism for complaints and for monitoring professional practice.

3. **Credentialing**. Physicians and recognized allied health professionals must be credentialed and privileged to practice in a number of health care settings, mainly acute care and managed care. They must apply for privileges through an extensive application-and-review process. They must document their activity from the time they enter their medical training to the time of their application for appointment, with no lapses in their experience unaccounted for. An extensive background check is done by requesting references from medical schools, teaching institutions regarding postgraduate training, all professional references and prior work settings, licensing, drug enforcement agencies (where applicable), etc. This credentialing process is a very time-consuming procedure that could take weeks to months to complete before an applicant is notified that his or her application and request for privileges has been approved.

In comparison, medical transcriptionists do not have direct patient-care responsibilities and are not recognized as allied health professionals. We do transcribe the patient's medical record and make every effort to produce an accurate document, but we cannot vouch for medical record accuracy. Only the physician, after reviewing his or her transcribed report, can do that. Therefore, why would we need liability coverage?

The "burden of responsibility" is central to any liability issue and where medical records are concerned, the physician's signature is still "where the buck stops." This is the accepted standard in health care, recognized through the health care regulating, accrediting and licensing bodies. Hospital surveyors will ask a physician if he reads the transcribed reports he dictates. If the physician answers "no" or "not always" the surveyor will remind him that he — not the transcriptionist! — is legally responsible for the content of that document. The burden of responsibility lies with the dictating physician when his signature is on that document.

Speaking with physicians regarding medical transcriptionists' purported need for professional liability insurance raises a lot of eyebrows and comments like "That is ludicrous!". . . "Ridiculous!". . . "Someone is hoping to dip into deep pockets!" More important, these doctors affirm that the accuracy of the health care records they dictate and which are subsequently transcribed is their responsibility.

It is interesting to note that the Joint Commission for the Accreditation of Hospitals (JCAHO) accreditation does not require a facility to carry liability coverage on health care practitioners credentialed to practice within the hospital setting. Some state regulating agencies do, but only for those groups noted above.

According to Link Resources, approximately 50% of the work force in this country is working from home, as an employee of others or self-employed. The insurance industry, which is satisfactorily meeting IMT insurance needs today, is well aware of this trend and will, we believe, anticipate and meet our future insurance needs.

WAIVER OF LIABILITY AND INDEMNIFICATION CLAUSES

All independent medical transcriptionists should be proactive in protecting their business and personal interests from the trickle-down effects of lawsuits. When negotiating a contract with a client, address liability issues and consider including a Waiver of Liability Clause or an Indemnification Clause (client agrees to hold you harmless against any claims which might be asserted by third parties arising out of the performance of this contract).

In addition, contact your insurance agent to discuss your present business coverage and evaluate possible additional coverage. Professional independent insurance agents have been trained in risk analysis and are familiar with insurance coverages. Your insurance agent should be able to assist you in obtaining appropriate protection from potential hazards resulting from your business operations.

COMPUTER SECURITY

In past years a computer system was an information reporting tool and sometimes a long term planning tool. Today, information technology has penetrated virtually every aspect of business operations and is an integral part of corporate service. It empowers companies to provide customers with timely, accurate information, which clients have grown to expect. Information technology enables companies to provide new levels of customer service and gain a competitive advantage.

Today's marketplace is information driven. If you lose your information, you lose your competitive advantage. However, information security specialists concur that security depends on people more than on technology. They note that employees are a far greater threat to information security than independents. Therefore, it follows that improving security depends on changing beliefs, attitudes and behavior of individuals and groups.

PROTECTING YOUR INVESTMENT

Every year millions of dollars of computers and computer equipment are stolen. You can protect yourself and your business by insuring your computer and regularly backing up your data, but there is little you can do to prevent an actual theft. Most desktop PC makers offer a Kensington Lock-like feature on their computers that stops unwanted users from booting up your system, and some manufacturers offer cable locks for securing a notebook or desktop to the desk. But what's to stop someone from stealing the desk, too?

Absolute Software (800-220-0733) has put viruses to good use by creating a user-friendly variety that tracks stolen PCs, much like the Lojack auto theft retrieval device. The company's CompuTrace TRS tracks down crooks when they hook up your stolen machine's modem to a telephone jack. CompuTrace TRS dials the modem to Absolute Software's headquarters to reveal the location of the guilty party, and Absolute Software officials notify the authorities. CompuTrace TRS runs in the background and disables your modem's speaker to ensure that the cons are clueless to when they are about to give themselves away.

Swap-Crypt from SCM Microsystems (408-370-4888) makes your PC's files and directories unreadable and useless to the PC thief. The Type II PC Card Encryption Card codes the original file to a temporary file, permanently deletes the original file, and then renames the temporary file with the name of the deleted file. Each file or directory can have five-character passwords and uses SCM Microsystems's One Time Pad encryption technique (patent pending).

Just think of the marketing possibilities! It will be exciting to tell clients of both new and old accounts about the new antitheft features you have added to your service, and clients will be favorably impressed with your knowledge of current technology and your commitment to maintaining patient record confidentiality.

BELIEFS AND ATTITUDES

Copying software without authorization is a felony. Nonetheless, some users have the attitude that it does not matter. The Software Publishers Association (SPA) training video *It's Just Not Worth the Risk* presents the issues involved in copyright infringement and warns that sooner or later software thieves will be caught and their careers devastated.

ANTIVIRUS TECHNIQUES

Currently there are a number of antivirus techniques available through vendors of antivirus products. As a personal computer user, you should have a practical, working understanding of computer viruses and how they can damage your PC. You can then evaluate the various antivirus products and decide which will best address your computer needs.

> *"As a personal computer user, you should have a practical, working understanding of computer viruses and how they can damage your PC."*

THE TARGET

The sole purpose of viruses, trojan horses, logic bombs, stealth viruses, and the myriad other malicious codes being unleashed upon the PC community is to wreak havoc on computer systems and programs. A representative of the National Computer Security Association (NCSA) in *Fighting The Virus Bulletin* stated, "There currently are anywhere from 2200-3000 known viruses worldwide. Between 50-60 new viruses appear each month and it has been this way for the last 18 months. There have been some months where the total has reached as high as 90 and the low has been around 25."

Techniques currently available that protect the PC environment from various virus exposures can be broken into two categories: software techniques and hardware techniques. There are three main software techniques employed within a number of vendor antivirus products:

1) Antitamper/integrity check

2) Signature scan

3) Use of activity monitors

Some antivirus products use combinations of the above. As with any other product, do your homework and talk with experts before purchasing.

The *advantages* of the antitamper/integrity check are these: the program and data files can be protected; no prior knowledge of the assailant is required to detect the change in the programs; and any change will be flagged. The *disadvantages* are the following: the technique is time consuming; the program must go through every program/directory to generate/check the checksums; and the checksum files themselves can become targets of attack.

The signature scan technique scans for specific code combinations, which may indicate that a virus is present. The *advantages* of this technique are these: a virus can be detected prior to execution of the program; the signature will identify the type of infection; and by identifying the virus the user may be able to reverse the damage of the infection or remove the virus.

The *disadvantages* of the signature scan technique are the following: it is time consuming; the software must search every file looking for all known signatures;

constant software updates are required to keep up with new viruses being created on a daily basis; as the number of signatures increases, the possibility of false alarms also increases; and the detection of a virus means the infection has already occurred.

The activity monitor is different from the previously mentioned techniques in that the software is loaded in the background and monitors system activity. If the application software executed an operation the monitor considers suspicious, the monitor will alert the user of a possible virus attack. The *advantage* of this technique is that it can detect and neutralize propagation. The *disadvantage* is that it can be bypassed. Because the monitor program resides in memory itself, it also may be subject to attack.

HARDWARE TECHNIQUES

Four types of hardware techniques are currently available. They include boot-up protection, command monitor, sensing, and sector-by-sector protection. The first two techniques do not involve protecting the actual physical drive. They set logically on the PC bus, which is the main information highway from the computer CPU to the peripheral cards. Access to the PC bus is through the PC card slots in the machine. (A PC usually has eight slots for cards.)

The last two techniques are physical drive protection techniques. They fit logically between the HD controller card and the physical drive. Boot-up protection is a hardware board that plugs into a PC bus slot and operates logically on the PC bus. This board prevents a boot from a floppy drive, thereby eliminating a major source of infection.

INFORMATION SECURITY BASICS

When computer users are asked to describe their computer security measures, many often respond, "Well, everyone seems to tell us to change our passwords, and that's about it." However, information systems security is more complex than a simple catch-phrase. Various computer crime techniques are called *sabotage, piggybacking, impersonation, data diddling, super zapping, scavenging, wire tapping, trap doors, trojan horses, salamis, asynchronous attacks and logic bombs, data leakage, simulation, viruses and worms*. Human errors, accidents or omissions are estimated to account for 50-80% of the annual dollar loss in computer data information destruction. Criminal hackers, although flashy and attractive to the news media, actually account for a small percentage of all harm to computers.

Investing in effective security policies and ensuring proper training are important factors to computer security.

PREVENTION

Even the best security measures cannot totally eliminate all human errors and accidents, but they can reduce the likelihood of such events by using several techniques:

- Eliminating access

- Providing audit trails

- Emphasizing accountability for actions

- Showing how important data is to the business

WHO ARE THE CRIMINALS

An American Bar Association study in 1984 found that 75% of computer offenders were insiders who had authorization to access data they mistreated. Employees were the third most costly threat to information security.

Because of the preponderance of insider "data diddlers," outsiders are probably an overrated threat. In the 1988 Internet worm case, a graduate student caused an estimated $96 million dollars of damage by introducing a program that replicated itself throughout the network and brought thousands of computers to a halt. One of the resources used by criminal hackers (a term that originally referred to dedicated programmers but now is used loosely to refer to anyone who tries to gain unauthorized access to computer systems) is public bulletin board systems (BBS). Hackers have shared a variety of illegally obtained information such as details of corporate security measures, dial-up-port telephone numbers, passwords, and even stolen credit card numbers for long distance phone calls.

HOW TO DISCOURAGE HACKERS

To make it more difficult for hackers to steal valuable information from computer records, try the following:

- Turn your modem off when the office is closed.

- Protect your passwords and access codes. Don't distribute that information to people.

- After hours, disconnect units with internal memories.

- Don't forget that digital copiers, laser printers and fax machines have internal memories that can be accessed by hackers.

- Read the security control sections of manuals that come with these units.

- Store sensitive data on disks rather than in the computer's hard drive and remove the disks from the computer drives at night.

SOFTWARE THAT COMBATS MALICIOUS CODES

Logic bombs, worms and viruses are among the most interesting forms of infosec attacks. Logic bombs are routinely and secretly inserted into programs. They check for conditions such as date of presence of the programmer's name on the payroll. Worms and viruses are programs that reproduce. The effects can include obscene messages on the screen, bizarre effects (e.g., having all letters on the screen drift slowly to the bottom of the screen like leaves in autumn), or random data modification, new errors in spreadsheets and outright data destruction (wiping out your hard disk).

NETWORKS

Another threat of growing importance in industrial espionage is telecommunications networks. Local area networks (LANs), which have been installed at a growing pace worldwide, are vulnerable to easy eavesdropping using "off the shelf" "sniffer" software available for about $1000 in stores but also available free on the Internet and from underground BBS.

SOME FINAL THOUGHTS ON COMPUTER SECURITY

For a number of years now, sophisticated antivirus software has been effective in the detection and removal of malicious codes that can infect PCs and networks. These antivirus software solutions minimize the amount of damage from both the cost perspective and the loss of information perspective; but antivirus software only identifies the infection the user ***already has***. Users must continuously update their antivirus software in order to keep up with the seemingly unending release of new viruses. Software solutions, while providing a limited level of effectiveness against viruses, requires users to actively monitor their systems. Newer systems have virus scanware that is activated when you boot up your computer.

Viruses released today are more sophisticated than viruses released in the 80s. They are now polymorphic viruses that continually mutate and create new signatures. They are viruses that target the actual hardware level of the PC, and they also appear at a much faster rate — fifty to sixty new viruses per month. This means, when looking toward the future, that software solutions alone may not be able to stop or detect all new viruses appearing on the market.

Currently there is no way a user can be certain that software is providing effective antivirus protection. The only way users will know why their software did not work is when something terrible happens. In order to maximize your protection, it is recommended that a top quality scanning software be used to check files for obvious known infections before activating hardware protection.

Experts agree that education is the key element to all computer crime prevention. To be most effective, it must begin during the earliest levels of academic education, continuing through high school and college and on into the workplace. It has been said that when revealing your password causes the same emotional response as pulling your pants down in public, we will be on the way to better computer security.

A very important point is that prevention is a form of insurance. Just as most organizations spend money on insurance policies to cover losses after an accident, you should spend money to prevent accidents before they occur. This approach is all the more sensible given reports of difficulties in collecting even coverage that was paid for.

THE UNLICENSED SOFTWARE POLICE

There is a significant amount of unlicensed software use occurring throughout the industrial workplace, including the health care industry. According to the Business Software Alliance (BSA), 26% of all software in use in the United States is pirated, accounting for vendor losses of about $2.9 billion dollars.

The BSA, an international organization, is funded by companies such as Adobe, Apple Computer, Autodesk, Bentley Systems, Lotus Development, Microsoft, Novell and Symantec. Since its inception in 1988 it has filed more than 600 lawsuits worldwide against suspected copyright infringers. Through public policy and education, the BSA seeks to control software piracy.

Making a copy of a software product is relatively easy, and frequently, people think of it as a victimless crime. However, no sector of the computer-using community is exempt from the Copyright Act or is protected against the unauthorized duplication of software. The BSA reports that the health care industry is particularly prone to this copyright infringement and has instituted an investigation of these crimes. The majority of tips regarding software piracy are received through the complaint hot-line.

The BSA operates 35 complaint hotlines around the world for callers seeking information about copyright matters or wishing to report suspected incidents of unauthorized copying of software. If you have concerns about software or want information about the Copyright Act, call the following number:

- **888-NO-PIRACY**
  (in the United States)

MAINTAINING FAX CONFIDENTIALITY

FAX machines are very effective in transmitting stat reports required for patient care. In order to maintain patient record confidentiality and decrease professional liability, we recommend the following guidelines for fax machine use:

- Locate the fax machine where access is limited and monitored at all times.

- Always use a fax transmittal sheet (cover page). Transmittal rates are determined by the amount of information on the sheets transmitted, so keep your fax cover page as simple as possible. After sending your transmittal, attach the fax machine's printout, which verifies the time of transmittal and the telephone number dialed, to the cover sheet, and file for future reference.

- Verify the recipient's fax number before transmitting transcribed material.

- Call ahead to notify recipient that information is being transmitted via fax.

- Identify the recipient on your fax transmittal sheet, and indicate the number of pages transmitted.

- Maintain a log, or copies, of information transmitted via fax machine. Many fax machines automatically record and print a copy of fax activity including date, time, and fax number accessed.

- Consider inserting a sentence on the transmittal sheet that states: "These documents are for the eyes of the receiver only."

- Stamp or write the word "COPY" on each sheet transmitted, so it will not be mistaken for an original document.

Protecting patient privacy remains our main concern as professional medical transcriptionists, whether we're an employee or are self-employed. When contracting our services to hospital accounts, most of us have been asked to sign nondisclosure agreement clauses, which state that if the confidentiality of any report is violated, our services may be terminated immediately.

By California law, health care professionals are required to maintain confidentiality of patients' personal and medical records. We are legally bound to limit discussions of patient information to health care professionals only for patient care purposes. We cannot legally discuss patient information with family, friends, insurance representatives, private investigators, pastors, newsmen, attorneys, etc.

When a medical report is faxed to either a hospital account or a physician's office, we do not know who is receiving that information on the other end. Could it be a family member of the patient whose report is being transmitted? If you think this could not happen, then you better think again. The pathology department of a hospital transmitted a biopsy report via fax to the surgeon's office. The diagnosis: terminal cancer. Imagine the shock of the physician's receptionist when she took the report from the fax machine and realized the patient in the report was her mother. It was an insensitive way to be informed of a loved one's brief life expectancy.

Although we cannot stand by each fax machine as reports are transmitted, there are steps independent home-based medical transcriptionists can take to minimize the threat to patient confidentiality. Each faxed report should include a cover sheet that includes the following:

TO: **FAX NUMBER:**   **DATE:**
FROM: **FAX NUMBER:**
NUMBER OF FAX PAGES:

Most fax machines include a "confirmation" feature that prints out everything you have faxed including phone numbers, time of day, and date.

Every faxed medical report should also include a disclaimer such as:

> *"The information contained in the transmission accompanying this notice is confidential and protected by the physician-patient privilege. It is intended only for the use of the individual or entity identified above. If the reader of this message is not the intended recipient, you are hereby notified that any dissemination or distribution of the accompanying communication is prohibited. The physician-patient privilege is not waived by the parties sending the accompany documents. If you have received this communication in error, please notify us immediately by telephone, collect, and return the original message to us at the above address via the United States Postal Service."*

You can have a rubber stamp made for this purpose and stamp it either at the bottom of each report or along the top. Keep in mind that although a report may be faxed, an original report must also be sent to the physician or hospital.

CONFIDENTIALITY AND THE CELLULAR PHONE

Everyone in the health care field is concerned about patient confidentiality. How many of you are transcribing for physicians who dictate their reports from car phones? We would venture to guess that 90% of you are. You might want to inform your doctors that there are scanners on the market designed to monitor car phone conversations. Imagine someone sitting in their living room listening to a history and physical, an operative report or a discharge summary being dictated on a neighbor or relative. No one is safe from the technobots, neither MTs nor MDs.

AUTOAUTHENTICATION

"The key issue is whether hospitals have adequate systems and appropriate policies to monitor and control document authentication by physicians — not by transcriptionists."

Autoauthentication has long been an issue of concern to health care professionals. Although many facilities have practiced auto authentication for years, recently, new and significant concerns regarding this practice have arisen. The problem involves the process of obtaining timely, accurate and complete patient-care documentation; authorship and authentication.

We differentiate authorship and authentication as follows:

- **Authorship:** The process of identifying the responsible health care practitioner who has released a health care entry for use. The identification process occurs in writing, by dictation, with keyboard or keyless data entry.

- **Authentication:** The voluntary, secondary process of confirming the content of the health care entry. Confirmation occurs by written signature, identifiable entry, biometric identifier or computer key.

The above definitions convey the differences between authorship and authentication and also address the responsibility of the health care practitioner who is documenting.

In autoauthentication, each doctor is routinely assigned an identification number for dictating. A file card with a handwritten signature indicates he or she "authorizes" use of their electronic signature, and they must also key in their assigned number for autoauthentication. The key issue is whether hospitals have adequate systems and appropriate policies to monitor and control document authentication by physicians — not by transcriptionists.

NOTE

In every authentication situation physicians have the option to review and personally sign transcribed documents. Physicians can also specify at the beginning of dictation if they feel it is particularly complex and should not be electronically signed.

The JCAHO requests that health care providers develop proposed scoring guidelines for documentation with second party intervention, with the provider demonstrating 98% documentation accuracy in cases where second party intervention was obtained prior to implementing authorship. JCAHO and Medicare Guidelines of the HCFA, of the U.S. Department of Health and Human Services (HHS), require that signatures, electronic or otherwise, be done by the practitioner and not be delegated.

It is the position of the American Association for Medical Transcription (AAMT) that the HCFA and JCAHO guidelines that permit the use of electronic signatures by physicians and other caregivers and require that signatures electronic or otherwise be affixed by the author of each entry *not* be delegated to anyone other than the physician who dictated the material.

Medical transcriptionists can attest to the quality of their transcription, that it is complete and is as correct as possible based on dictation provided, but we cannot attest to the accuracy of the dictation itself, including but not limited to the identity of the dictator and of the patient, dates given, history and treatment recorded, and the physician's conclusions. Only the direct caregiver can attest to the accuracy of patient-care documentation.

The patient should be a primary concern to all parties when signature policies are established because the patient's medical record will be a primary source of his or her future medical care. It will, of course, also be the primary source of documentation for legal, reimbursement, and statistical purposes. Thus, the accuracy of the patient record is appropriately the responsibility of the health care provider. Therefore, we believe it is not appropriate for health care providers to delegate persons other than physicians the authority to affix signatures that authenticate documents.

AUTOAUTHENTICATION —
AN ACCIDENT WAITING TO HAPPEN

Throughout the United States, hospitals are facing severe shortages and cutbacks by most insurance programs, especially government-sponsored programs like Medicare. Time is of the essence in documenting patient care for the purpose of reimbursement. The faster a chart is completed, the faster the institution will be paid by the insurance carrier. In eliminating the need to confront doctors about signing charts and/or completing their records, many hospital administrators have begun to implement autoauthentication, even though such programs are discouraged by many regulating agencies.

This shortcut is an added liability to medical transcriptionists and is one we should not be asked to assume. We all know that most doctors hate dictating almost as much as they loathe reading their dictation. As seasoned veterans in the war of words, we know, too, that the quality of dictation is often lacking in clarity. Dictating stations are invariably located in recovery rooms, emergency rooms, and physician lounges, where it is not uncommon to hear the cries of a screaming child awakening from anesthesia, the sounds of CPR in progress, or the latest Osama bin Laden joke. We also know that while dictating, doctors have an affinity for chewing gum and/or food, taking big gulps of liquid, yawning, snorting, burping, whistling, singing, playing musical instruments, talking to peers, and even snoring! By adding the phrase "DICTATED AND AUTHENTICATED" after the dictating physician's name, we are attesting to 100% accuracy in the medical record. We should not, indeed we cannot, do that. How can we verify that the patient was in stable and satisfactory condition upon arrival in the recovery room or that medication was administered to the patient? We weren't there. The only person who can, and should, attest to the accuracy of transcribed physician dictation is the physician himself.

Medical transcriptionists must not give in to those who urge us to cooperate with autoauthentication, arguing that there is no risk. **There is risk — to our individual services and to our profession — and the risk is great**.

AAMT POSITION SUMMARY*

Medical transcriptionists are medical language specialists who transcribe dictated patient reports. They interpret and edit raw data and dictation as completely, clearly, consistently and correctly as possible. MTs can attest to the accuracy of their transcription; they cannot attest to the accuracy of the dictation on which it is based. Patient care and well-being are at risk if health care providers do not give proper attention to the content of the patient record before the provider's signature is affixed. The provider's signature communicates accuracy of record content that only the provider can give. Thus, delegation of authority to affix signatures is inappropriate and should not be allowed.

This position summary was adopted by the AAMT House of Delegates, August 4, 1993.

CONFIDENTIALITY

Consultation and documentation are the twin pillars of malpractice prevention. Like all sensible approaches to risk management, good documentation is also good clinical practice. Integrally linked with consultation and documentation is confidentiality, which is also of central importance to quality care and malpractice prevention. The medical record is relied on heavily during the investigation of potentially compensable events and lawsuits. Often, medical malpractice suits can be eliminated or mitigated through accurate documentation, medical record security, and adherence to patient record confidentiality.

Every independent medical transcriptionist needs a basic understanding of risk and how to manage it. In the health care field the patient record is the medium of exchange. Our business is information and this information becomes a permanent part of the patient record. When developing our medical transcription business strategy, it is essential that we take into account the significance of the information we move in our business; how fast we turn it around, our work capacity, and the quality of our work.

The movement to electronic information is taking place in two specific segments. One segment is on the financial side. To promote standardization of the medical record, health care reform is proposing that each health care facility be able to access a record of all health information for any given person. We believe such a level of access is an intrusion of patient privacy. The inability of computer systems to communicate is perhaps the greatest vanguard of privacy individuals have. Thus, the development of a standard record will have serious confidentiality and privacy implications.

It is up to those of us working in the health care field to determine how much privacy we are willing to risk for an automated health care system. Those setting standards for automated patient records must realize there is more at stake than just confidentiality issues. The electronic medical record will also be used by attorneys, for peer reviews, and during other proceedings.

AHIMA has established a position paper on disclosure of health information. They maintain that health records, regardless of the media in which they are maintained, are the property of health care providers, but the health information contained in the records belongs to the patient. Disclosure of health information must be handled prudently to protect the patient's right to privacy.

The issue of confidentiality is a hot topic today. In our business, maintaining confidentiality is of utmost importance. Those of us in the health information field have a responsibility to help guard health information. A breach of confidentiality, invasion of privacy, and defamation of character can have major legal and financial impacts. We all know that humans err, and no individual or facility can fully guarantee confidentiality. A breach can occur from within or without a facility, and the system is especially vulnerable as a result of the communication technology we use. Now, more than ever, we need to establish guidelines for a program to protect confidentiality.

Guidelines for facsimile transmission should be established, and access procedures for files and users should be protected. We can start as follows:

- Determine state and federal regulations, agency standards and local precedents affecting confidentiality and release of information.

- Identify all manuals and computer sources of patient-specific information within the business and retention methods.

- Establish safeguards for appropriateness of information retention.

HOW TO MAKE TOUGH DECISIONS

Be aware that you cannot control the outcome of a decision. All you can do is control the decision-making process. Start by identifying your wants and needs, and jot them down on paper — even if they appear to be contradictory. Rank things you want and need in order of importance. If some items are contradictory, ask yourself, "Which would I choose?" Gather all the information necessary to make the decision. Look at your alternatives, consequences, advantages and disadvantages. Be as objective as possible, and don't let your emotions interfere with the decision process.

Determine how much risk you are willing to take, and once you have done this consider the following strategies:

- Choose the safest alternative — the one that can't fail.

- Pick the option with the best odds for success. Select the alternative with the most desirable outcome — despite the risk.

- Eliminate any option that might present a loss you won't be able to live with — despite high odds for its success.

- Picture how you would deal with negative consequences.

AVOIDING "RISKY BUSINESS" — DEVELOPING A RISK MANAGEMENT PLAN

It seems that every time we turn around there is another merger or acquisition in the medical transcription industry, and keeping up with the new venture names is nearly impossible. Nonetheless, this changing health care landscape does not spell doom and gloom for the independent transcriptionist. Indeed the solo practice is a very viable option in the sea of mergers and acquisitions, but it will take good risk management practices to keep the ship afloat.

Large or small, we all want to provide the best service possible in the most cost-effective manner. High quality and reasonable cost are not mutually exclusive goals, and quality need not be sacrificed for cost. Because of the technology available, IMTs are able to provide high-quality service and find a niche in the market, but this is not done without taking some risks.

In every business, large and small, there are risks — some expected and others, unpredictable and beyond control. Risk management is the practice of identifying, analyzing, managing and minimizing risk in your business. To remain competitive in the industry, it is essential that independent and solo transcriptionists focus on good risk management. Because you work alone without a workforce to back you up, you are more vulnerable to economic downturns, and an unexpected loss could prove catastrophic.

Taking the time to develop a risk management plan could very possibly save your business. Large companies hire risk managers or teams to carry out this function. Because of the cost involved, the independent transcriptionist does not generally have this luxury and must take responsibility for this task.

To the IMT the most common concerns in our business are the day-to-day operations of our service: operating costs, taxes, salary expense, equipment and supplies, fee-for-services and often (but not always) volume of work. When we think of the risks involved, we generally think of the most predictable risks, which are fire or injury, for which we purchase insurance to protect us. However, there are many unpredictable events or effects we tend to overlook or ignore, often because we do not understand the full scope of a possible loss. Without recognizing potential problems and their repercussions, it is difficult to develop a realistic strategy to avoid or minimize catastrophe.

How would you manage your business if you experienced smoke and water damage to personal property, damage or loss of equipment in your home office, and/or damage to leased equipment on your premises? Think about the business you might lose during the time it takes to return your business to normal, and the potential (perhaps permanent) loss of clients to competitors? Remember, during the downtime not only will your income be reduced or eliminated, but your business expenses — taxes, loan payments, etc. — will continue.

An interruption in your business could also trigger other expenses. To retain your client base you may have to use subcontractors (other IMTs) to service your clients. This will put an added strain on your finances at a time when you are able to generate little if any income yourself.

What about an unexpected illness? Have you thought about the impact your absence would have on the volume, productivity and costs of your business? If an accident should make it impossible for you to work, how would you reassign your duties to cover this period? What would be your replacement costs to cover the operation of the business? What would be your replacement source of income? Who would continue your business if you are not able to work? Would you leave your family with a source of income?

Other risks might result from liability and/or contract violations, loss of a good client, competitors' actions, changing technology and trends and their resulting effect on your market and clients, and in the current health care environment, the economy and its impact on your client base.

Without understanding the full scope of a possible losses incurred from catastrophes such as fires, floods, hurricanes, and earthquakes, you would not be able to develop a realistic strategy for dealing with such events. It is important to carefully analyze your business operations and identify what potential losses would cost. Although your standard insurance provides money for repairing or rebuilding property damaged, most policies do not cover indirect losses such as income that is lost while the business is interrupted for repairs. You must plan ahead if your business is to survive a catastrophe.

Any loss can directly affect your day-to-day operations, reduce profits and result in unexpected financial losses serious enough to cripple or even bankrupt your business. Using insight, you can develop good risk management practices in your business. Here are some things to think about:

There are two ways to manage risk. One is to limit exposure to loss by avoiding risk. This can be done through professional business practices and work ethics, having a good quality improvement plan, and technology security. Make sure you are operating your business with the proper licenses and permits, carry required insurance, and pay your taxes. As a professional, have a good business plan in place. List references and resources available in your area. Develop a step-by-step plan to doing the right things the right way. Implement the new process, eliminating inappropriate variations from the established standards. Be aware of and make a directory of all the referral networks available to you and your business. Make sure all your technology is registered and software is stored in a secure place.

The second way of managing risk is to transfer the risk. This is done through the purchase of insurance. There are the required insurances such as fire, liability, automobile and disability. In some areas crime insurance is also essential. There are specialized policies to cover full replacement cost of equipment and software, personal disability for the home-based independent medical transcriptionist, additional home-business coverage, and business life insurance. There probably is such a thing as "overkill" when it comes to the types of insurance available, but underinsuring can be hazardous as well. Be sure your equipment is insured to cover full replacement costs, not for what it was worth at the time of the loss. Most independent insurance agents are trained in risk analysis and will help point out exposures you may overlook.

Along with your insurance coverage there are other services your insurance company should provide to the policyholder and these include legal defense (liability insurance usually includes legal defense), rehabilitation (disability policies) and claim management services for loss analysis.

Business interruption insurance: I recommend this type of coverage, which reimburses policyholders for the difference between normal income and the income earned during the shutdown period. You will be required to furnish proof of income through tax documents and bank statements. Unfortunately these policies will not reimburse 100%, but many will reimburse up to 70% of your monthly income, which for an independent could still be much more than any unemployment policy would pay.

For the independent medical transcriptionist, a personal disability policy is a must, especially if your business income is the major supporting income in your family. As home businesses are becoming increasingly recognized as viable work options, more insurance companies such as Massachusetts Mutual are offering very comprehensive personal disability policies for home-based business owners.

If you are not sure about developing a solid plan for your needs, let your business planner, attorney, accountant and insurance agent help you develop a risk management plan to protect your business.

Finally, there are risks you probably haven't even considered:

- You are not sufficiently disciplined to do the work.
- You are not being paid — a very real risk.
- You don't like being in business.
- You are unable to retain clients.
- You are charging too little.

Remember that your business is your financial life support and a good risk management plan isn't difficult to set up. Consider the following guidelines:

- Recognize the risks — the ways you can suffer loss.
- Develop professional business practices and work ethics.
- Have a good quality improvement plan to monitor your processes and measure outcomes.
- Practice good technology security.
- Keep a list of resources and networks to fall back on.
- Follow the guides for buying insurance economically.

- Organize your insurance management program.
- Get professional advice.

Outsourcing (Subcontracting)

"In golf and in life, it's the follow through
that makes the difference."

—Anonymous

As your business grows and you add new clients, there will be ebbs and flows in the volume of dictation. This fluctuation occurs for a variety of reasons, and although low volume probably creates greatest concern, high volume can result in problems, too.

Sometimes a hospital or clinic's transcription department is short-staffed and must contract with a service to process overflow. If you take on such an account, you may be delighted to have the extra volume of work and added income but find yourself unprepared and unable to personally fulfill the transcription demands. You need help to meet your deadlines. The solution lies in backup transcriptionists with whom you can outsource work when the need arises.

Through networking, you can easily accumulate a list of transcriptionists in your area who will take on overflow transcription. These are generally individuals who have full-time jobs but enjoy moonlighting occasionally.

Many independent transcriptionists also use outsourcers (subcontractors) to cover them while taking days off or vacations, and outsourcers are lifesavers in the event of illness or other emergency.

EVALUATING OUTSOURCERS

After developing a list of potential outsourcers, your next step is to request resumes and review those submitted to you. Always interview the best prospects as if you were employing them for a major company. Some professionals like to interview at this time; others prefer to wait until after reviewing "test tape" transcription.

"Test tapes" are a common practice with larger transcription services and are an excellent tool for accurate evaluation of a potential outsourcer's technical skills. Send test tapes to all transcriptionist candidates and review the tapes carefully when they are returned. You will know immediately if the transcriptionist's skills are not up to your standards or if the candidate is trainable. If the work is satisfactory, you will schedule an interview, or a follow-up interview, with the applicant.

It is important to be selective in your choice of outsourcers. Remember, it is your account and your reputation that are ultimately on the line. Regardless of who actually transcribes, the end product is your responsibility so make your outsourcing decision wisely.

Before delivering work, verify that the outsourcer has adequate and appropriate transcription equipment, and make it clear that the working relationship is on an as-needed basis. If completed work is satisfactory, let them know. If not, briefly explain why and then locate a more skilled outsourcer.

It is also important to be certain that you are not the only source of income for outsourcers. Like you, they are independents and fall within the same guidelines as "independent contractors," so you should ask them to sign an outsourcer agreement.

Medical transcriptionists' work styles are as different as their personalities. When interviewing, it is important to determine a potential outsourcer's technical skill level, work style, workplace, and attitudes. If the work you release through your service is to be uniform and of consistently excellent quality, which you want it to be, outsourcers will have to conform to your standards. Some transcriptionists find this difficult; others find it impossible. You will eliminate many future problems by carefully evaluating potential subcontractors, avoiding any medical transcriptionist who is unwilling to forego an old style and conform to your standards.

PAYING OUTSOURCERS

You will pay your outsourcers so much per line or page, and keep a percentage for yourself. Be sure that your percentage covers your administration time.

It is wise to have enough cash reserve to pay your outsourcers on a regular basis, usually once or twice a month, even though it may take longer for your accounts to pay. It is difficult to keep good transcriptionists if they never know when they are going to get paid. Even if your accounts do not pay you promptly, you still have an obligation to your outsourcers.

TERMS OF AGREEMENT

The terms of agreement between you and your outsourcer can be spelled out in a contract, which might include performance, equipment/supplies, pricing/payment, communication with clients, non-compete clause, scope of work, termination, etc. There is a sample contract included in the appendix of this book. Have the contract reviewed by your attorney.

When working with outsourcers, schedule ahead of time, well in advance of the actual outsourcing work date. Outsourcers have other personal and professional commitments, frequently work with more than one transcriptionist, and usually have calendars that fill up as quickly as your own. Advance scheduling gives you more flexibility in selecting an outsourcer and helps prevent last minute frustration.

Communicate periodically with outsourcers and potential outsourcers to verify their continuing availability and to discuss any status changes.

WHEN YOU ARE AN OUTSOURCER

Newly independent transcriptionists frequently work as outsourcers while establishing their businesses and building a solid client base. Even after they are well established, many independent medical transcriptionists continue to accept outsource assignments when work is slow.

If you decide to take on outsource work, carefully consider all factors involved. Be sure to discuss job requirements in full and verify payment arrangements. If you disagree with the work plan or have questions, suggestions or requests, speak up before signing a contract.

OUTSOURCER UNDERBIDDING

Unfortunately, outsourcers have been known to "go in the back door" and "underbid," or, as some put it, "steal" accounts from others. This is generally considered unethical, but it happens.

If you are the outsourcer, resist any temptation to underbid. Respect the service you are working for and maintain professional transcription standards. The transcriptionist who resorts to unethical practices usually ruins his or her professional reputation and finds a career as an independent short-lived.

OUTSOURCERS AND THE IRS

Those who use outsourcers must complete an IRS Form 1099 on each noncorporate subcontractor to whom you pay more than $600, and these must be mailed by January 31st to the outsourcers, with a copy to IRS and the State Franchise Tax Boards where applicable, along with Forms 1096 and 596, by February 28th. If you outsource your services, you should expect a 1099 from the service you worked for.

OUTSOURCING ISN'T FOR EVERYONE

Outsourcing on a wide scale has drawbacks, and we do not recommend it for every independent transcriptionist. It is rarely appropriate for new independents, and experienced transcriptionists do not always find outsourcing a suitable option.

Outsourcing requires a great deal of administrative control, a level of responsibility that many independents cannot manage. It requires relinquishing a substantial percentage of standard fees, which many cannot afford.

If you choose to work with outsourcers, you will be responsible for the quality of your transcription and for the quality of their transcription, which must meet your standards and those of your clients. As a quality control measure, you will spend many hours distributing work, proofreading and verifying that work is done to specifications. Other responsibilities will increase, too. You will spend more time billing and paying bills, handling additional telephone calls, maintaining more complex public relations, and dealing with a greater number of unanticipated problems.

If you work with more than one outsourcer, you may find that you are spending the majority of your day administrating instead of transcribing. You must schedule pickup and deliveries, sort and arrange the work load for each day, estimate and know how much volume each outsourcer can handle.

You will provide formats and samples for new accounts, help with transcription difficulties, and when the outsourcer does not follow through or complete assigned work, be prepared to pick up the pieces until the job is completed. Soon you may discover that you are managing a "transcription service" and have lost the freedom and flexibility of independence.

Overcommitting is always a risk in outsourcing. If outsourcing with one transcriptionist works well for you, you may be inclined to accept greater volumes of work and outsource more frequently, which may present difficulties for you and your subs.

Spurred by enthusiasm for increased business, you may develop an inappropriate dependence on outsourcers. Likewise, outsourcers whose service is used frequently may grow to depend on your overflow for their primary source of income. If your volume drops off or you lose accounts, you will be responsible for breaking the news to the outsourcer, which is a very unpleasant task.

On the other hand, if your volume suddenly expands by leaps and bounds, you may find yourself with inadequate people-power to meet deadlines. Or you might lose an outsourcer and, even with standard levels of work, be unable to fulfill your commitments.

The Independent Contractor

"The secret of happiness is not doing what one likes,
but in liking what one does."

—Logan Pearsall Smith

INDEPENDENT CONTRACTOR

A person hired to perform a service with responsibility for the end results of the effort. The hirer has no control over the independent contractor's methods of performance or details of work such as one would have over an employee's labor.

On the surface, the definition of an independent contractor seems simple, but in working-world reality, it is actually quite complex. Our government has established very specific rules and regulations regarding who and who cannot legally call themselves independent contractors. Even with rules, however, there are gray areas, and some "independent contractors" have found themselves in legal limbo. Others, of course, are in hot water because they have made no attempt whatever to follow the rules. Don't let this happen to you.

Anyone desiring to be an independent contractor should clearly understand the following four points:

1. Government rules determine if a worker is an independent contractor. The IRS and state laws determine whether a worker is an independent contractor or an employee — not the written or oral agreements between you and the person you contract with. A contract in a file is not proof of an independent contractor relationship.

2. Workers are employees unless the hiring firm can prove otherwise.

3. Independent contractor status has nothing to do with job titles or type of work. Two people can do exactly the same job. One can be a true independent contractor, and the other can be an employee. It all depends upon how the hiring firm treats each worker.

4. One mistake can cause an independent contractor to be converted into employee status. Independent contractor status is not static. Any action by the hiring firm or its employees to control independent contractors can convert them into employees.

State and federal rules concerning independent contractors come from two sources: direct legislation and court decisions.

Court decisions or legislation may significantly alter the validity of this information. It is wise to periodically consult an attorney or other tax professional who monitors independent contractor rulings.

The key issue in determining whether or not a worker is an independent contractor is this: Who has the right to control the worker and how the work is accomplished. If a hiring firm controls the means by which work is done, the worker is automatically an employee. If the hiring firm can exercise control only on results of the work, the worker can be an independent contractor. It is the right to control, not the actual exercising of control, that is important.

The hiring firm cannot control an independent contractor's work. If it does, the worker's legal status will automatically be an employer-employee relationship and the hiring firm will be liable for employment taxes and benefits.

The hiring firm does have the right to exercise control as to the results of the work; it can provide job specifications to the independent contractor.

A hiring firm can only terminate independent contractors if it breaches the contract or if completed work is unacceptable. If a hiring firm claims the right to fire a worker at will, the worker's legal status usually is an employee.

BENEFITS TO INDEPENDENT CONTRACTORS

- Personal flexibility

- Being your own boss

- Business expenses are tax-deductible

BASIC CHARACTERISTICS OF INDEPENDENT CONTRACTORS

> Independent contractor status has nothing to do with job titles or type of work. Two people can do exactly the same job. One can be a true independent contractor, and the other can be an employee.

- Hired on a job-by-job basis

- Operate as a separate business

- Offer their services to the general public

- Hired to perform a specific task with no ongoing relationship or obligation by the hiring firm

HOW FIRMS BENEFIT BY HIRING INDEPENDENT CONTRACTORS

Firms that hire independent contractors benefit in significant ways. They avoid responsibility for the following:

- Social security taxes or Medicare premiums

- Workers' compensation insurance premiums

- Unemployment insurance (2001 and 2002 state and federal rate for new businesses is 6.2% on first $7000 of wages, up to $434 per employee)

- In some states, employment training taxes

- Health insurance and retirement benefits

- Long-term employee commitment

- Liability for the worker's action (with exceptions)

- Dealing with labor unions and their accompanying demands for union scale wages, benefits, and hiring/firing practices

RISKS TO THE INDEPENDENT CONTRACTOR

- **No disability or workers' compensation insurance**
  If the independent contractor is injured, they cannot collect disability or workers compensation insurance.

- **No unemployment insurance**
  Independent contractors are not eligible for unemployment insurance.

- **Can be held liable**
  Independent contractors can be held liable for their actions, instead of being protected by the hiring firm or its insurance coverage.

- **May develop tax troubles**
  Independent contractors must pay quarterly income tax and social security

self-employment taxes (15.3% on first $80,400 net taxable income for 2001 and $84,900 for 2002) — a big shock to those who do not plan ahead. When you add federal income tax (15%-39.1% for 2001 and 10%-38.6% for 2002) and state taxes, the total tax bill can be huge. If independent contractors spend that money elsewhere before tax time, they can get into significant trouble with the government.

> *"The key issue in determining whether or not a worker is an independent contractor is this: Who has the right to control the worker and how the work is accomplished."*

INDEPENDENT CONTRACTING AND THE TWENTY COMMON LAW PRINCIPLES

When the IRS audits a company and spot-checks for fraudulent independent contractors, it relies on these twenty "common law" principles:

1. **No Instructions**
   Contractors cannot be required to follow instructions to accomplish their tasks.

2. **No Training**
   Contractors rarely receive training to perform a task.

3. **Service can be rendered by others**
   Contractors can hire others to do the work for them.

4. **Own work hours**
   Contractors set their own work hours.

5. **Nonessential work**
   Contract work is not essential to the company.

6. **No day-to-day working relationship**
   Most contractors do not have a day-to-day relationship with their employers.

7. **Control of assistant**
   Contractors can hire, supervise and pay assistants independent of their employers.

8. **Time to pursue other work**
   Contractors should have enough time to pursue other work.

9. **Job location**
   Contractors decide when and where the work is done.

10. **Order of work set**
    Contractors control the sequence of tasks that lead to finishing the job.

11. **No progress reports**
    Contractors are not required to submit interim reports to employer.

12. **Paid for the job**
    Contractors are paid for the job, not for the time spent doing the job.

13. **Working for multiple firms**
    Contractors should have time to do work for more than one employer.

14. **Business expenses**
    In most cases, contractors should pay their own expenses involved in doing a job.

15. **Own tools**
    Contractors usually furnish their own tools.

16. **Significant investment**
    Contractors' investment in their trade must be significant enough to make them independent of employer's facilities.

17. **Services available to the public**
    Contractors must show that they make their services available to other employers.

> "To determine independent contractor status, you must
> look at **all 20 common law factors.**"

18. **Potential profit or loss**
    Contractors are liable for any expenses and liabilities they may encounter in performing their jobs.

19. **Limited right to discharge**
    Contractors cannot be fired at will so long as they produce a result specified in their contract.

20. **No compensation for noncompletion**
    Contractors cannot be paid for partial completion of a job.

Failure to satisfy all 20 principles may result in an Internal Revenue Service audit on the past three years with the business owner penalized for each misclassified worker, whether they were deliberately misclassified or the misclassification resulted from an honest mistake. One mistake can easily cost a business $25,000.

The 20 common law factors described above were developed by the IRS. There are at least five other government agencies in California involved with determining whether workers are independent contractors or employees:

- Employment Development Department (EDD)

- Workers Compensation Appeals Board

- Immigration and Naturalization Service

- U.S. Department of Labor

- Labor Commissioner

These governing agencies will vary from state to state.

Like the IRS, all these agencies consistently agree upon one key determining factor: In a true independent contractor relationship, the hiring firm has no right to control the work of the worker.

However, each agency has developed its own "factor list" to show right to control. For the most part they parallel the IRS factors. Here are the most important factors common to all these agencies:

1. Hiring firm does not have the right to control the worker

2. Type of work is not the hiring firm's primary business

3. It is not a continuing relationship

4. Payment is made by the job

5. Worker has own tools

6. Worker cannot be fired at will

7. Worker determines job location

8. Worker has a distinct occupation or operates a separate business

The U.S. Department of Labor uses a six point "Economic Realities" test to determine if a worker is an independent contractor. Reference: *Employment Relationship Under the Fair Labor Standards Act*, Publication 1297, U.S. Department of Labor.

SIX FACTOR "ECONOMIC REALITIES" TEST

1. Work should not be part of the hiring firm's regular business

2. Working relationship should have a degree of non-permanence

3. Worker should have invested in equipment, materials, or assistants

4. Hiring firm should have no right to control work

5. Opportunity for profit or loss exists, depending on the worker's managerial skills

6. Work should require initiative, judgment, or foresight to successfully compete with others

Regarding homeworkers, the IRS and California have ruled that homeworkers are statutory employees if the hiring firm gives them specifications, provides them with materials or goods, and requires them to return the finished goods to it and the following conditions exist:

1. Substantially all work is performed personally

2. Worker does not have substantial investment in facilities

3. Work is not a single transaction

4. Worker does not offer services to the general public

5. Worker does not keep records

6. Worker sometimes uses hiring firm's facilities and equipment to perform the task

7. Worker is paid hourly

THE BOTTOM LINE

To determine independent contractor status, you must look at **all 20 common law factors** to form a total picture. Do not rely on any one factor. Aside from determining which factors are the most important, examine the factors that you cannot meet and ask yourself why. Then, work on meeting all of those factors before you classify yourself as an independent contractor.

You must be willing to be an entrepreneur and take business risks (make a profit or loss on jobs), assume liability if the work is faulty, hire assistants, invest in your business, advertise, and be able to conduct business even after losing a client. If you are not willing to do that, then you cannot classify yourself as an independent contractor.

Educate yourself. In California there is an Independent Contractor Package designed to make it easier for independent contractors to comply with government requirements and plan for unexpected illnesses, injuries, or unemployment. This package is available through the state chamber of commerce and through some local chambers. If you don't live in California, check with your state or local chamber of commerce to see if a similar independent contractor package is available.

- **The California Chamber of Commerce**
  P. O. Box 1736
  Sacramento, CA 95812-1736
  916-444-6670

For those outside California, locate your state's chamber of commerce in the resource section at the back of this book.

ADDITIONAL PROTECTION FOR THE INDEPENDENT CONTRACTOR

To protect itself, the hiring firm may ask you for the following items:

1. Contractor's business license

2. Contractor's fictitious name statement (if applicable)

3. Evidence of insurance (business liability coverage)

OFFICE RECORDS

Most medical transcriptionists enjoy transcribing, and independent transcriptionists sometimes wish they were free to concentrate entirely on that responsibility, focusing all their attention on producing the quality work that results in an excellent income. For independent transcriptionists, such a wish will never be realized because they must also carefully and conscientiously administer their business — organizing, restoring and retrieving, and taking care of accounts receivable and accounts payable. A well-organized office is essential to success.

To maintain accurate and organized records in your office, we recommend the following:

1. **Clients**
   A file for each client.

2. **Physician lists**
   If you are dealing with hospitals and large clinics, you must keep a physician

directory. Each hospital has a directory of active staff physicians, consulting staff, courtesy staff, and temporary staff physicians.

It is also a good idea to keep a directory of physicians from the area you are servicing. This can be obtained by copying the yellow pages of the local telephone directory, or by requesting a physician directory from the local medical society (not all physicians belong to medical societies, but most do). These lists should include not only the names, but addresses and phone numbers as well. You must keep the lists updated yearly as new physicians are added.

3. **Daily work log sheets**
Logging in jobs daily is very important if you are dealing with several clients.

This log can identify the work you take in daily by date, client name, minutes; and upon completion you can log the lines. We find a daily log reference invaluable, especially when the schedule is very busy and there isn't always time to transfer information to a ledger. We often catch up on paper work on weekends or in the wee hours of the morning before starting work the next day. Establish good daily logging habits in the beginning, and you won't regret it.

4. **Service contracts**
We have a file for equipment service contracts that are renewed yearly. If there is a problem with equipment, the information is readily available when calling for service.

5. **Rolodex® - Business Cards**
Keep these handy, and collect them from other transcriptionists at seminars, meetings, trade-shows, etc. Also collect business cards of book and equipment vendors, and any other appropriate contacts.

6. **Continuing education**
As a certified medical transcriptionist, you must obtain a certain amount of continuing education credits (CECs) to maintain your certification.

For many chapter meetings, seminars, and symposiums, certificates are given to attendees verifying the number of CECs earned. If no certificate is available at an event you attend, save your program and place that information in your file. Even if you are not certified, continuing education is important, so we suggest you maintain this file, because your ultimate goal should be to become certified in the future.

Your continuing education credits will also prove impressive to prospective clients and employers, and you can include this information on your resume or curriculum vitae. This helps to build credibility and to attract more clients for your business.

7. **Outsourcers lists**
   If you have occasion to use outsourcers, and even if you do not, it is still a good idea to keep a list of other self-employed transcriptionists that you can call upon if needed — to cover your vacation time, for emergencies, or for unexpected overflow. This list should be updated at least yearly.

8. **Calendar/meetings**
   Keeping a daily planner at your desk is very handy. You can pick these up at a local office supply store. The calendar can be filled in monthly, weekly, or daily, as you see fit, and is an ever-present reminder of your daily, weekly, and monthly schedule.

9. **Correspondence**
   Be sure to keep a file of your correspondence. You may not think this will be necessary, but the paperwork just seems to accumulate!

10. **Formats/transcription samples**
    Keep a file of your client formats and transcription samples. If you have several clients, it's usually a good idea to keep an individual file, or a binder with dividers for each client, to avoid confusion.

11. **Contracts/agreements**
    You should have copies of all contracts and agreements you enter into with clients, other services, and outsourcers.

12. **Word lists**
    From medical lectures, magazines, newsletters, and a variety of other sources, you will accumulate many new word reference lists. These lists will be handwritten, photocopied, and printed — not in book form. You'll want to keep these handy references in a readily accessible place. A file or binder is convenient. Maybe someday you will write your own word book but in the meantime, never throw away a word list!

LOG SHEETS

Every transcriptionist must keep a record of what was transcribed on any given day. If your software program offers the capability of constructing a daily log, all the better.

Why is a daily log necessary? Simply put, to increase efficiency. Here is a typical scenario: An account calls asking if and when you transcribed an operative report on Mr. Blank, which was supposedly dictated three months earlier. If you don't keep a daily log sheet, how are you ever going to find that work?

First, you check your computer files, which indicate that you did not transcribe dictation on Mr. Blank during the specified three month period. Your log sheet backs you up.

A sample of a daily log sheet appears on the following page of this book. It should include the name of the account, the date transcribed, number of tapes received and returned, and the total line count for that date. It should also include the patient's name, the dictating physician's name, type of report, date dictated, number of lines for that report, and any problems associated with the dictation.

Of course, a log sheet can be designed to fit your style and mode of work, but it is a necessary tool in the field of transcription. Many line count software programs include generated transcription report logs similar to the one shown on the following page.

RECORDS

In addition to retail books and forms, free or low cost reference materials are also abundantly available. Use resources at your local library or order government publications from the Internal Revenue Service (IRS), the Small Business Administration (SBA), the Department of Commerce, and your state resources.

> Cardinal rule: keep your personal assets and liabilities separate from those of your business.

TRANSCRIPTION LOG SHEET (SAMPLE)

Minutes of dictation _____   Total lines _____

Tapes picked up _____   Date _____

Page _____   Transcriptionist: H1

Account name _____

DATE DICTATED	CONTROL #	PHYSICIAN	PATIENT	REPORT	TOTAL LINES

SEPARATING YOUR PERSONAL AND BUSINESS CHECKING ACCOUNTS

There are three important reasons for opening a separate banking account for your business:

- It will provide you with a complete record of your income and expenditures for tax purposes, and at tax time, you won't waste hours separating personal from business expenses. Also, if you are ever audited by the IRS, the auditor may be less likely to look into your personal finances.

- Using personal checks for your business expenses suggests that you are a small-time operation and your credibility may suffer. On the other hand, if your business checks are embossed with your business name and logo, you will enhance your professional image.

- It is much more difficult to unravel your business and personal finances if they are kept in the same account.

When opening your business checking account, the bank clerk will ask you for your business license and your fictitious name statement (if you have one), as well as your social security number. We recommend that you ask to have your check numbers start at 300 or above. This will give the image that you have been in business for awhile. This may be helpful because some suppliers are reluctant to extend credit to a new business that has no track record of reliability or success.

APPLYING FOR A BUSINESS LOAN

In order to qualify for a small business loan, you must provide the lender with information regarding your business. You will need a business plan describing your product or service, your target market, your financial projections, and your current financial statements.

The SBA (U.S. Small Business Administration) offers excellent references for the small business owner. One publication is called *ABCs of Borrowing* (FM-1). This publication covers what lenders will require, what type of financial information you will have to provide, collateral, the loan application and agreement, types of loans and much more.

The Small Business Association also offers an extensive selection of information on most business management topics. All of this information is listed in *The Small Business Directory*. For a free copy of the directory, write to SBA Publications.

- **SBA Publications**
  P. O. Box 1000
  Fort Worth, TX 76119

THE SMALL BUSINESS ADMINISTRATION (SBA) AS A BUSINESS ALLY

According to the National Association of Women Business Owners, 32% of small business owners are women; however, only 8-10% of women entrepreneurs receive SBA loans. Why the disparity? According to the National Association of Women Business Owners (NAWBO), ". . . personal or commercial bank loans are the number one type of short-term financing among all businesses, but credit cards are clearly the number one funding source for women. Most women probably have one or two cards and they see them as readily available sources of cash. They also don't have to supply the two years of financial statements required for most bank loans." Why are women having to turn to alternative types of financing in order to keep their businesses alive?

A study by the National Association of Women Business Owners indicates that attitudes and practices of loan officers are a significant barrier to many women seeking business loans. The NAWBO study noted that common complaints among women business owners include bank requirements for more assets or collateral and a longer business track record, and the banks' own limited experience in dealing with service businesses.

There are other reasons why businesswomen turn to credit cards. In the past, Small Business Administration requirements for obtaining business loans were extremely stringent and only the fittest survived the loan application process. All too frequently the process required many months of paperwork and meetings with lenders before approval could be obtained from the SBA. Most women business owners, who became frustrated with the interminable process and the lack of progress, turned to other sources — primarily credit cards — to finance their businesses.

Until 1994, 90% of all loans given by the SBA were covered under the 7 (a) Guarantee Loan Program. The purpose of this loan was to assist the new or growing business with its financial needs. Eligibility was restricted to manufacturers with up to 500 employees; wholesalers with up to 100 employees; agricultural businesses up to $500,000 in annual sales; retail businesses with a maximum of $5,000,000 in annual sales; service industries with a maximum of $5,000,000 in annual sales; contractors up to $17,000,000 in annual sales; and special trade businesses with a maximum of $7,000,000 in annual sales. Proceeds from the loan were to be used strictly for working capital, acquisition of machinery and equipment, purchase of inventory, business buy-outs and start-ups, debt refinance, purchasing land and buildings, construction including land acquisition, improvements and renovations. To obtain a 7 (a) loan, collateral was needed such as mortgage on land, building and/or equipment, assignment of warehouse receipts, mortgage on personal property, guarantees and assignments of current receivables and assets of the business. This loan was for a maximum guaranty of $750,000. As you can see, most IMTs would not meet the eligibility requirements for securing such a loan.

SBA SMALL LOAN "LOW DOC" PROGRAM

In 1996 the SBA made available a Small Loan "Low Doc" Program to women business owners. The process is very simple. The applicant meets with an SBA advisor for screening at a local Small Business Development Center or at another organization designated by the SBA. After screening, a "pre-qualification" letter is issued. The applicant takes the letter to the lender of her choice for an SBA loan. The letter assures the lender that a loan made to the applicant will be guaranteed by the SBA up to a maximum of $250,000.

The "Low Doc" program is designed to reduce the paperwork and cost of providing loans of $150,000 or less and to increase the availability or such financing to small businesses. Emphasis is placed on the applicant's character and personal and business credit history rather than on traditional credit criteria. No predetermined percentage of equity injection is required.

SBA "LOW DOC" PRIMARY CREDIT CONSIDERATIONS

- Willingness to repay debts, as indicated by a good credit history; a cosignor may be considered if applicant has no credit history.

- The likelihood that expected earnings will be sufficient to pay obligations.

- With the requested financing, the business has a good chance of achieving success.

SBA "LOW DOC" LOAN
APPLICATION REQUIREMENTS

In order to apply for an SBA loan you must provide the proper documentation. This includes the following:

- Personal financial statement: Within past 60 days current.

- Personal tax returns: Prior three years, all schedules.

- Credit report: Get your own copy free from TRW 1-800-682-7654.

- Company's financial history: Business financial statement (Balance Sheet and Profit and Loss Statement) — as current as possible, no older than most recent quarter end.

- Accounts payable and accounts receivable aging statements (same date as financial statement).

- Business tax returns: Prior three years, all schedules. If your business is a sole proprietorship, the business's "tax return" is your Schedule C in your personal tax return.

Find out the location of your SBA Administration Development Center (most every town has one). Before seeking loans from lenders, make an appointment with an SBA advisor to see if you qualify for one of their new programs. In addition to being an excellent resource center, these development centers are wonderful for networking. Most of them provide a resource library, which can be used for free, as well as monthly workshops, which are usually less than $10 each, on a variety of business topics.

Business funding opportunities are opening up for women in other areas, too. Two of the nation's largest banks are now embracing female business owners by aligning themselves with major women's business organizations. Wells Fargo

Bank has teamed up with the National Association of Women Business Owners, a Washington-based group with 60 chapters, while Bank of America recently linked up with Women Inc., a Sacramento-based trade association.

Wells Fargo and NAWBO: Wells' loans are unsecured and require a one-page application form with no tax returns or financial statements. The minimum loan amount is $5,000. To qualify for a loan, women must have good personal and business credit, have been in business for two years and be profitable. For information, call 888-767-2444.

B of A and Women Inc.: Bank of America recently jumped into the market with its own lending program targeted toward women. B of A's alliance with Women Inc., which provides a variety of services and discounts to members, makes sense because both organizations share the goal of financially empowering women business owners. Women Inc.'s members benefit from a 50% discount on setup fees for new Advantage Business Credit loans up to $100,000. The bank also offers a one-page loan application.

- **Women Inc.**
  310-815-0975

> **A Note To Men:** For our male readers, we certainly hope the previous section on business loans for women does not offend you. It is not our intent to do so. It is unfortunate that we even have to include this in the book, but the fact remains that for many years there has been an almost impenetrable barrier in the banking world that has kept a large segment of our society from participating. If we are to achieve true parity in the business world, we need a level playing field.

DECIDING WHETHER TO KEEP GROWING

For those who resolve the difficulties encountered in running a home business and enjoy its advantages, the ultimate challenge becomes controlling growth. Many healthy home businesses begin to outgrow their settings after a few years, at which point one must decide whether to give up the benefits of working at home or scale back and keep the business small.

At this juncture, some businesses outsource work in order to stay small. Others choose to expand into office space and hire employees. If you are successful in your business, be prepared to think about this because you will be faced with this decision sooner or later.

As an independent you have the opportunity to make a great deal of money, but you probably will not make an annual income of $30,000-$60,000 during the first two or three years. For a few, financial security comes soon, but it is rare.

The length of time it takes to become financially secure depends on the individual. For many, it is reached at the point when they are no longer spending excessive time using reference materials, and this usually takes a number of years. There is no way to hurry becoming a good transcriptionist — no crash course. Excellence takes time. Medical transcriptionists get paid for what they know as it relates to quality production. The more we know, the more we can produce, ergo, the more we get paid.

Many successful independents eventually discover they have more work than they can handle. Some enthusiastically decide to find other MTs to help them . . . and soon they have several people helping them. Because their business has a reputation for excellence, they must utilize ICs or employees who conform to excellent standards, and the overhead creeps up. Even more work is accepted and more helpers employed . . . and then the process is repeated. Naturally, with all this work, increased deliveries must be scheduled, new equipment must be purchased and old equipment must be upgraded. The overhead climbs higher while the successful (although no longer so enthusiastic) MT's percentage of profits goes lower as she administers the business operations more and more and transcribes less and less. In addition, Uncle Sam always wants a bigger share.

When the time comes, carefully weigh the pros and cons of expanding. You may discover you had a lot more money when it was JUST YOU!

> *"The trouble with life in the fast lane*
> *is that you get to the other end*
> *in an awful hurry."*

EXPANDING TO A MEDICAL TRANSCRIPTION OFFICE

If the idea and challenge of expanding your service beyond independent freelancing appeals to you, perhaps you should consider opening an expanded medical transcription office in a commercial area.

NOTE: Although much of the information contained in this book will prove helpful to you in developing a successful medical transcription office, we do not address this subject specifically and recommend that you seek counsel elsewhere in this pursuit.

BURNOUT

Hopefully your business will soon grow beyond your wildest expectations, which is terrific if you are able to maintain a balanced life. However, beware if you discover the following symptoms: you are working your fingers to the bone; your eyesight is fading due to screen fatigue; your mind is filled with medical terms and nothing else; you can't sleep without your fingers and right foot moving; you are developing a wrist drop, a hunched back, and saying to yourself, "Is this all there is?" These are the first signs of burnout!

Perhaps it's time to learn how to erase old mental tapes and redictate new ones for your life. Work should not be your primary source of self-esteem, nor should it be used to escape from the outside world. When either occurs, burnout is inevitable.

Workaholism in our society today is rewarded. Corporations encourage employees to fill their off-time by traveling from one assignment to the next and attending self-improvement seminars. Workaholism leads to burnout.

Burnout is easy to spot. It occurs when one gives more than one has to give and there is nothing left. Frequently, the first signs of burnout are depression and an inability or unwillingness to get out of bed in the morning, by sleeplessness at night or waking every couple of hours, and wanting to eat everything in sight or nothing at all. Physical symptoms can be characterized by tightening of the jaw, neck, shoulders and chest; palpitations, ringing or buzzing in the ears, and a general sense of unease.

Once you are able to realize that there is a big world outside of transcription, which is meant to be enjoyed, you can start making some changes. The term "work" must be redefined. It is necessary to conclude that it is just a job and nothing more, an activity to be performed for a prescribed amount of time per day that allows you to pursue other interests. To many medical transcriptionists — and other professionals as well — being "unproductive" translates into "worthlessness." Have you ever felt that if you said "no" you would be replaced and if you did not do everything perfectly, you were not good enough? Beware burnout!

Remember, the main reason for becoming independent is to work smarter not harder. Of course one's best laid plans can fall by the wayside. After a few months at home, you might realize that you are working harder than ever before and definitely enjoying it less. There is always work to be done and you can no longer leave it at the office. Your clients are demanding more and more of you.

Many transcriptionists overwork because they are not making enough profit. If this is your situation, evaluate your transcription rates and if they are low, consider raising them.

Without work limits and lacking confidence to say "no," it is easy to fall into a workaholic rut. You fear saying "no" will send clients scurrying elsewhere, leaving you to pound the pavement in search of accounts.

It is important to set limits for yourself and do only what is acceptable to you. Start by really communicating with your accounts, telling them what you feel is practical and what is not. Tell them emphatically how much work you can take per day and that if they give you more, they cannot expect a fast turnaround time. Explain to them that when you decline to take work on any given day, it is because you are running behind and know you will not be able to make the delivery within the time limit already agreed upon.

The first time you use the NO word, your hands might be clammy, your brow beaded with sweat, and your voice no bigger than a squeak. You will probably be pleasantly surprised to find that instead of rushing out to find another service, the client will actually call you back the next day. By setting limits for yourself, your clients will respect you for your honesty. They will know what they can expect from you, and you will know what to expect from them. What a professional concept!

Following are ideas we have found useful in developing good work habits.

- **Know your performance style and accept it.**
  Independent contractors are usually very goal-directed and like to get work out as fast as possible in order to have time for themselves. Whether you are a person who likes to work from 9 a.m. to 5 p.m., do your best work at night or wait until the last moment, do it. Individual work patterns are neither right nor wrong. The power comes in acknowledging what works best for you as an individual and accepting it.

- **Be aware of your priorities and live by them.**
  It is easy to give everything equal priority; working, doing laundry, watering the garden, filing income taxes. Make a priority list every morning and attempt to complete the list in order of priority. Some days, you might be able to accomplish everything on the list and some days not, but the structure will keep you from feeling overwhelmed and panicky.

- **Discover your limitations.**
  No matter how much you try, you cannot do everything. Everyone has limitations. Be aware of how much you can comfortably transcribe in a given day. By knowing this and accepting it, you will have eliminated much stress from your life.

- **Build in time for yourself.**
  It is essential that we have balance in our lives: work, family, friends, and hobbies. Allow yourself time to play and enjoy this wonderful life and the fabulous people in it. Set aside one hour each day just for yourself. Go for a long walk, ride a bicycle, take a long, hot luxuriating bubble bath, read, or go out to dinner or to a movie with friends. When you know there is a block of time set aside just for you and only you, the day goes smoother and faster.

> *"Long-range planning does not deal with future decisions, but with the future of present decisions."*
> —Peter F. Drucker

HIDEY-HO! THE LONG RANGER!

An Option for Long-Range Planning — Working for an MT Service

*"Most services recognize and appreciate the benefits of utilizing
the talents of highly trained, experienced IMTs
who are already successful independents."*

Remember when a mouse was something that got caught in a trap, or sent granny squealing with her petticoats flying everywhere? When our tools of the trade were typewriters, one transcriber and two or three books? The future seemed so uncertain, we barely communicated with each other, and new technology was a scary thing! That seems like a lifetime ago. Now, the mouse has a whole new meaning and the tools of the trade have advanced so rapidly that we are outdated before we get the latest gadget paid for. It's a race out there. We have spent a lot of time remembering when, but how much time should we be spending making our long-range plans for the future? A lot.

In years gone by, we worked alone and we weren't known as "independents." There were a few large transcription services that dominated the field, just a few. When the evolution of many MTs from the work place into independence began to gain momentum, some of the large transcription services promoted themselves through smear campaigns, their ads showing the independent worker at home with the computer/typewriter set up in the kitchen, the baby crying in a nearby playpen, dirty dishes in the sink, the MT in curlers and a bathrobe, gossiping on the phone to a pal about what she was transcribing, cup of coffee in hand and puffing on a ciggie. The caption said something like "do you want your medical records transcribed in this environment? At our company, all service is provided in a **professional** office environment."

When the ad appeared in a very well known and respected professional journal, a resounding and unanticipated protest erupted from the previously unrecognized IMT work force, and letters of protest went flying. The ad was abruptly pulled and a public apology was made to IMTs by the publication, explaining that it had been unaware that such as strong workforce of independent workers existed. During that period, IMTs felt that working for a service was like scraping the bottom of the medical transcription barrel. The pay was insultingly low, and many stories circulated that described the service environment as much like the old sweatshops at the turn of the 20th century. This too has changed.

As an example of how the industry has evolved, in just a few years, the "service" has done a complete about face and taken on a new image. Because of industry standards — the method of counting lines/characters, quality, confidentiality, knowledge and technology — many services today are very well organized, and their benefit packages are gradually becoming more attractive. In addition, there are more large-service players, and they use IMTs . . . lots of them. In fact, the majority of transcription done in big services is by IMTs, working remotely throughout the globe as telecommuters. Most services recognize and appreciate the benefits of utilizing the talents of highly trained, experienced IMTs who are already successful independents. These skilled, dependable workers provide a solid work force and increase the services' bargaining power as they seek to expand their markets. Today, services are an attractive work option for IMTs. Still, it's wise to be alert and cautious. Although most services are ethical, there are some unethical operations out there.

As part of your long-range plan, at least consider the option of working for a global service. Making the connection to work with a service is fairly easy and does not necessarily mean that you will have to buy another piece of equipment. Generally, services require that you have or incorporate equipment to download from their system, or from the client's system directly. This can be done through the general Lanier, Dictaphone C-phone or the basic $35.00 Radio Shack "special." Other services may require a system such as a PC Dart board installed in your computer, which is easy to do, or the service will provide its own technology and technical support to help you get set up. You will telecommute through communications software such as ProCOMM, or a system that is compatible with the service's or client's system, which a computer tech can set up .

Usually, services provide you with a list of equipment needs and all necessary instructions, which you must follow carefully. You needn't be a rocket scientist. I remember being terrified at the thought of taking my computer box apart to install a new piece of hardware. That wasn't in my area of expertise, and I felt so stupid I actually took a computer class called "What's In A Box." I experimented first by taking my old computer box apart, which was pretty cool. I felt like I had just conquered a new horizon. Now, that's history. Getting used to the Windows environment was not bad at all. As a DOS die-hard I was totally resistant to changing over to the windows environment, but now I love it. However, many services still use the faithful WP5.1, which is great for what we do — process words. I use both DOS and Windows now. It's very efficient, I might add . . . you could, too.

If you are interested in connecting with a service to supplement your slow time with your own clients, shop around. Here are a few things to look for, and some questions to ask:

Research Reputable Services: Look for services that are promoted in professional journals, those you may hear about through networking with other MTs at meetings, conventions, and through networking on the Internet. Often, there will be comments from MTs who have experience working for services. If you are curious, follow up and get additional information. Remember, though, ask respondents to address their comments to you through private e-mail, not publicly. For a broader perspective, contact more than one individual who has experience with a particular service

When you have selected the services you want to follow up with, call them . . . if their telephone numbers are available. Some services only publicize their fax numbers so resumes can be relayed; others do mass mailings to medical transcriptionists when they want to add MTs to their work pools; and still others buy space at conventions and seminars to market their services to prospective MTs.

Target market and required MT qualifications: To be well-informed, ask basic questions about services you are evaluating: Where is the home office located? What is their target market /client base (hospitals, clinics, physician accounts, etc.)? What type MT experience is required (CMT, acute care, etc.)? What work production requirements are they looking for (MTs who produce at least 100 minutes of dictation per day, MTs who are available on specific days, etc.)? If you apply to a service, they may ask you how many minutes of dictation you routinely produce and when you are available, which helps them evaluate where you would fit in their transcription pool.

What are the service's quality standards? This is very important because as medical transcriptionists we are committed to quality and need to know whom to access if there are problems with transcription and whether there are editors who monitor and conduct quality control checks on transcription. As IMTs we are responsible for doing quality control on every document we produce. If you work for a service, your quality control responsibilities will not change. Not only will you be required to meet your own quality standards but theirs as well. Your work will be screened and reviewed through their quality control system. Some services provide editors who routinely monitor work for accuracy on certain transcription accounts.

What is your rate of pay, when, and how? In order to understand and evaluate how you will be paid, you need to know specific details about how, when and how much each service compensates its transcriptionists. Ask when and how you will be paid, if direct deposit is available, and if taxes are taken out? Often, pay formulas are complex, so request a detailed description. The pay formula may vary depending on your experience and qualifications. CMTs, high volume/ high quality producers, and those who work at an advanced level of complexity often command higher pay. And remember, you will not be paid as much as you can make as an IMT; be prepared for half as much. Even so, service work can supplement your income during downtimes when your own work is slow.

What role do MTs play in your business operations? Many of the key player services now recognize the value and potential of utilizing experienced CMTs and qualified IMTs for many aspects of their business, not just keyboarding. Many transcriptionists work in service operations as partners, advisors, consultants, technicians, educators, editors, and instructors. Others are utilized as telemarketers to access clients and potential MTs.

What benefits and incentives are offered? Some services offer attractive benefit packages to home-based MTs, which was unheard of five years ago. Many services pay taxes, provide direct deposit of pay, offer company stock options, and other benefits and incentives to participating MTs. Currently, some services are considering offering health care packages, too.

How and with what frequency do you communicate with your MTs? Useful communication resources include newsletters, updates on equipment, laboratory, terminology and medication lists, and open communication and networking between MTs. Some services communicate very well with their MTs through Intranet e-mail and Internet connection, and often praise transcriptionists for their efforts in keeping work backlog up to date and clients happy. This is important when you are working remotely. A little praise goes a long way.

What MT training is required? Some services require a period of on-site training for newly recruited MTs but this, too, is becoming more convenient. Instead of requiring that new MTs go back to the service's head office for training, which is often not feasible for the MT, many services are sending their trainers to you, arranging a date and region that is convenient.

If you are interested, do your homework; you may not be disappointed. As IMTs we have gained a new respect for the medical transcription services of the

21st century. They are going global and, as part of effective long range planning, independent medical transcriptionist should consider what they have to offer in this global economy as a potential option to our own medical transcription businesses.

The authors of this book have worked long and hard as IMTs, and have seen many changes in the industry. Years ago we dreamed of eventually gassing up the motorhome and traveling together across our great nation. After that, we'd relocate to a cottage in some far away, exotic locale — perhaps the South of France or a tropical island paradise. There, occasionally gazing at the shimmer of sunlight on a sapphire blue bay, we'd spend our work days humming away at the keyboard, secure in the knowledge that the check was in the bank.

Independents' dreams can come true. Both authors of this book have recently made happy personal and career moves. Mary Glaccum, with her newly adopted son, relocated to a cozy suburban cottage in Southern California, where their life together is blossoming; and Donna Avila-Weil, with her youngest son, now lives and works in Hawaii, where they enjoy endless sunshine, palm trees swaying in the tradewinds, and ocean waves lapping at their ankles. As to their future, both Mary and Donna are planning ahead for further adventures. As independent medical transcriptionists, the possibilities are limitless.

THINKING GLOBALLY

At the dawning of this new century, we look back on an era that has been filled with change and uncertainty for our industry. The global economy continues to explode even through occasional recessionary periods, and we are swept up in growth. Throughout the world, MTs are providing their services as advisors and consultants, educators, reviewers and even as part of the worker-bee forces that keep our industry humming along at an incredible pace. Numerous articles have been written about these changes, which have already and will continue to impact our industry and the way in which we perform our jobs. There are, however, some things that have not changed, which are still very much a part of what we do and how we do it.

Those of us who have been a part of this industry before it became a profession — or even a job description — know that certain key issues have spanned three decades. Now, as in the past, our main concerns are recognition and compensation.

Technological Leaps: Technology has made great leaps in shortcutting and even bypassing the much-needed skills of medical transcriptionists, whose role has historically centered around helping provide health care providers with quality documents. Some years ago, technology was introduced which many thought would soon replace medical transcriptionists. In fact, promoters of the new technology, which utilized either voice activation or point-and-click systems, or both, touted it as a cost-effective way to eliminate the need for MTs.

As it turned out, this technology turned out to be a great disappointment to would-be users because it was too archaic, slow, complex, and time-consuming to train providers to use the equipment. Enthusiastic health care providers jumped on the technology, confident doctors would use it and that it would be a great time- and money-saver. Eventually, however, they tossed out the equipment or shoved it in a dark corner because health care professionals, especially doctors, did not have the time or patience to try to comprehend, let alone master, its complexities and foibles. Health care providers returned to MTs, who were able to take in garbage and turn out top quality, enduring bad dictation while producing excellent documents. Technology has not been able to replace our minds and bodies to meet the needs of the dictators and their scheduling demands. This same technology, however, is now being utilized to "enhance" the skills of the MT, and it is working very well in that capacity.

Capitation Complexities: Today in the managed care setting, health care providers are required to care for patient populations at a capitated fee, regardless of the condition or length of illness (e.g., $246.00 a year per head). This means that their performance must be geared for optimum productivity (just like medical transcriptionists) and now physicians and other health care providers are accountable to organizations they contract with to provide medical care for a negotiated dollar amount. If they do not, they may lose their contract! This situation impacts the entire industry. Capitation does not stop at the physician. The trickle-down effect impacts every health care provider, including medical transcriptionists. As physicians are required to accept capitated fees for patient "populations," many MTs are being approached by their clients to do the same.

The Bottom Line: Various reporting agencies, MCOs and HMOs require physicians and other health care providers to provide printed documentation to health care networks in order to get reimbursement for services. This is important to medical transcriptionists because our knowledge of medical language and keyboarding skills are necessary to provide timely, legible, quality documents that are utilized not only for patient information but to guarantee reimbursement for services provided. This also creates additional pressure on transcriptionists to provide timely turnaround of these documents. Once again, the bottom line is the almighty dollar. As long as quality and turnaround remain key issues, there will be a demand for our astute mind and body skills.

Monetary Compensation: Being compensated for what we do has always been and continues to be a serious issue. Some will argue that MTs should not be paid on a fee-for-service (by production) basis. Often, those who take this stand are salaried employees or former-employees-turned-consultants who believe fee-for-service demeans the value of the service we are providing. However, I have never talked with a single MT who works independently or for a service who is of this opinion. We are very proud of the service we provide and WE WANT TO BE COMPENSATED FOR IT. In our 65-plus years of collective transcription experience there has never been another way derived that can provide appropriate compensation for the MT, other than by what he or she produces. Other professionals who charge on a fee-for-service basis include lawyers, physicians, consultants, and many others.

Collecting Payment: Collecting payment from clients is still a challenge. We must be more assertive in negotiating with clients and developing skills needed to accomplish this. We must also recognize our worth. Many transcriptionists undervalue the skills we possess and the significance of our physical and monetary investments, so we hesitate to make demands for better work standards and compensation. To produce the highest quality transcription and remain competitive, we make significant investments in and utilize the most advanced technological upgrades, highest quality educational and reference materials, and network and communicate with health care professionals. Nevertheless, we are now paid less now than we were five years ago. What's worse, we are doing nothing about it.

Dictation Quality: Over the years, the way physicians dictate has not changed. Even with encouragement and coaxing, there are as many poor-quality dictators today as there were more than 30 years ago. Even though a few (and we emphasize the word *few*) medical programs briefly touch on communication skills and a few dictation how-tos, most do not. Most physicians learn about the requirement to dictate when they walk into their first hospital. Communication skills do not come naturally to most people, so why do we expect physicians to be different? Rumor has it that a medical transcriptionist is writing a book on how to teach physicians to dictate. Our question is . . . who will read it? If they don't have time to read their own dictation, what would inspire them to read a basic how-to book?

Once upon a time in health care, transcriptionists had to follow doctors from room to room taking shorthand notes, which would be transcribed later. Understandably, transcriptionists were thrilled when the first magnetic loops, or dictation belts, appeared on the scene. These were scratched on once like a phonograph record, transcribed and then tossed. Not all magnetic loops were tossed immediately, however. Because they came in pretty red and blue transparent colors, they were often used to make Christmas bows.

In bygone days we transcribed through static and scratching, echoes and various background noises, plus the not-too-good dictators and ESL physicians. In the 70s and early 80s, there were lots and lots of ESL MDs. So, we had to deal with not only the quality of the dictator's speaking, but the tape quality as well. Then came cassette tapes, which were a whole new world . . . so clear and precise. Now we can enjoy analog or digital, with sound quality so great we feel like we are in the same room as the dictator. To those transcriptionists who complain about not being able to hear or understand dictation, we say, today's quality is FABULOUS compared to what it was years ago!

Respect Is a Two-way Street: Don't take inept dictators personally. These guys are really getting beat-up on the Internet. In fact, doc bashing seems to be the main course in MT newsgroups these days. It is disappointing that real issues are being either overlooked or ignored because insulting doctors is so much easier. Sometimes, I think, it is difficult to see the big picture, to admit that there is so much more than medical transcription going on in medicine. Let's show a little more professional respect for what MDs and other health care providers endure. We want their respect; well, it's a two-way street.

We transcriptionists should be focusing on how we are doing our job, just as physicians are focusing on how they are delivering patient care, not on how they sound on a recording. Medical transcription plays a key role in the delivery of health care, but physicians play a vital role, accountable for hands-on quality patient care and the risks involved in the delivery of that care. They have good days and bad days just as we do. They have difficult, complex patients. We endure difficult and complex dictation.

Professional Recognition: This brings us to another issue that has not changed. Professional recognition. For decades we have encouraged our professional organization to pursue AMA recognition for medical transcription as an allied health care profession, yet we still go unrecognized. Until this happens we are virtually nonexistent to physicians as "health care professionals." Without official recognition, we are viewed as medical secretaries or typists, or transcriptionists, but not professionals.

Physicians are very aware of the importance of accurately transcribed medicolegal documents, but most are still oblivious to the professionalism of the staff producing and delivering these documents. Have you ever thought what would happen if every MT in the nation, or even in the acute-care setting alone, stopped doing transcription on a Wednesday morning at 8 a.m. and our keyboards were silent for the remainder of that week? By JCAHO standards, no H&P in the patient's record means the patient does not roll into the operating room. STOP. No H&P on the patient's chart within 24-hours of admission means that the health care standard is not being met . . . an operative report dictated and transcribed immediately following the procedure is standard . . . transcribed documentation that is utilized for coding and billing purposes would not be available . . . and the beat would continue to fade. The impact would be paralyzing to the health care industry. We are not getting the right people to listen!

Mandating Change: We can carry a lot of clout if we choose to take a stand, but it doesn't do us any good simply to think of ourselves as abused little children whose skills are unappreciated by the physicians we continually chastise for their wretched dictation and thoughtlessness. We don't have time for this. We should be mandating change for ourselves.

As the health care economy grows globally, our skills will be in more demand internationally. MTs now come from diverse backgrounds and potential candidates entering the field have so much to offer. Changes will continue, but the fact remains that the demand for timely documentation of health care records is growing throughout the world. We can provide positive support services to our clients. Transcriptionists who are strong and confident make a positive, competent impression on clients, who, in turn, will depend more readily on us to deliver quality service.

We must work harder at supporting each other individually and our profession as a whole. It is time we took a united stand, not presenting ourselves as a number of segregated entities. The focus on standards of style, line definition, education, and exposure are all of value, but as an IMT, there are issues that have never been adequately addressed. These include professional allied health care recognition, compensation for our professional skills and knowledge to produce quality health care documentation that is essential for quality of care, reimbursement and statistical data. We also need health care coverage, and many other benefits that we as a profession are entitled to.

Global Demand: The demand for MTs in the U.S. and abroad continues to increase steadily. According to D.P. Bhatt, Director of Cbay Systems, this increase was 20% in the last decade. As IMTs we must set our own standard in the industry as highly trained, skilled, competent and caring professionals. Our professional organization was founded to achieve professional recognition for the MT and it has accomplished much toward this goal. However, compensation needs are still not being addressed.

MTs United: Some have suggested forming another professional organization for independent MTs, but it would serve no purpose other than to segregate our industry even more. It would not carry any clout because our numbers are few and we are so specialized. The only organizational structure in the history of our nation that has been successful at addressing compensation for other industries is the union. Today increasing numbers of physicians are joining unions in an effort to take a stand against managed care and capitation cuts which have impacted their freedom and earning power tremendously. Perhaps the time has come for the MT industry to collectively address this as a viable option. Let's talk about it . . . we are nearing the state of a union!

Finances

"Money, which represents the prose of life, . . .
is in its effects and laws, as beautiful as roses."
—Ralph Waldo Emerson

Setting up an independent medical transcription business requires an investment of time and money. In the beginning, your dollar investment need not be great, but it must be managed well if you want your business to survive. As your business grows, consistent and regular money management will bring you not only economic success, but professional respect, too.

FINANCIAL NEEDS AND CAPITAL INVESTMENT

A home-based business can be established with little or no start-up capital. Your business is a labor intensive business — you provide a service. Initially you will need only a modest monetary investment in facilities and equipment. The greater investment will be the labor involved; that is, the service you offer which you will personally provide.

You will need little in the way of office facilities, and you may provide your services in facilities provided by your clients — on-site, on the client's premises — where you have free access to computers, copying machines and other equipment.

Perhaps you have enough personal working capital to get started on a modest scale, but you may soon find that you do not have enough operating capital to pay expenses right away or draw even a modest salary while your business is growing. This is a cash flow problem to avoid if possible.

Many entrepreneurs do not recognize the need for up-front operating capital. They assume that income will begin to flow as soon as they begin their business. There are two serious flaws to this line of reasoning:

1. **Your business may not start with a rush.** Most new businesses get off to a slow start. It usually takes time to develop business to the point where income exceeds expenses. This is especially true for a home-based venture.

2. **Cash may not flow in immediately.** Even if you acquire clients quickly and business is very good, it will still take some time for collections, or cash inflow. It depends on your billing practices and the length of time it takes clients to pay. Let's assume you bill on the 1st of each month.

If you start your account on the 10th of the month, you will work 20 days before you can bill, and the client will likely take another 15 or more days to pay the bill. On a full month, from the date the billing period starts until the time you receive payment could be 45 or more days.

Some of your clients may deliberately delay payment to you to enhance their cash flow. Soon, you may have a great deal of "billed out" money owed to you ("accounts receivable"). You need to collect that cash in order to pay your bills.

Instead of using personal savings, you may choose to take out a loan to get started. Do a monthly cash flow projection to forecast the cash you expect to receive and disburse during your first year or two.

It has been said that the little guy who can least afford to wait gets paid last — even by the federal government. Be prepared for slow collections at first, until you become established and develop some collection leverage with your clients.

WATCH YOUR COSTS AND EXPENSES

Cost reduction is important and cost avoidance even better, especially for a start-up business. The typical mistakes made by many novices are understandable.

You start out in business with enthusiasm, cheered on by friends and relatives. With this solid base of self-assurance and confidence, you begin with great style: handsome new furniture, shiny new equipment, expensive stationery, loads of office supplies, and a few extra goodies you could not resist. Almost all of this expense is not absolutely necessary!

You can do as much business at a secondhand desk, using modest stationery. If you purchase a computer and word processing system, think twice before you invest $3000 in a copier. A fax machine might prove a better value for you.

USING A BUSINESS CREDIT CARD

I don't know about you, but every year at tax time I find myself inundated with little bits and pieces of paper detailing my business expenses. Well, I have found the perfect solution . . . the American Express Gold Card.

Ten years ago, AMEX began offering its customers an end-of-year summary, detailing all transactions made on the card per year by categories (e.g., airline, travel, restaurant, merchandise, service fees, entertainment, health-related, etc.). I made the decision at that time to use this card only for business expenses. Don't get me wrong, I still save all my receipts. But, at the end of the year when I'm gathering and organizing financial data, it's so much easier to refer to my AMEX summary for itemizing tax deductions. Since almost all businesses accept the AMEX card, it is a very easy way to keep track of business expenses.

The annual fee for the AMEX card is $75/year, which is quite a bargain when you consider all the time spent, and time saved, getting paperwork ready for your accountant.

One special benefit to AMEX card users is a warranty extension on equipment. When using the AMEX card for equipment purchases, the company will double the warranty agreement. For instance, if you used your AMEX card to purchase a computer which came with a one year warranty, AMEX would extend the warranty for another year so the equipment would be covered for two years.

There is one major drawback in using the AMEX card, however. You must pay all charges as they are billed. There are no monthly installments. Therefore, before making any purchase, you must make sure you will have money in your business account to cover that expense when it becomes due and payable the following month. For more information regarding the credit card, call American Express.

- **American Express**
  800-635-5955

EQUIPMENT: LEASING OR RENTING VERSUS BUYING

"The primary benefits of renting office equipment are conserving up-front cash payment, potential cost savings, and convenience."

You can rent most equipment needed for a business including computers, printers, modems, copiers, or fax machines. The rental agreement may be for a period as short as a single day or for a year or more. If your need for computer equipment is short-term, it usually costs far less to rent than to buy.

Renting can serve as a low-cost way of sampling various pieces of equipment. If you are unsure about the features you need in a computer system, fax machine or copier, short-term renting is a good way to evaluate new or different technologies. If you need to upgrade your equipment within the first year of business, renting will probably offer greater flexibility to acquire equipment.

When starting your business, you may have enough money saved to cover the first three months of your new venture, but that money may be needed for operating expenses — not for purchasing equipment. Even if you want to make an equipment loan from a bank, local bankers may be wary of lending money to your new business.

Rental agencies retain ownership of rented equipment. The renter merely pays for the privilege of using it for a period of time. During the period of the rental agreement, the rental agency is usually obligated to service the equipment if it becomes inoperable. When necessary, the agency is also responsible for replacing the equipment in a timely fashion.

The primary benefits of renting office equipment are conserving up-front cash payment, potential cost savings, and convenience. You pay only for what you use, and may save money by avoiding a large purchase price. Renting should also save time. Rental agencies often have fairly extensive inventories, so they can promptly deliver what you need.

For tax purposes, rental fees, like lease payments, are considered business expenses and are fully tax-deductible. You won't be bothered with complex records of fixed assets and depreciation calculations at tax time.

If you think you will need temporary equipment beyond a few months, determine the most economically advantageous rental period. Monthly payments for personal computer rentals typically hover between 8-11% of the average retail price of the equipment. However, payments can go higher. After eight months to a year of renting, your rental payments will total approximately what you would have paid to buy the system.

Many computer stores offer computer systems for rent. Don't assume that local dealers will be cheaper or more efficient than national chain stores. Prices can vary greatly, so shop for the best bargains.

Don't hesitate to ask questions. Does the quoted price include a complete system? For a computer, will the necessary cables, monitor, video card, or keyboard cost extra? Does the quoted price include delivery and installation of the equipment at the beginning of the rental period and its dismantling and removal when the agreement expires? Does installation service include loading software onto the hard-disk? Does the quoted price include normal maintenance and emergency services?

The level of service offered may differ from vendor to vendor. Do you get prompt on-site service or is the service limited to a technician guiding you through a troubleshooting routine over the telephone?

LEASING EQUIPMENT

When building your business, it is helpful to know how to acquire the equipment you need when you need it. Although you may not have cash or credit to buy equipment outright, you may be able to lease equipment and create an efficient and cost-effective office.

A lease arrangement, with affordable monthly payments applied to the purchase price of equipment, is a viable option for many business owners on a limited budget. At the end of the lease agreement period, the business owner may own the equipment.

Large corporations frequently lease all or part of their office equipment. Among other things, they appreciate the increased flexibility and the convenience of equipment and financing neatly wrapped in one payment package.

The main advantages to leasing equipment are financial. Even though leasing is usually more expensive than buying outright, the ease of tax-deduction from lease expenditures may be more desirable than purchasing and depreciating equipment.

NOTE

IRS rules and regulations change frequently, so check with your accountant for specific information regarding depreciation.

Even though you may have ready cash to pay for office needs, leasing offers the advantage of cash conservation. In the beginning, you may need or want to put some of your cash to work in areas that will help generate profit. Instead of buying equipment, you may invest in advertising — business cards, fliers, and space advertising. Leasing allows you to manage cash flow, paying for your equipment over time.

Leasing equipment also gives you a little more leverage with the vendor if a piece of equipment is a "lemon."

In addition, leasing also offers you greater flexibility in terms of payment plans and equipment updates. Because the computer industry is changing at such a rapid pace and new technology is offered with incredible frequency, leasing minimizes your risk of having to use obsolete technology. If your business needs change mid-lease, you may be able to get more powerful equipment with little or no financing penalty. However, this depends on the specific type of lease.

Fixed monthly payments over time represent some savings in real dollars (i.e., your lease payments are made in increasingly devalued (inflated) dollars). In contrast, if you choose to purchase your equipment outright, every dollar you recover through depreciation is worth less due to inflation. Let's look at your leasing options.

- **The closed-end lease, or finance-lease**, allows you to actually purchase the equipment after the last installment has been paid. Generally the purchase price is either a percentage (often 10%) of the original price or a pro forma amount (usually $1). A closed-end lease is nothing more than a disguised loan.

- **An operating lease or open-end lease** offers you three options at the end of the agreement. You can purchase the equipment at its fair market value or blue book value. You can renegotiate and extend the lease, usually with new equipment. Or you can simply terminate the lease and the equipment reverts back to the lessor.

You must decide which type lease is best for you. If financing is your primary reason for leasing because you want to eventually own the equipment, the closed-end or finance lease may meet your needs. However, if your goal is to upgrade equipment conveniently and economically, your best bet is the open-end or operating lease. Consult your accountant before making a final decision.

Be aware that you will be paying more by leasing your equipment than by buying it outright. Like credit card loans, you are paying for the privilege of paying over time.

There is a simple formula used by lessors for calculating the monthly cost of a lease, applying a "rate factor" to the purchase price of the equipment. For example, if the rate factor on a three-year finance lease at $5000 were 0.035 or $35 per $1000, monthly payments on this lease would be $175 or five times $35. The rate factor can vary slightly depending on other provisions in the lease, such as payment timing and end-of-lease purchase agreements.

When shopping for a lease, look for one in which the total cost is as close as possible to the equipment's purchase price. Expect to pay a 33% premium if you lease instead of buy.

With a finance lease, shop for the lowest rate factor. To get the maximum benefit from an operating lease, consider the economic life of the equipment and your projected need for equipment upgrades. The ideal operating lease is one whose term actually coincides with the economic life of the leased equipment (the point when the equipment ceases to depreciate any further). At this point you can purchase it at the lowest possible price. If the lease term also corresponds to the "useful life" of the equipment (expiring at just about the time you would be upgrading your equipment), it gives you maximum flexibility in renegotiating the lease for new equipment.

WHEN NOT TO LEASE EQUIPMENT

Currently, Internal Revenue Code Section 179 allows immediate deduction for up to $24,000 per year of equipment purchases, and in 2003 the amount will increase to $25,000. With this immediate deduction, you can reduce your income taxes and thereby keep more of your hard-earned cash. Section 179 requires that you use your equipment for five years, so if you plan on trading in your system in three years, you may have to pay the IRS taxes related to the unused portion of the five-year depreciation period. So, generally, you are likely better off purchasing equipment and deducting it under Section 179 instead of leasing the equipment and taking the deduction over the lease period.

In general, leasing makes the most sense when you buy expensive equipment. A $2000 PC won't be worth the effort and expense of setting up a lease agreement. When computers first became affordable for home businesses, the technology was changing rapidly — by the micro-minute it seemed. Just when you thought you had purchased the latest turbo-driven computer, it seemingly became obsolete overnight. Leasing computers at that point made sense. For a very small outlay of cash, one was able to keep up with expanding technology. Now, however, computers have become very upgradable and it is not hard to keep up with the Jones'. However, in any case, always check with your tax adviser for advice on purchasing versus leasing in the context of your business situation.

There are other situations when leasing might not be a viable equipment option.

- You may not qualify. Some computer equipment lessors want to do business strictly with registered companies, preferably corporations with credit histories, and not with individuals.

- Some leases have riders that prohibit you from moving the equipment out of the state in which you received it. If relocation is a possibility within the next few years, leasing should be avoided.

- A leasing company lien may prevent you from selling the equipment before the lease has expired, even though, with a finance lease, you may eventually own the equipment.

You can't "prepay" a lease. Whereas most bank loans and mortgages allow the borrower to prepay without penalty, with leases you must pay your installments every month whether your business is thriving or floundering. This is generally no great risk to your business, but it is something you should be aware of.

PAYING YOURSELF

As a sole proprietor, how much are your services worth? Well, that depends on your gross receipts. As pointed out earlier in this book, you must save a portion of your gross income to pay such mundane things as self-employment (FICA) taxes, state and federal income taxes, health insurance, disability insurance and all business related expenses. According to most financial experts, your salary could be between 10-45% of your gross receipts. Being home-based medical transcriptionists, our overhead is fairly low once the large expenditures for equipment have been made. Therefore our percentage would be greater than that, say, of a building contractor who needs equipment and supplies and may be at the lower end of the pay scale.

Without question, it's tough to figure out your pay when you're self-employed. Take too little from the business and you begin to wonder why you ever kissed off that hospital job and its sweet biweekly paycheck. Take too much and your business may slowly go bust. That's why, according to most financial experts, it is better to err on the side of paying yourself too little. You can always give yourself a bonus at the end of the year.

One way to gauge your pay is to look at the age of your business. IMTs just starting in business shouldn't expect to draw a paycheck from the get-go. Financial experts advise that first-year owners take just enough to cover personal expenses, keeping the remaining revenues for business expenses. In general, it takes six months of steady cash flow — a sign that your business is viable — before you can cut yourself a monthly paycheck.

For service businesses such as ours, a good rule of thumb is to divide gross income into thirds. One-third goes to pay business overhead, one-third goes home, and the other third goes for taxes.

Unfortunately, accounts payable sometimes exceed receivables. Those of us who have been in business for awhile understand the fickle nature of medical transcription. Come flu season or Joint Commission, we are inundated with work and find ourselves sitting at our computers fourteen hours a day, seven days a week. Then comes summer vacation, and it seems that no one is dictating. Always ensure that you have enough cash in the bank to cover expenses in down times.

When money piles up in your account, don't be lulled into thinking you can cut yourself a bigger monthly paycheck. If there's one thing you can always count on, it's unexpected expenses, and a little spare cash may mean the difference between making it through a rocky period or folding up your headset.

TAX INCENTIVES: BUSINESS TAXES

*"A primary goal of any business should be
to operate in such a way as to avoid (legally!)
as many taxes as possible."*

Smart home-based medical transcriptionists should learn all they can about different types of business taxes in order to take advantage of tax savings opportunities. In reality, this can mean the difference between success or failure.

Learning all about taxes is not an easy task. In fact, one independent transcriptionist colleague recommends that anyone considering self-employment should investigate this area first. She recommends, "Go to the nearest IRS office and ask for information regarding self-employment. That alone may make you return to your previous job pleading temporary insanity when you gave your notice."

A primary goal of any business should be to operate in such a way as to avoid (legally!) as many taxes as possible. Appropriate deductions may be taken for home maintenance and improvements, automobile expenses, telephone expenses, office and work space, and major purchases, as well as for items like safe deposit rental, stationery and business cards. As a business owner you can also take advantage of tax-deferred retirement plans and tax-deductible medical insurance.

This chapter has been written to give you an overview and simplified understanding of tax law and practice. However, as stated before, it is imperative from the outset that you seek the counsel of an accountant who can guide you through specific tax issues and help you plan and implement strategies to minimize taxes.

Always bear in mind that being aware of how the tax system works, and paying only those taxes legally required, will be to your advantage. Knowing the facts about tax breaks will save you tax dollars, help you avoid unwise purchases, and guide you in better record keeping.

NOTE: Tax laws change frequently. What holds true today may not necessarily be the case in future years. Consult your accountant about tax law changes that may affect your business.

TYPES OF TAXES

"Business owners must pay taxes to federal,
state, and local governments."

Independent medical transcriptionists should never forget this old saying: "In this life you can be sure of only two things — death and taxes?" Well folks, you can run but you can't hide from the IRS.

There are home-based medical transcriptionists, as well as other independently employed professionals, who have not filed a tax return in years. Many feign ignorance of tax law; some have convinced themselves they don't owe any taxes and, therefore, are not required to file; others have procrastinated filing a return to the point of embarrassment, fear and denial; and a few simply think they can outsmart Uncle Sam.

However, the majority of tax evaders are caught and penalized heavily for not filing a proper return when it was due. Today's IRS computer system is very efficient in cross-checking earnings records in detail.

For most people, tax evasion also takes a personal toll in terms of physical, mental, and emotional stress. The longer the evasion, the greater the tension. After a time, personal and professional relationships, as well as business activities, may suffer.

Business owners must pay taxes to federal, state, and local governments. The following are the most common types of taxes.

FEDERAL TAXES

Federal taxes that apply to sole proprietors, partnerships, and S corporations, and their appropriate tax forms, are listed below. For **free** forms and publications, call your district IRS office, write to the government printing office or access them online at www.irs.gov.

Another terrific resource is the free CD called *The Small Business Resource Guide* (which is IRS Publication 3207). It is produced by the IRS and the U.S. Small Business Administration (SBA). There are versions for Windows or MacIntosh. This guide contains all of the business tax forms, instructions, and publications needed by small business owners. In addition, the CD provides an abundance of other helpful information with links to many resources provided on the Internet by IRS, SMA, U.S. Department of Commerce, U.S. Department of Labor, U.S. Social Security Administration, U.S. Census Bureau, OSHA, and other government agencies.

- **IRS District Office**
  800-TAX-FORM

- **U.S. Government Printing Office**
  Superintendent of Documents
  Washington, D.C. 20402

Or, particularly brave souls can call the IRS at the 800 number listed in the Government Pages of your telephone directory under "United States Government, IRS Forms."

- **1040** Individual Income Tax Return 1040C *Profit or Loss from Business or Profession*: This form is used to report the revenue, detailed deductible expenses, and resulting net income of your business.

- **1040ES** *Estimated Tax for Individuals*: This form is used to report quarterly best estimates of income tax you will owe for the calendar year, and to calculate amounts to pay quarterly.

- **1040SE** *Computation of Social Security Self-Employment Tax*: Your estimated tax payments will also include payment into your social security fund.

- **4562** *Depreciation and Amortization.*

If you have employees, you will also need to submit the following forms:

- **SS-4** With Circular E. This is the *Application for the Employer Identification Number (EIN)*: Circular E, the Employer's Tax Guide, explains the federal income and social security withholding requirements.

- **940** *Employer's Annual Federal Unemployment Tax Return*: This form is used to report and pay the Federal Unemployment Compensation Tax.

- **941** *Employer's Quarterly Federal Tax Return*: Use this form to report income tax withheld from employees' pay during the previous calendar quarter and social security tax that was withheld and matched by you, the employer.

- **W-2** *Employer's Wage and Tax Statement*: This form is used to report to the IRS and to your employees the taxes withheld and compensation paid to employees.

- **W-3** *Reconciliation/Transmittal of Income and Tax Statements*: This form is used to summarize information from the W-2 and is sent to the Social Security Administration.

- *Index to Tax Publications* (No. 048-004-01596-B)

- *Your Federal Income Tax* (Publication 17)

- *Tax Guide for Small Business* (Publication 334)

- *Starting a Business and Keeping Records* (Publication 583)

- *Business Reporting* (Publication 937)

- *Business Use of Your Car* (Publication 917)

- *Business Use of Your Home* (Publication 587)

- *Employer's Tax Guide* (Circular E)

- *Self-Employment Tax* (Publication 533)

- *Tax Information on Depreciation* (Publication 534)

- *Business expenses* (Publication 535)

- *Retirement Plans for Self-Employed* (Publication 560)

- *Information on Excise Taxes* (Publication 510)

- *Tax Withholding and Estimated Tax* (Publication 510)

- **U.S. General Services Administration**
  Consumer Information Center
  P.O. Box 100
  Pueblo, CO 81002

- *Financial Management: How to Make a Go of Your Business* (Publication 130Y)

- *Starting and Managing a Business from Your Home* (Publication 132Y)

FORM 1099 AND YOUR BUSINESS'S INCOME TAXES

If you work as a noncorporate independent contractor for hospitals, clinics or physicians and are paid more than $600 in commissions, fees or other compensation including payments to outsourcers, you should receive a 1099 form in February or March of each year. Form 1099 is like the W-2 form that employees receive. Copies are sent to the IRS, to the state taxing agency, and to you.

If you are a sole proprietor, you must report your 1099 income on form 1040, Schedule C, *Profit or Loss From Business or Profession*. Your business expenses are also recorded on this form. You should consult a tax adviser and read the book *Smart Tax Write-offs* to make sure you are taking all business deductions you are entitled to. You will also have to attach 1040, Schedule SE — *Computation of Social Security Self-Employment Tax*.

TAX DEPOSITS

Independent contractors must deposit three taxes each quarter:

- federal income tax

- social security self-employment tax

- state income tax

The deposits must be carefully calculated or the IRS and state taxing agency (Franchise Tax Board in California) will assess fines. As a self-employed individual, you will have to pay estimated taxes quarterly.

If in doubt about how much to pay, you should pay at least as much as you paid the previous year, and in most cases the IRS cannot penalize you for underpayment of estimated tax. When your clients pay you, be sure to set aside money for taxes, including self-employment tax (in 2001, 15.3% of the first $80,400 of income plus 2.9% of the excess; in 2002, 15.3% of the first $84,900 of income plus 2.9% of the excess). If you have any questions, it would be wise to talk to a tax consultant or call the IRS.

- **IRS**
  800-829-1040

The three taxes are paid with two forms: the federal 1040 ES (for federal income tax and social security self employment tax) and California's 540 ES (for state income tax). Tax deposits are due on April 15, June 15, September 15, and January 15.

NOTE

To avoid income tax penalties, you must prepay as estimated tax payments 90% of the taxes owed for the current year or the equivalent of 100% of your tax liability of the previous year, or 110%* if your previous year's adjusted gross income exceeded $150,000. (*112% for 2001)

Independent contractors pay taxes on their net income, which is gross income minus business expenses. An expense must be "reasonable and necessary" for it to be deductible. Exact deductions vary for each type of business and are continually changing. When estimating your business expense deductions it is wise to remember that the expenses must be "reasonable and necessary." Generally, the more you can prove something was used exclusively for your business, the easier it is to prove it is a legitimate deduction.

If you don't use equipment, car, or other items exclusively for business, you should keep records which clearly detail tax-deductible use: specific equipment used, dates of use, time, and purpose.

SOCIAL SECURITY TAXES (FICA)

All self-employed people must file a self-employment form when the annual profit claimed on Schedule C reaches $400. At this point, the self-employed person starts to pay into a personal social security account at a rate specified by the government. In 2001 the rate is 15.3% of the first $80,400 and 2.9% on any amount over $80,400. In 2002, the rate is 15.3% of the first $84,900 and 2.9% on any amount over $84,900.

Social security benefits are available to the self-employed just as they are to wage earners. Your payment of self-employment tax contributes to your coverage under the social security system, which should eventually provide you with retirement benefits and medical insurance benefits (Medicare). To learn the amount in your account, contact the Bureau of Data Processing.

- **Bureau of Data Processing**
  Social Security Benefits
  Baltimore, MD 21235

Paying this tax can be quite a shock, especially for those of us who worked as employees in the past. When working as an employee, the employee and employer each pay half of the social security tax. That advantage is lost, however, when a self-employed medical transcriptionist becomes solely responsible for payment of the entire tax.

The independent does get a break though since half the social security tax may be deducted from the self-employed's gross income.

CHECK YOUR SOCIAL SECURITY RECORD

The Social Security Administration (SSA) has thousands of uncredited earnings reports totaling hundreds of millions of dollars. If three years pass, the statute of limitations may prevent otherwise eligible recipients from correcting a mistake in their earnings records, and their social security benefits may be reduced as a result. Check your earnings record by filing SSA Form 7004 with your local SSA office. This is a free service and one which all independent MTs should take advantage of, especially since we are paying **all** our FICA taxes.

EMPLOYER'S IDENTIFICATION NUMBER (EIN)

Partnerships, corporations, and sole proprietors that have employees are required to have an Employer's Identification Number (EIN). Sole proprietors without employees have the option of using their social security number or obtaining an EIN number.

The purpose of the EIN is to facilitate record keeping by the government. Failure to use the number on the appropriate form can result in a fine of $50 each time it is omitted.

An EIN is obtained by filing IRS Form SS-4, which is available from the IRS.

ESTIMATED TAX PAYMENTS — A HORROR STORY!

Taxes are withheld throughout the year from wages earned by employees. However, as a self-employed individual, you are responsible for making periodic payments of your estimated federal income tax.

A case in point: When one of the authors went into business, she was naive about tax law. At the end of her first year, she dutifully met with an accountant to discuss taxes. She was horrified when he informed her that she owed $14,000 in federal and state taxes on April 15th — all because she had not been making quarterly tax payments.

To avoid such a catastrophe, have your accountant set up a schedule of quarterly tax payments, which are due April 15th, June 15th, September 15th, and January 15th. These will include payment of federal income tax, social security tax or self-employment tax, and state income tax. This procedure will help you avoid a shock to your system and your checkbook when April 15th rolls around.

To avoid penalties in most cases, you must prepay at least 90% of the taxes owed for the current year or the equivalent of 100% of your tax liability of the previous year. You can request estimated tax payment forms from the IRS. As stated above, your accountant will also be able to give you the needed forms and advice, calculating the amount you owe each quarter.

STATE TAXES

Taxes vary from state to state, but most have an income tax. This tax is calculated on net income and is usually due at the same time you file federal tax returns. In some states, the tax is calculated on gross income, less certain qualified deductions.

Some states require employers to carry Workers' Compensation Insurance for all employees. Even though it is called insurance, it feels like a tax. The program can be managed by the state or by the insurance agent who carries your other business insurance. Contact your state administrators to research this issue.

HOW TO EARN $40,000 NET INCOME

"Net income is determined by deducting from gross income the allowable expenses of doing business."

Earlier in the book we talked about netting $40,000 per year. As you will recall, we also stated that in order to do so, you would need to **gross** $80,000 for that year. Net income is determined by deducting from gross income the allowable expenses of doing business. Following is a scenario showing estimates of typical business expenses and how they contribute toward "netting $40,000" from an $80,000 gross income.

Remember that these are just your business expenses. In order to determine your personal taxable income, you also need to consider your itemized deductions, personal exemptions, and your personal income from other sources, such as interest income, etc.

NET INCOME CALCULATION

Gross income	$80,000
Less expenses	32,660
Taxable business income	47,340
Less self-employment tax	7,240
"Net"	40,100

BUSINESS INCOME TAX DEDUCTIONS

- **Automobile** $ 3,000
  The greater of 34.5 cents for 2001 (36.5 cents for 2002) or actual expenses, which includes DMV, maintenance, insurance, gas and oil.
- **Office Supplies:**

Laser printer cartridges	750
Laser toner	260
Printer paper	460
Fax paper	100
File folders	30
Tape cassettes	60
Pens/pencils	50
Pencil sharpener	50
Appointment book	30
Dot matrix printer ribbons	310
Ledger book	50

• **Convention/trade shows**	1,200
• **Courier** ($15 per day)	3,900
• **Gifts to business organizations**	300
• **Dues & fees to professional organizations**	260
• **Education**	150
• **Entertainment of clients**	300
• **Insurance**	
Health	1,270
Disability (incorporated businesses only)	1,580
Life insurance (incorporated businesses only)	2,500
Special rider for home business ($50 per month)	600
• **Cleaning person** ($30 per week)	1,560

- **Legal/professional fees**
  - Computer consultant   300
  - CPA   200
  - Lawyer   500
- **Licenses/permits/fees**
  - Business license   100
  - DBA   100
- **Service contracts**
  - Digital systems   85
  - Transcribers   ($250 each)   500
  - Fax machine   225
- **Mail box rental**   55
- **Outsourcers (Subcontractors)** (overflow)   1,800
- **Postage**   150
- **Print communications**
  - Stationery   225
  - Business cards   50
  - Fliers   145
  - Brochures   225
- **Promotional costs**   225
- **Repairs to business equipment**
  - Computer   225
  - Printer   500
- **Safe deposit box**   75
- **Subscriptions/reference material**   500
- **Tax preparation fees**   300
- **Travel for business only**
  - Plane   750
  - Car rental   200
  - Auto storage   100
  - Parking   75
  - Meals   175
  - Tips   50
  - Telephone & fax   30
  - Hotel room   1,050
  - Laundry   75
- **Rent/lease expenses**   1,900
- **Depreciation** (including Sec. 179 expense)   2,500
- **Interest on business loan**   500

TOTAL EXPENSES   **$32,660**

HOME-SWEET-TAX-DEDUCTION

*"**You** have to do the thinking and recordkeeping in order
to maximize your tax deductions. Do not assume
that your tax-return preparer will think of
all of **your** potential deductions. "*
—Norm Ray, *Smart Tax Write-offs*

As a home-based business owner, you qualify for tax deductions for your home office — either as a portion of your rent or as depreciation. The amount of the allowable deduction is based on the percent of the home used for business purposes. For tax deduction purposes, the home-based office must meet the following criteria:

- Clearly separated from family living space

- Used exclusively for business purposes

- Used on a regular basis for business purposes

- Used as your principal place of business or used as a meeting place for you to interact with clients.

Keep in mind, however, that any business deduction taken for depreciation of your home office reduces the tax basis of your home and normally must be "recaptured" when you sell your home. "Recaptured" means you will pay income taxes at your regular rate instead of at the lower capital gains rate on that portion of your home sale profit represented by your home office depreciation.

There are two ways to calculate the percent of your home used for business purposes:

- One method is to divide the square feet in the home by the number of square feet used for business purposes. Thus, if in a 3000 square foot home, 1000 square feet of space is used for business, 33-1/3% of applicable home expenses can be claimed as a tax deduction.

- The other method for figuring space is to count the number of rooms (if they are nearly equal in size) and divide the number of rooms used for business purposes by the total number of rooms. If one room is used in a five-room house, then 1/5 or 20% of the home expenses are legitimate home-use business deductions.

Either method is acceptable, so use the one that results in the best benefit to you.

A percentage of the expenses listed below can be deducted from income as business expenses:

- Rent

- Mortgage interest

- Insurance premiums on home

- Utilities, including gas, electricity, and water

- Services such as trash and snow removal, house cleaning, and yard maintenance expenses

- Home repairs, including labor and supplies

The TOTAL amount of the following expenses are also tax-deductible:

- Decorating, painting, and remodeling costs for the part of the home used solely for business purposes.

- Telephone — all long distance business calls and charges for extra business related services.

WHEN THE HOME OFFICE DEDUCTION IS NOT THE BEST OPTION

According to stringent IRS rulings, any home office that qualifies for the deduction must be a distinct space that is specifically used for business. If you qualify for and take the deduction, when you subsequently sell your home, you may be forced to shell out income tax on the business portion of your gain instead of rolling all the profit into a reduction of the tax basis of your new home.

Here's how the IRS sees it: If a taxpayer claims a deduction for an in-home office, he or she has changed that portion of the property to a commercial tax status. So in the year the taxpayer sells the property, the business portion may not qualify for the much easier rules that allow rollover of the gain from the sale of the residential portion. Depending on your individual tax situation, you may want to plan ahead concerning the sale of your home and make sure it's considered a 100% residential property by claiming no home-office depreciation deductions.

> *"Taxes are what we pay for civilized society."*
> —Oliver Wendell Holmes, Jr., 1904

AUTOMOBILE EXPENSES

The legitimate business use of a car can generate significant tax deductions for small-business owners. Commuting is not deductible, but other business travel is: picking up and delivering work, client meetings, trips to the post office, trips to office supply stores, etc.

Keeping a mileage log in your car to document business use is still a smart idea. In addition to keeping a log book, keep the first and last repair bills of the year. If the car's mileage has been noted at the time of repair, you can present the bills to the IRS as proof of the number of miles you drove through the tax year.

The IRS offers two alternative methods for calculating the amount of automobile expenses:

1) **Standard mileage rate** method provides an umbrella deduction equal to the number of business miles you have driven during the year multiplied by 34.5 cents per mile in 2001 (36.5 cents per mile in 2002). The standard mileage rate covers the cost of operating the car, including depreciation, maintenance and repairs, gasoline, oil, insurance and vehicle registration fees. Under this method, those expenditures are not separately deductible, but you can deduct tolls and parking fees in addition to the standard mileage rate calculation.

2) **Actual car expenses** method allows you to deduct the exact costs of each of the above items, as well as tires, garage rental fees, lease payment and even rental car costs. However, you can deduct only the percentage related to the business use of the car. If your records show that you drove 10,000 miles during

the year but only 4000 miles were business-related, you can deduct only 40% of actual car expenses.

The IRS lets you choose whichever method will lead to the higher deduction, so it is in your best interest to do both calculations. Remember, if you use a car primarily for business, the actual car expenses method may provide a significantly better deduction.

There are exceptions to the rules, most of which impact the deductibility of your car expenses, including lease payments and depreciation. The first "gotcha" is that if you use the standard mileage rate method the first time you report business use of your car to the Internal Revenue Service, you cannot subsequently depreciate that particular car using the accelerated depreciation method. However, if you calculate your first deduction using the actual expense method, you are allowed to toggle between the two methods in subsequent years.

Under the actual car expenses method, the total amount you can include for depreciation has IRS limitations. These are varying limits based on the year you start using your car for business and on the specific year of the depreciation.

Depreciation deductions apply only to cars you buy outright. If you lease a car, still more rules and exceptions apply. Lease payments are fully deductible if the car is used solely for business. If not, the deductible amount is in proportion to the percentage of miles driven for business. But Section 280F of the IRS code stipulates an add-back, an amount keyed to the value of the car, that you must declare as taxable income. The government's intent is to place a cap on the lease deduction that is equivalent to the ceiling on a depreciation deduction.

It is best to sit down with your accountant while you are shopping for that new car, not after you buy it. The two of you should calculate the tax deductions for both buying and leasing based on the assumed business use percentage including the add-back.

> *"The legitimate business use of a car can generate significant tax deductions for small-business owners."*

INTEREST ON CAR LOANS

You can deduct interest on the business use portion of a car loan. The nonbusiness use percentage is considered nondeductible interest on a personal loan.

WHO SHOULD LEASE AND WHO SHOULD BUY?

Consider leasing a car if you:

- enjoy having a new car every 2-3 years
- want to drive a more expensive car and still have lower monthly payments
- enjoy having the option of not making a down payment
- enjoy having a car that's always in warranty in case something goes wrong
- hate having to sell or trade your old cars
- don't like tying up your money in depreciating assets

Consider buying a car if you:

- typically drive your cars for several years or until they fall apart
- drive more than 15,000 miles a year on average
- usually sell or trade your cars before they are fully paid for
- drive your cars hard or under rough conditions
- typically buy fad cars that quickly lose their resale value
- like to know you own your car

BUSINESS-RELATED TRAVEL EXPENSES

Whether you travel by air, rail, bus, or personal automobile, your expenses associated with travel for business purposes are tax-deductible. Make it a habit to save your ticket stubs, credit card slips and checks to present as evidence of travel expenses, and make notes on items to document the business activity.

EDUCATION EXPENSES

An added benefit of joining a professional association is that expenses incurred in attending meetings, including travel expenses, symposium or convention fees, and books can be tax-deductible.

Education expense is deductible if the education improves or maintains a skill required in your business. However, if the education is required to meet minimum education requirements of your present business, or if the education will qualify you for a new trade or business, the expense is not allowed. Incidentally, any self-employed medical transcriptionist can take a course in bookkeeping, computers or any other course that helps you run your business better and deduct the cost as a business expense.

EXPENSING AND DEPRECIATION

Expensing means taking an income tax deduction for the entire cost of an item in the year it is purchased, up to a current limit of $24,000 per year in 2001 and 2002 ($25,000 in 2003). *Depreciation* is taking a deduction for business property ratably over its useful life of more than one year — usually at least five years.

Expensing is usually preferable to depreciation because a tax write-off (resulting in cash in your pocket instead of Uncle Sam's pocket) is more valuable earlier than later. However, under certain circumstances, depreciation may be preferable. Remember that the IRS does change depreciation rules periodically, so it might be wise to expense while you can. Again, check with your accountant and refer to IRS Publication 334 for small businesses.

RECORDS NEEDED FOR TAX PURPOSES

Keep all receipts for business expenses and keep all miscellaneous receipts for out-of-pocket purchases, noting what was purchased on the back of the receipt. Use an accordion file for storing all your receipts and checks for the year. This will help tremendously around tax time.

Your business checkbook will also be a valuable resource at tax time to calculate tax-deductible expenditures. The IRS can investigate a return for up to three years after it has been filed, so keep all records for at least three years. In fact, it wouldn't be a bad idea to keep them for seven years or as long as you operate the business.

> *"Keep all receipts for business expenses and keep all miscellaneous receipts for out-of-pocket purchases."*

388

TAX SHELTERING THROUGH RETIREMENT PLANS

*"Tax sheltering is an excellent way to protect
your hard-earned money."*

As your business grows and prospers, you should consider tax sheltering as a way to better protect your hard-earned money. A retirement plan tax shelter allows you to reduce taxes by investing a portion of your pretax income in special programs designed to defer payment of taxes. Taxes are not avoided but simply postponed until you withdraw money from your fund at a later time, usually during retirement, when, presumably, you will be in a lower tax bracket.

Popular tax sheltering plans include the Simplified Employee Pension (SEP), Individual Retirement Account (IRA), and Qualified Profit Sharing Plans (Defined Benefit or Defined Contribution).

SIMPLIFIED EMPLOYEE PENSION (SEP)

A Simplified Employee Pension (SEP) is a retirement program whereby an employer makes contributions into employees' IRA accounts. For your one-person business, the pretax contribution is into your IRA. The SEP plan allows a higher contribution than an individual IRA and can be made to owner/employees over 70½ years old. The maximum contribution to a SEP is the lesser of 15% of employee compensation or $35,000 for 2001 ($40,000 for 2002). For the owner of a sole proprietorship the maximum contribution is limited to 13.043% of net Schedule C income less one half of self-employment tax percent.

SEPs are attractive for the following reasons:

- They are simple and easy to establish

- They can be established after the close of your business year and after April 15th

- They don't require IRS filing or Form 5500 reporting (which are required in profit sharing plans)

- There are no administration costs

- Contributions are tax deductible and elective (they do not have to be made every year)

- Contribution amount may vary from year to year, from zero to 15%

INDIVIDUAL RETIREMENT ACCOUNT (IRA)

The Individual Retirement Account (IRA) provides an opportunity for you to establish a personal retirement program using pretax dollars. There are two conditions that must be met in order to qualify for this plan: 1) You must not participate in any other type of retirement plan (other than social security), and 2) your adjusted gross income must be less than $43,000 in order to have full deductibility.

If you meet the above criteria, the amount saved and earnings generated by an IRA are not currently taxable. The tax-free status continues until you retire. Even if you do not meet the above qualifications, you can put money into an IRA although the money deposited is not fully tax-deductible. However, the income earned on the account's investment is not taxed until withdrawal. The maximum amount you can contribute yearly to an IRA is $2000 for 2001 ($3000 for 2002).

Although the IRA is not taxed until payments are received, after age 59½, IRA funds may be withdrawn without a 10% penalty should you become disabled. In the event of your death, the funds are paid to your beneficiary. You can also withdraw IRA funds without penalty in order to pay some medical expenses.

IRA plans are available through banks and savings and loans (certificates of deposit), money market and mutual funds, stockbroker-managed or self-directed IRA accounts, insurance companies annuity plans, and United States minted gold.

HEALTH INSURANCE

If you are a sole proprietor, partner in a partnership, or owner of an S corporation, you are allowed an income tax deduction of 60% of the cost of health insurance in 2001, 70% for 2002, and 100% after 2002. According to *Smart Tax Write-offs*, Rayve Productions, there is a way to make your personal health insurance premium 100% deductible now. Your business can enroll your employee-spouse as an insured employee in your business's health insurance plan. The insurance premium for this employee is fully deductible, and you can then be covered in the plan as his or her spouse.

SHOULD YOU HIRE AN ACCOUNTANT, BOOKKEEPER OR TAX PREPARER?

Most of us have had experience balancing our own checkbooks and know some basic bookkeeping principles. However, business bookkeeping is much more detailed, and savvy professionals seek the best possible counsel affordable when establishing an accounting system.

We recommend that you work with an accountant and/or a tax adviser. A knowledgeable bookkeeper may also be capable of setting up a basic system.

An accountant should be consulted a minimum of once or twice a year to analyze the books, prepare and analyze financial statements, and help with tax returns. The accountant can also advise you on financial decisions and help to chart the future course of your business based on an analysis of your financial records.

It is unfortunate, but true, that many businesses fail because of inadequate financial planning and visibility. It is crucial to set up and maintain a system that will be comfortable for you to maintain and use as a tool for running your business smartly.

Do your homework. Review a book such as *Easy Financials for Your Home-based Business* in order to get a basic understanding of your available choices. Then confer with a knowledgeable professional to help you set up your system. It is well worth your investment in time and money to set up a system that will give you the visibility to manage your business successfully. And these professional expenses are tax-deductible.

Beware of hiring a tax preparer instead of an accountant. This could cost you considerable money in the long run. Tax preparers may only be capable of working with the numbers you provide them and may not have the experience to pursue available tax breaks aggressively.

On the other hand, an accountant who is knowledgeable about your type of business will be aware of tax advantages, suggesting desirable business actions. It is likely that the accountant will save you more money than his or her fees.

How do you select an accountant or a bookkeeper? Ask professional associates for recommendations. Carefully evaluate training, experience and references.

It is important to find an accountant or bookkeeper who has experience working with small businesses. To prevent any unpleasant surprises, be sure to discuss fees in advance with the bookkeeping or accounting service.

Why Businesses Fail

"When all is said and done,
there's much more said than done."

—Anonymous

Businesses fail for a variety of reasons, most of which are not extraordinary. If you plan your business carefully, learn from the wisdom (and mistakes) of others, and consistently and regularly manage well, your chances of business success are greatly increased. From time to time, you should evaluate your business, and if you find weak areas, correct them immediately. Following are basic weaknesses usually found in troubled businesses.

LACK OF PLANNING

Poor planning, or no planning at all, results in hit-or-miss control of your business. Work out a plan of operation, develop measurable goals and objectives, and monitor your progress.

INEXPERIENCE

Managing yourself as an independent requires skill and knowledge. You must devote time to studying good business practices, consult experts frequently for advice and guidance, and follow through with continuing education. This is how professionals succeed.

INSUFFICIENT FINANCIAL RECORDS

Without complete daily figures showing the financial condition of your business, you are working in the dark. With proper financial records you can spot excessive costs, waste, and other drains on your profits. Keep figures current — old figures are worthless. It's also important to monitor industry trends and manage your business accordingly.

INADEQUATE CASH RESERVES

Put money aside regularly into a savings account, even if only a small amount. A cash reserve will provide needed working capital, act as a hedge against unexpected income declines or unexpected emergencies, and enhance your credit rating.

EXCESSIVE OVERHEAD

The steady trend toward higher costs and prices makes control of overhead doubly important. Budget your operating expenses. Carelessness, waste, errors, and general inefficiency may account for 10-20% of your overhead.

OVEREXPANSION

Enthusiasm is a vital ingredient in the growth and progress of a business, but slow, steady growth is safer than rapid, uncontrolled growth. Try not to take on more than you can handle.

COMPLACENCY

Do not allow yourself to become too content with the status quo. To maintain a competitive edge, always look for ways to improve your service and efficiency and reduce overhead costs.

> *"Most people don't plan to fail; they fail to plan."*
> —John L. Beckley

IGNORING COMPETITION

Some of your competitors are more successful than you; others are not. Study their methods and operations and make a conscious decision to avoid known pitfalls while moving forward with successful endeavors. Become a leader, not a follower, and try to understand that there is strength in competition!

POOR SALESMANSHIP, POOR SERVICE

Be aware of new technology and focus on continuing education to provide optimum service. Know how to effectively present yourself and your product, and consistently provide excellent service and follow-up.

What's Ahead?

"Champions keep playing until they get it right. "

— Billie Jean King

Throughout this book, we have discussed how technology and the home-based workplace have changed the way we do business. Working from home has been and is still the hot topic as we move into the new millennium. Medical transcription is a multibillion-dollar industry that continues to evolve along with technological advances. Telecommunication and the utilization of Web-based service providers continues to make access to a global client base even more efficient even for the independent transcriptionist. Clients benefit from reduced turnaround time and medical transcriptionists benefit from increased productivity and more flexible working conditions. It's a win-win situation for all.

According to the Information Technology Association of America (ITAA), 346,000 information technology jobs are vacant in the United States; and only about 40,000 students graduate in computer science per year. According to the U.S. Department of Labor, medical transcriptionists, court reporters and stenographers held about 110,000 jobs in 1998 in the United States. More than one in four were self-employed. About one in four worked for hospitals and physicians' offices, reflecting the concentration of medical transcriptionists in health care services. And, this does not include the global pool of medical transcriptionists that now are employed by medical transcription services and other health care entities.

The overall demand for medical transcriptionists, court reporters and stenographers is projected to grow about as much as the average for all occupations through 2008, and it is projected that the employment growth among medical transcriptionists may be offset by the decline among stenographers.

The demand for medical transcriptionists is expected to increase due to rapid growth in health care industries spurred by a growing and aging population and the continued demand for more detailed documentation of every aspect of the patient care experience.

Speech recognition technology has made more advancements in the last two years than in the past 20 years. However, these advancements are not projected to reduce the need for medical transcriptionists but will modify the role of the MT in some respects to include editing skills for reviewing document accuracy generated by speech recognition technology. Growing numbers of medical transcriptionists will be needed to amend patients' records, edit grammar, and discover discrepancies in medical records.

Medical transcription is now a global enterprise. Many services are now utilizing medical transcriptionists in other countries, there are international medical transcription services accessing health care clients globally, and the beat goes on. This trend opens many doors for experienced MTs, who now have alternative career paths in the global market, traveling to provide their expertise as consultants for new services and clients starting medical transcription careers.

Each of us has, in large measure, control of our destiny, and it is up to us to evaluate and decide which of the myriad career opportunities we will follow in the years ahead. Then, to achieve the greatest success in our endeavors, we must strive to remain on the cutting edge of information and technology.

Periodically take time to re-evaluate your skills, reposition your career and modify your thinking. It is the knowledge of the medical language that sets the medical transcriptionist apart from all other health care professionals — that undeniable quality that can turn a health provider's thoughts into clear, concise, legible medical language — and it will be this knowledge, in conjunction with excellent transcription skills, that continues to set us apart in the years to come.

By focusing on the cornerstone of knowledge, we have positioned ourselves to quickly adapt to the dizzying array of new technologies that are either here or in development, including speech recognition, Web-based services, digital and wave technology, hardware and software, and technology will only be successful if the medical language it produces is of high quality that meets the standard of excellence. That standard can be reached only under the judgment and careful eye of the medical language expert.

Will Technology Replace Medical Transcriptionists?

"Destiny is not a matter of chance,
it is a matter of choice;
it is not a thing to be waited for,
it is a thing to be achieved."

—William Jennings Bryan

It is highly unlikely, even with advanced technology and sophisticated software, that medical transcriptionists will become obsolete. The complexity and variety of patients, medical conditions, and physicians will continue to require the human element — especially intelligent, well-trained medical transcriptionists — in medical record quality management.

No two patients are exactly the same. "Routine" procedures and "standard" treatment plans are diverse. Physicians will continue to dictate with accents, rapidity, mumbles, missing and incorrect words, inappropriate comments, sneezes and coughs.

Human intelligence and logical thinking will be necessary to transcribe correct medical terms when dictation isn't clear — "Metatarsal" or "metacarpal?" "Atherosclerosis" or "arteriosclerosis?" Medical transcriptionists have the skills to do this.

Medical treatments and technology will continue to grow more complex, requiring flexibility and continual information updating. Computer systems alone will not be able to meet the medical record requirements of the future.

The refinement of voice-activated technology is on the horizon, and the role of the medical transcriptionist will undoubtedly change with the advent of more sophisticated technology. As medical language specialists, transcriptionists will be a vital link in editorial and quality assurance activities, developing or assisting with development of hardware and software, and taking on new career challenges as opportunities arise.

CHALLENGES, CHOICES AND CHANGE

As medical transcriptionists we are a profession of high achievers, obsessive and compulsive about our work. At times we overcommit and can't say "no" and knock ourselves out to be the best that we can be. We are justifiably proud of the service we provide. We like to control our work environment, but our environment is changing. Like many others before it, the medical transcription industry is going global; it is, in fact, now a reality.

Transcription services are sending transcription overseas to countries such as India and the West Indies. The concern, of course, is loss of jobs in the U.S. This is a burning issue. It is creating a division in the medical transcription industry between those who feel threatened and are resisting change and those who realize that changes represent additional resources and opportunities to fill needs on a global scale.

The trend toward globalization of medical transcription, which many are not prepared to face, has created an atmosphere of anger and insecurity in our industry. Each of us wants to have control of his or her destiny. That is why we choose to remain independent. However, sticking our heads in the sand will not make inevitable industry changes disappear. Instead, when we pull our heads out of the sand, we'll discover even greater changes and, because we will have fallen so far behind, we will be lost.

Why are services seeking offshore transcriptionists? Because there have never been enough "qualified" hospital-level medical transcriptionists to fill the need. There are plenty of entry-level transcriptionists and qualified clinical transcriptionists, but training entry-level and hospital-level MTs has always been a problem. Transcription programs and schools can pump out graduates in twelve-week to two-year programs, but even after completing a two-year program, MTs have great difficulty finding a hospital that will offer them entry-level positions. Acute-care facilities, which are usually already backlogged and do not have staff available to train new recruits, want "experienced" MTs. It is a catch-22 situation. Unfortunately, as multitudes of health care facilities continue to restructure and downsize, training programs for MTs are simply not viable options within those settings.

Twenty-five years ago there was no medical transcription industry as we know it today. It was a profession striving to be recognized. There were true pioneers like Bob Seale and Sally Pittman, one who built a transcription service empire and the other with a vision of a professional medical transcription organization that would offer membership and certification and be dedicated to promoting our profession through creativity, resourcefulness and innovation.

Visionaries like Bob Seale and Sally Pittman never promised that the world of medical transcription would remain the same forever; they realized that change is an inevitable fact of life. Their innovations grew and expanded, and there were more that followed. The "profession" became a business and evolved into a multibillion dollar industry in which there have been divisions, reorganizations, mergers and affiliations.

The medical transcription industry playing field is very different today than it was 25 years ago, especially for independent medical transcriptionists. Twenty-five years ago there was no such thing as an IMT. We were hidden in the closet, a virtually silent work force, like wine tasting in the Napa Valley used to be. Now it is the rage. We have arrived! Thousands are striving to homebase. This is no cottage industry. It is a revolution into independence. But, each day holds a challenge, and there are many changes yet to come. The biggest challenge is to remain competitive in today's marketplace.

POSITIONING YOUR BUSINESS IN THE GLOBAL MARKETPLACE

How do we position ourselves to compete successfully in the global marketplace? We continue to work on our image and our service. Ask yourself these questions:

- What is special about the service I provide my clients?

- What professional image do I reflect? A business image is every bit as critical to your success as your skills.

- What is my strategic plan for providing the best service to my clients?

- What makes my service stand apart from my competitors?

Have you evaluated your business services recently? You should do this at least biannually. Remember, nothing lasts forever! Clients who are here today may be gone tomorrow. What is your strategic plan when you lose a client? How will you market your services to potential clients? Building and operating your business is an ongoing process, just as your processes for improvement should be ongoing. Your goal is to be the best that you can be. Your objectives should include vision, commitment and persistence. Be proactive in your plans for improving your business and your own professional development. Have some processes in place in the event of possible loss of a client or revenue. Constantly seek out and research new industry trends that may affect the way in which you do your work. Have access to technical support in the event of unexpected equipment failure. Keep your technology up-to-date so that your business will remain competitive.

Take responsibility as an independent business owner. Be accountable, consistent, reliable and qualified in the work you are committing to. Follow through with this image in your physical appearance, the physical appearance of your office and how you present yourself to your clients. Your answering machine message should project professionalism, as should your stationery and business cards. Your voice should always be positive and professional.

Be consistent in your project follow-through. When business is slow keep up a positive appearance, even when you're feeling low. Use your downtime to do quality audits of your work and pay attention to details. This can be done by reviewing a number of reports selected randomly within a selected time frame (e.g., 15 days, 30 days). Review the documents and point score errors for punctuation (.25), grammar (.75), dropped letters (.50) typos (1), wrong words (1), etc. Grade yourself. Keep audit logs and quality/productivity reports at designated times during each quarter cycle. Review what can be improved upon. You may find from these self-audits that you can benefit from improving your technical skills and knowledge base. Catch up on reading about industry trends, and attend trade shows and workshops. The more exposure you get the more informed you will become.

Be smart about your business investments. Cost containment is important. Avoid investing in equipment and technology that is just a "fad." Research the market. Don't run out and buy the latest and the greatest just so you can brag about it on the Internet or keep up with the Joneses. Carefully evaluate your options, network with others regarding what is working for them. It's okay to step back for a time and see which way the tree is going to fall. Products are not always what they are touted to be. The true test is in the hands of the user. Your safest bet is to go with a product that has been established in the marketplace and will suit the needs of your clients. Research technical support and make sure you have a backup for downtime that might occur with equipment failure.

As far as the services you provide your client, the trend is toward service, service, service. Tailor your services to suit your client's needs, not yours. This is an area where you can truly stand out from competing businesses by offering your client the best of the best.

Marketing is still a serious issue for many independent medical transcriptionists. There are those who have only targeted local resources, which is okay, but this could change suddenly. With a change of office staff, a new office manager, new medical director, or often the chief financial officer may make the decision not to use your services and/or to go with a larger service whose bid is lower than what your are charging. Suddenly, with scarcely any notice, you could find yourself without a client. It is never wise to put all your eggs in one basket. This cannot be emphasized enough.

To remain competitive, you should continually improve your knowledge base, flexibility and diversity. Continuing education is key. You will also benefit by mastering the ability to be flexible and adapt when necessary to changes in the work schedule. Peaks and valleys occur often. Have a backup plan in place. The more diverse your talents as an MT, the more valuable you will be. You should continue to build on your transcription base whenever possible.

If you fear being without a job because transcription work is going offshore, then quit whining and do something about it. Most of those jobs are hospital-level transcription positions. The good old U.S. of A. isn't the only country where there are highly educated and qualified people, and in some countries they are better educated! You still have the choice to be the best that you can be. In our 60-plus years as MTs, we have never ever been without work. More often than not, there is more work than there are qualified MTs. Are you threatened because you are underqualified? Or are you threatened because you do not see the "big picture" and are lacking full awareness of what is going on within the medical transcription industry. You have choices. Do something about it. Think about improving your knowledge base, take that anatomy/physiology course, English grammar course, and advanced terminology course. Attempt to attain a higher level of expertise not only in medical transcription but about technology, because the most technically savvy will merit higher pay. Learning everything you can about telecommuting will improve your position in the market. There are educational opportunities through local, state, regional and national programs. Organizational membership is not required for attendance. If you have no telecommuting experience, network with other telecommuting MTs. This is an area you must pursue. Telecommuting is no longer the future . . . it is the NOW. Limiting yourself to your little comfort zone may lead to your demise in the current global industry environment.

We still have choices. The future holds many opportunities. Even though medical transcription is just one piece in the very complex health care puzzle, it is a very important piece.

There are many avenues that we independent medical transcriptionists can pursue to expand our horizons and offer greater diversity of services to our clients. Coding and billing services are viable options, and there are now services and courses that provide training for transcriptionists who wish to pursue these paths.

There are exciting and challenging years ahead. As medical transcriptionists, we need to make wise and healthy choices in our professional and personal lives. We are in an excellent position to thrive and excel as we move into the 21st century. We chose this profession with its pleasures and perils. If we are to be players, we must walk the walk and talk the talk. We should embrace change because change is progress. Someone once said, "If you can't change it, change the way you think about it."

Summary

"Do not delay; Do not delay;
the golden moments fly!"
—Henry Wadsworth Longfellow

Lao Tzu is quoted as saying, "The journey of a thousand miles begins with a single step." If after reading this book you find yourself intrigued with the idea of self-employment but are apprehensive about taking the steps necessary to become a home-based medical transcriptionist, take that first experimental step anyway.

Go to a local print shop or desktop publisher and have business cards made. Action always boosts self-esteem; so take action.

You can succeed in anything you attempt by defining some healthy lifestyle patterns for yourself, along with specific goals and objectives, and consistently following through on them. When things don't work out exactly as planned, be gentle with yourself. Don't be afraid to make mistakes; we have all made them and have learned and grown from each experience.

Don't let fear stand in your way. The key to overcoming fear is knowing our enemy (usually oneself). Take risks, minor ones at the start, and graduate to larger ones. Eat a balanced diet, get enough sleep, exercise regularly, and see how much better you feel about yourself and your environment. Meet each negative situation with a positive response and you will surely become a winner.

Reward yourself at the end of a long day of transcription. Be your own best friend and the type of boss you always wished you had. Take pride in your finished product and be the best you can be.

Our hope is that by reading this book, you will avoid many of the stumbling blocks and pitfalls we have encountered on our journey toward professional freedom.

Problem Solving — Questions and Answers

The following questions are frequently asked at workshops we present. Each subject is covered in more detail elsewhere in this book. Check the index for specific pages.

Q: How do you become a CMT?

A: Call AAMT 800-982-2182. They will send you information regarding certification through the American Association for Medical Transcription.

Q: Can you send brochures/advertising to all doctors without stepping on toes of fellow transcriptionists?

A: Yes, you can. You have the right to make a living just like everyone else. If another transcriptionist is worried, maybe she has reason to be. If clients are happy with the service you provide, they will not shop around.

Q: What turnaround time constitutes "STAT" in regard to charging extra for this type of service?

A: The word "Stat" means different things to different clients. One may consider 24-hours "Stat," another, immediately, and another, 12-hours. The term "Stat" must be clarified with your client. If you are going to charge an additional fee for "Stat" work, you should inform the client of your fee schedule for different types of turnaround.

Q: If you are working in your home as an employee for a service, do you need a business license?

A: No. You are an employee, not a business.

Q: What is the best source for learning about word processing/computer equipment?

A: Others in the field, trade shows, conventions, product suppliers, computer publications, online bulletin boards and networking.

Q: How do you find out the standard rates in your area?

A: Network with others in the field. Approach the subject by asking what is the range (low-high). Do not ask someone directly what they charge as this approach sometimes offends and may put the individual you ask on the defensive.

Q: When working for a service as an independent contractor, how are you paid?

A: The service generally accepts your fee at a rate that is determined by your level of technical expertise. If you are very diversified, you can demand a high rate of pay. If you are limited in your specialties, expect to be paid less for your services.

Q: When working from home, what is the proper disposal method for rough drafts to ensure confidentiality? In other words, can I throw them in the recycling bin?

A: Dispose of drafts by shredding or burning them. **DO NOT** throw them in the recycling bin.

Q: What is the current standard for billing on character count?

A: At the current time, there is no set standard. You will have to network and find out what the standard is in the area you work in. Currently, several industry groups are attempting to standardize character count measurements, but the groups have not yet been able to agree on a standard. Your standard will be what you negotiate with your clients.

Q: How much does the FDA bulletin board cost?

A: The FDA bulletin board is free. You need a computer and modem. Modem settings: Baud 1200, E, 7, 1, N. For more information, call 800-222-0185.

Q: How do I handle a client who requests daily pickup and delivery, yet many times has no work or only one letter on a tape?

A: Perhaps you can renegotiate your agreement/contract with the client and include a clause for a minimum dollar amount for pickup and delivery. Since they insist on daily service, a minimum of $25 would at least compensate you for your time and overhead. The client could go for it, or reconsider whether daily pickup and delivery is really necessary and/or cost-effective.

Q: I was told "no compete clauses" are definitely unenforceable and that it is illegal to deprive anyone the right to do business. Please comment.

A: We would not use the word "definitely." It depends upon the facts and circumstances of the situation. Always remember that you are the negotiator when it comes to the contract. You cannot deprive one of the right to make a living, but if you sign that contract, you are agreeing to what is in it. If it is a reasonable restraint — encompassing a reasonable period of time — it could hold up. **Always** seek legal advice before signing an agreement with this type clause. We have been encouraged by our legal adviser not to sign a contract with a no compete clause. Check with your attorney.

> *"Many transcriptionists work in service operations as partners, advisors, consultants, technicians, educators, editors, and instructors."*

Q: How do you arrange for vacations?

A: This depends on the terms and agreements you maintain with your clients. If they expect coverage from your service whether or not you are the one doing the work, you will have to arrange backup transcriptionists to cover for you. If this is the case, make sure they have the appropriate credentials to be operating a business, and if your backups are your employees, they should also have sufficient skills to manage the client's work. If your client does not expect coverage, they may hold the work until you return (if it's a short vacation). It will take serious planning to arrange vacation plans if you are running a full-time business. For many independents, vacations are few and far between.

Q: What do you do if payments aren't made on time?

A: Assuming that you have set your terms for payment in an agreement with your client, you will have to follow up. Call the accounts payable department and ask if your invoice has been processed. Remember to always include an invoice number at the top of your statement. This expedites processing and tracking for the client, as well as the vendor (you). If your statement has not been processed, kindly ask when it will be. Go from there. You may have to remind them of your payment agreement and make sure that you both had the same understanding of the terms.

Q: How many hours do you work to do 10,000 lines per week?
A: On an average eight-hour day, 2,000 lines per day x 5 days per week.

Q: In what way is a contract binding? If they don't want you anymore, they will simply have no work for you.

A: A contract basically states **how** the work is done. Specify in a contract the volume of work you will be receiving (minimum/maximum), and perhaps a termination or renegotiation date.

Q: Where can I obtain more information about working for outside services? Do they deliver tapes to you? Is there extra cost? Do they pay to deliver and pick up transcription?

A: Check the local yellow pages, also local trade publications. Network with other MTs. Call the service directly and ask them questions. Every service is different and may not provide the same benefit package, etc. If you are considering working for a service, you are looking for employment. Interview them to see if this is the type service you want to work for. If they are a reputable company, the service will interview you and request a resume of your qualifications.

Q: How are you paid when telecommuting? Do you invoice telecommuting clients the same way you invoice clients where you pick up and deliver tapes?

A: Telecommuting offers many advantages in terms of turnaround schedules, confidentiality, and reimbursement. Turnaround is virtually instantaneous. There are no delays with pickup, deliveries and arranging courier schedules. There are fewer people handling documents, which assures patient confidentiality. Some offices are virtually paperless, and all records are sent via modem. No paper is printed in the transcription office; it is printed out in the client's office. The client can be invoiced via modem or fax, which guarantees delivery to long-distance clients.

Q: I recently heard that the SBA has done a home-based business study. Do you know the results of their findings?

A: The study commissioned by the SBA was titled *Myths and Realities of Working at Home: Characteristics of Homebased Business Owners and Telecommuters*. The research was conducted by Joanne H. Pratt Associates.

The findings of the study included:

- Homebased businesses have a greater net worth than non-homebased businesses.

- There is little difference between the hours working in a homebased business versus a non-homebased business.

- Telecommuters tend to have more positive attitudes towards their jobs than non-telecommuters. They like the kind of work they do, they do not feel isolated from their peers, and they enjoy considerable job stability.

Pratt predicts that home-based businesses will increase in the future. "Because of technology, home-based businesses can contract for what megacorporations, in the process of downsizing, no longer do themselves."

Resources

ASSOCIATIONS, ORGANIZATIONS, NETWORKS

- **American Association of Home-based Businesses**
  P. O. Box 10023
  Rockville, MD 20849
  Voicemail: 202-310-3130

- **American Association for Medical Transcription**
  P.O. Box 576187
  Modesto, CA 95357-6187
  209-551-0883
  fax: 209-551-9317
  E-mail: aamt@sna.com

- **American Federation of Small Business**
  150 West 20th Avenue
  San Mateo, CA 94403
  415-341-7441

- **American Health Information Management Association**
  (formerly) American Medical Record Association
  919 North Michigan Avenue
  Chicago, Illinois 60611-1683

- **American Home Business Association**
  397 Post Road
  Darien, CT 06820

- **American Medical Writers Association**
  9650 Rockville Pike
  Bethesda, MD 20814
  301-493-0003

- **American Woman's Economic Development Corporation**
  60 East 42nd Street
  New York, NY 10165
  212-692-9100

- **Association for Women in Computing, Inc.**
  407 Hillmoor Drive
  Silver Springs, MD 20901

- **Association of Enterprising Mothers**
  914 S. Santa Fe Avenue, Suite 297
  Vista, CA 92084
  619-434-9225

- **Center for Entrepreneurial Management**
  83 Spring Street
  New York, NY 10012
  212-925-7304

- **Council of Smaller Enterprises**
  690 Union Commerce Building
  Cleveland, OH 44115
  216-621-3300

- **The Encyclopedia of Associations**
  Fifteenth edition
  Gale Research Company, 1981

- **Feminist Computer Technology (FCTP)**
  Erin Computer Systems, Inc.
  4412 Jutland Drive
  San Diego, CA 92117

- **Homebased Businesswoman's Network**
  5 Cedar Hill Road
  Salem, MA 01970

- **Home-Workers on the Move to Economic Success**
  (H.O.M.E.S. Guild)
  31255 Cedar Valley Drive
  Westlake Village, CA 91362
  818-707-0008

- **International Information/Word Processing Association**
  1015 North York Road
  Willow Grove, PA 19090
  215-657-6300

- **Keyboard Connection**
  P. O. Box 338, Dept 12
  Glen Carbon, Il 62034

- **Medical Transcription Industry Alliance (MTIA)**
  1-800-543-MTIA
  E-mail: kcameron@ainet.com

- **Medical Transcription Student Network**
  Health Professions Institute
  P. O. Box 801
  Modesto, CA 95353-0801
  209-551-2112
  Fax: 209-551-0404

- **Mother's Home Business Network**
  (A national organization dedicated to helping mothers work at home).
  P. O. Box 423
  East Meadow, NY 11554

- **National Alliance of Home Based Business Women**
  P. O. Box 95
  Norwood, NJ 07648

- **National Association for Public Continuing and Adult Education**
  1201 16th Street, NW
  Washington, D.C. 20036
  202-833-5486

- **The Association of Business Support Services International, Inc. (ABSSI)**
  (Formerly National Association for Secretarial Services—NASS)
  Lynette M. Smith, CPS, Executive Director
  5852 Oak Meadow Drive
  Yorba Linda, CA 92886-5930
  714-695-9398; 800-237-1462
  Fax: 714-779-8106
  E-mail: abssi4YOU@aol.com
  www.abssi.org

- **National Association for the Cottage Industry**
  P. O. Box 14460
  Chicago, Illinois 60614
  312-472-8116

- **National Association for the Self-Employed**
  P. O. Box 345749
  Dallas, TX 75234
  800-255-9226 (in Texas 800-442-4733)

- **National Association for the Self-Employed**
  2316 Gravel Road
  Fort Worth, TX 76118

- **National Association of Home-based Businesses**
  1045 Mill Run Circle, Suite 400
  Owings Mill, MD 21117
  410-363-3698

- **National Association of Professional Consultants**
  20121 Ventura Blvd., Suite 227
  Woodland Hills, CA 91364
  213-703-6028

- **National Association of Women Business Owners (NAWBO)**
  200 P Street, NW
  Washington, D.C. 20036
  202-338-8966

    or

  1100 Wayne Avenue, Suite 830
  Silver Spring, MD 20910
  301-608-2590
  Fax 301-608-2596

- **National Business League**
  4324 Georgia Avenue, NW
  Washington, D.C. 20005
  202-638-3411

- **National Computer Security Association**
  10 S. Courthouse Avenue
  Carlisle, PA 17013
  717-258-1816
  Fax 717-243-8642

- **National Federation of Independent Business**
  150 West 20th Avenue
  San Mateo, CA 94403
  415-341-7441

- **National Small Business Association**
  1604 K Street, NW
  Washington, D.C. 20006
  202-296-7400

- **New Families Work Options Network**
  P. O. Box 41108
  Fayetteville, NC 28309

- **Rural Women Cottage Industries**
  505 Linder Street
  Friday Harbor, WA 98250

- **Small Business Administration (SBA)**
  800-827-5722

- **Small Business Administration (SBA) Office of Women's Business Ownership**
  202-205-6673

- **Small Business Development Centers (SBDC)**
  (Every state has one or more SBDC branches.
  Check the telephone directory for your closest SBDC office)

- **Small Business Foundation of America**
  69 Hickory Drive
  Waltham, MA 02154

- **Women in Information Processing, Inc.**
  1000 Connecticut Ave., NW
  Washington, D.C. 20036

INFORMATION RESOURCES FOR BLIND AND VISUALLY IMPAIRED INDIVIDUALS

This list contains useful sources of information for computer users with blindness or visual impairments. The list is divided into four sections: organizations, newsletters/journals, networks, databases/bulletin boards, and books/pamphlets. No recommendations or endorsements are implied by inclusion on this list. Contact each resource for more specific and up-to-date information.

ORGANIZATIONS

- **American Foundation for the Blind, Inc.**
  11 Penn Plaza
  Suite 300
  New York, NY 10001
  212-502-7642
  Fax: 212-502-7773
  E-mail: afbinfo@afb.net

Conducts product evaluations of assistive technology including Braille technology, optical character readers, speech synthesizers, screen magnifiers, and closed circuit televisions.

- **American Council of the Blind**
  1155 15th Street, Suite 720
  Washington, DC 20005
  800-424-8666
  202-467-5081
  Fax: 202-467-5085

  Publishes a computer resource list about various devices and where to buy them. Visually Impaired Data Processors International, a computer users' special interest group, is part of ACB.

- **American Printing House for the Blind**
  P.O. Box 6085
  1839 Frankfort Avenue
  Louisville, KY 40206-0085
  502-895-2405
  800-223-1839
  Fax: 502-899-2274
  E-mail: info@aph.org

  Producers of software for users with visual impairments. APH also produces user manuals in Braille for Apple computers, instructional aids, tools, and supplies. Four-track recorder/players available. Tutorial kit for Microsoft Windows available for users with visual impairments.

- **Braille Institute**
  741 N. Vermont Avenue
  Los Angeles, CA 90029
  800-272-4553
  323-663-1111
  Fax: 323-663-0867
  E-mail: Info@BrailleInstitute.org

  This is an educational organization for persons who are blind, deaf-blind, or partially sighted. It has technological resources, a talking book library, and a large community outreach program. A subsidy program for funding equipment is available to persons who are currently employed and legally blind.

- **Carroll Center for the Blind**
  70 Centre Street
  Newton , MA 02158
  800-852-3131
  617-969-6200
  Fax: 617-969-6204
  E-mail: intake@carroll.org

Through this center for the blind various publications and rehabilitation and educational programs are available for persons who are blind or visually impaired. A computer-training program, Project CABLE, provides computer assessment, training on adaptive devices and software, as well as word processing training. Summer training courses for youth are also offered.

- **Central Blind Rehabilitation Center**
  Veterans Affairs
  Edward Hines, Jr. VA Hospital
  PO Box 5000 (124)
  Hines, IL 60141-5000
  708-202-2271

The Central Blind Rehabilitation Center provides information on various types of computer access devices for men and women who have visual impairments.

- **Centre for Sight Enhancement**
  School of Optometry
  University of Waterloo
  Waterloo, ON N2L 3G1
  CANADA
  519-888-4708
  Fax: 519-746-2337

Centre for Sight enhancement is a clinical, teaching, and research facility which provides assessment, prescription, instruction and/or rehabilitation by a multidisciplinary professional team. The Centre also provides sight enhancement devices under the Provincial Ministry of Health's Assistive Devices Program.

- **Helen Keller National Center for Deaf-Blind Youths and Adults**
  111 Middle Neck Road
  Sands Point, NY 11050
  516-944-8900
  Fax: 516-944-7302
  E-mail: hkncdir@aol.com

The Helen Keller Center is the only national program that provides diagnostic evaluation, short-term comprehensive rehabilitation and personal adjustment training, and job preparation and placement for Americans who are deaf-blind. Local services provided through regional offices, affiliated agencies, a national training team, and a technical assistance center for older adults.

- **The Hephaestus project**
  E-mail:neohephaestus@geocities.com

The Hephaestus Project is one of many efforts around the world which is trying to help those who are blind and vision impaired. This page links to Web-hosted directories of websites and databases of tools related to this effort, but inclusion here does not necessarily indicate endorsement. Listing order is arbitrary. The Project solicits nominations for additional entries.

- **International Braille and Technology Center for the Blind**
  National Federation for the Blind
  1800 Johnson Street
  Baltimore, MD 21230
  410-659-9314
  E-mail: nfb@iamd.igex.net

This organization provides demonstrations, comparative evaluations, cost comparison, ADA compliance assistance, personal and telephone consultation pertaining to assistive technology for the visually impaired, as well as tours, meeting and conference facilities. Resource for blind persons and sighted individuals. Overnight and dining accommodations may be available for a fee.

- **National Association for Visually Handicapped**
  22 West 21st Street
  New York, NY 10010
  212-889-3141
  Fax: 212-727-2931
  E-mail: staff@navh.org

  or

  3201 Balboa Street
  San Francisco CA 94121

  This organization deals with the needs of people who are partially sighted, and provides information about computer access.

- **National Braille Press, Inc.**
  88 St. Stephen Street
  Boston, MA 02115
  617-266-6160
  800-548-7323
  Fax: 617-437-0456
  E-mail: orders@nbp.org

  National Braille Press offers publications on personal computer technology for people who are blind. Many printer and modem manuals transcribed in Braille.

- **National Eye Health Education Program**
  National Press Club Ballroom
  529 14th Street, N.W.
  Washington, DC
  E-mail:nehep@nei.nih.gov

  The National Eye Institute, a component of the National Institutes of Health, is the Federal government's principal agency for conducting and supporting vision research. The National Eye Health Education Program (NEHEP) is coordinated by the National Eye Institute in partnership with public and private organizations who plan and implement eye health.

- **National Federation of the Blind**
  1800 Johnson Street
  Baltimore, MD 21230
  410-659-9314
  E-mail: epc@roudley.com

The National Federation of the Blind programs include: Committee on Evaluation of Technology (which evaluates current and proposed technology for people who are blind or visually impaired); International Braille and Technology Center for the Blind (a demonstration and evaluation center for computer technology for blind and visually impaired users); and NFB in Computer Science (a nationwide computer users' group which publishes an annual newsletter for people who are blind or visually impaired).

- **Recording for the Blind and Dyslexic (RFBD)**
  20 Rozel Road
  Princeton, NJ 08540
  800-803-7201
  E-mail: webmaster@rfbd.org

Recordings for the Blind and Dyslexic provides academic textbooks and other educational textbooks to people who cannot read standard print because of physical, perceptual, or other disabilities. Must be a registered member in order to borrow materials; call for details. Also sells reference books on disk and related software products.

- **Sensory Access Foundation**
  1142 West Evelyn Avenue
  Sunnyvale, California 94086
  408- 245-7330
  408-245-1001 (TDD)
  Fax: 408-245-3762

The Sensory Access Foundation compiles and publishes consumer information on technology updates, including computer adaptations, for blind and visually impaired people. Assists in career placement for people who have visual impairments. Career services are only available within California; information services available worldwide. Publishes a magazine and has a technology training center.

- **Smith-Kettlewell Eye Research Institute**
  Rehabilitation Engineering Center
  2318 Fillmore Street
  San Francisco, CA 94115
  415-345-2000
  Fax: 415-345-8455
  E-mail: webmaster@skivs.ski.org

Smith-Kettlewell Eye Research Institute is a respected research and development center that provides information on assistive technology (including work on computer access devices) for people who are blind or visually impaired.

- **Upshaw Institute for the Blind**
  16625 Grand River
  Detroit, MI 48227
  313-272-3900
  Fax: 313-272-6893
  E-mail: webmaster@upshawinst.org

The Upshaw Institute for the Blind provides adaptive technology information, occupational information, mobility information, education information, and much more.

NEWSLETTERS AND JOURNALS FOR BLIND AND VISUALLY IMPAIRED INDIVIDUALS

- *Braille Forum*
  American Council of the Blind
  1155 15th Street
  Suite 720
  Washington, DC 20005
  202-467-5081
  Fax: 202-467-5085

  The *Braille Forum* offers a publication dealing with a variety of blindness-related issues, such as legislation, technology, and product/service announcements.

- *Journal of Visual Impairment and Blindness*
  The Sheridan Press
  450 Fame Avenue
  Hanover, PA 17331
  717-632-3535
  E-mail: pubsvc@tsp.sheridan.com

  This research journal features issues related to visual impairment and blindness. Includes research reviews, application papers, and articles on special topics (including assistive technology). It is published monthly, except July and August.

- *Tactic*
  Clovernook Center
  7000 Hamilton Avenue
  Cincinnati, OH 45231
  513-522-3860 x294
  E-mail: clovernook@clovernook.org

  This international quarterly offers information and reviews on technology for people with visual impairments. It is published in Braille, large print, and diskette (IBM compatible) formats.

- *Technology Update*
  Sensory Access Foundation
  1142 West Evelyn Avenue
  Sunnyvale, California 94086
  408-245-7330
  408-245-1001 (TDD)
  Fax: 408-245-3762

  This bimonthly newsletter contains information regarding technology and vision impairment. It also includes new product announcements, product reviews, and consumer information. It is available in print, large print, cassette, and diskette.

- *Visual Field*
  Florida Instructional Materials Center
  5002 North Lois Avenue
  Tampa, FL 33614
  813-872-5281
  Fax: 813-872-5284

  Visual Field is a biannual newsletter on products, projects, conferences, etc., related to education of students with visual impairments.

NETWORKS, BULLETIN BOARDS, & DATABASES FOR BLIND AND VISUALLY IMPAIRED INDIVIDUALS

- **Louis Database**
  American Printing House for the Blind
  Attn: Paul Brown
  PO Box 6085
  Louisville, KY 40206-0085
  800-223-1839
  Fax: 502-895-1509
  E-mail: info@aph.org

  An online database that lists materials in media accessible to people who are visually impaired. Over 120,000 records including Braille books, large type materials, music scores, electronic books, sound recordings, software programs, and tactile graphics. Contact APH for billing and access information.

- **The Family Village**
  Waisman Center, University of Wisconsin-Madison
  1500 Highland Avenue
  Madison, WI 53705-2280
  E-mail: familyvillage@waisman.wisc.edu

  The Family Village provides chat rooms and discussion boards, as well as other information and resources, for many different types of disabilities.

BOOKS AND PAMPHLETS FOR BLIND AND VISUALLY IMPAIRED INDIVIDUALS

- **CD-ROM Advantage**
  D. Croft, D. Kendrick, and A. Gayzagian, 1994
  National Braille Press
  88 St. Stephen Street
  Boston, MA 02115
  617-266-6160
  Fax: 617-437-0456
  E-mail: orders@nbp.org

  Answers commonly asked questions about CD-ROM technology and how it works with speech and Braille. Includes practical advice from users, profiles blind users of CD-ROM, and lists over 100 CD-ROM titles.

- **Computer Access, Resource Manual**
  Rosenbaum, et al., 1987
  Carroll Center for the Blind
  770 Centre Street
  Newton, MA 02158
  800-852-3131
  Fax: 617-969-6204
  617-969-6200
  E-mail: intake@carroll.org

Resource manual and curriculum for setting up an evaluation and training center in assistive technology applications for blind and visually impaired individuals.

- **Customer Service Representative Training Manual**
  Ferrarin, Rosenbaum, et al., 1994
  Carroll Center for the Blind
  770 Centre Street
  Newton, MA 02158
  800-852-3131
  617-969-6200
  Fax: 617-969-6204
  Email: intake@carroll.org

  A comprehensive curriculum for creating and providing job readiness skills for employment in customer service jobs to individuals with visual impairments utilizing assistive technology. For rehabilitation agencies, secondary institutions, or career counselors.

- **Extend Their Reach, 1990**
  Electronic Industries Association
  2500 Wilson Boulevard
  Arlington, VA 22201
  703-907-7500

  Gives an introduction to the types of products available to overcome impairments of sight, speech, hearing, motion, etc.

EDUCATIONAL OPPORTUNITIES FOR MEDICAL TRANSCRIPTIONISTS

- **Andrews School for Medical Transcription**
  Medical transcription home-based distance learning course. Educational skills and job training for MT careers as home-based or office-based medical transcriptionists.
  www.braindevelopers.com

- **Brain Developers**
  Medical transcription and training in India for doctors in the United States of America.
  www.braindevelopers.com

- **CAI Medical Transcription Training**
  Home study medical transcription course based in Barnegat, NJ.
  www.caitranscription.com

- **Career Step, Quality Medical Transcription Training**
  Distance medical transcription training and education for MTs who want to work at home.
  www.careerstep.com

- **Global Medical Transcription (GMT) School**
  Distance learning center for medical transcriptionists who want to learn at home. The school offers interactive, on the job training and placement for graduates.
  www.medicaltrans.net

  GMT Distance Learning Center
  P.O. Box 1421
  241 Beach Place
  Kaunakakai, HI 96748
  toll free: 877-779-8779
  E-mail: info@medicaltrans.net

- **ITES Horizon Pvt. Ltd.**
  Offers a six-month medical transcription training program and services in various specialties. Located in New Delhi, India.
  E-mail: ites@iteshorizon.com
  www.iteshorizon.com

  (Corporate Office)
  ITES Horizon (P) Ltd.
  C-3/7 Prashant Vihar
  Rohini, New Delhi—110085
  India
  phones: 91-11-726-8876; 786-8876

- **Lairds Medical Transcription School**
  At-home medical transcription training since 1980. Also provides mentoring services. Approved by the United States of America Department of Education.
  www.lairdsschool.com

- **Latter Day Saints (LDS) Business College**
  Two-semester educational programs in medical transcription and coding. Taught at a private, two-year college in Salt Lake City, Utah.
  www.ldsbc.edu

- **Medical Transcription Education Center, Inc.**
  A premier home-based distance learning medical transcription program.
  www.mtecinc.com

- **Medical Transcription Institute**
  An at-home course using the SUM program. Includes course catalog, how to enroll and contact information. The institute is located in Salt Lake City, Utah.
  www.medicaltranscriptioninstitute.com

- **Medi*Script Careers**
  Offers a self test to become a medical transcriptionist. Includes details about the course, materials, the instructor, testimonials and ordering instructions.
  www.mediscriptcareers.com

- **Meditech, Inc.**
  Medical transcription home training program, medical coding training, medical billing training.
  www.meditec.com/mt.html

- **MediTrans**
  Private vocational school for medical transcription, insurance billing/coding, medical terminology.
  www.medi-trans.com

- **MT Support Services, Inc.**
  Medical transcription distance learning course. Train to work from your home or from a clinic or hospital. Approved home study program.
  www.mtsupport.com

- **Review of Systems School of Medical Transcription (ROS)**
  Since 1995, ROS has utilized the SUM Program, college textbooks, extensive references, and experienced instructors to provide thorough home-based training and internship opportunities to students across the U.S.
  www.mtmonthly.com/ros

- **Sunrise Enterprises**
  Classes and instruction in medical records coding and health care information management. Based in Cheyenne, WY.
  www.sunrisent.com

- **Transcription Services**
  Step by step home study business package for professionals interested in starting their own medical transcription business.
  www.transcriptionservice.net

- **TransNet Medical Transcription School & Service**
  TransNet offers both remote and on-site educational courses.
  www.Transnet87.com

MEDICAL TRANSCRIPTION RESOURCES ON THE INTERNET

- **American Association for Medical Transcription (AAMT)**
  The mission of AAMT is to represent and advance the profession of medical transcription and its practitioners. This site includes career information, related Internet links, and more.
  www.aamt.com

- **At-Home Professions**
  Medical transcription training.
  1-800-347-7899 (Tues-Fri)
  E-mail for information on programs: enroll@at-homeprofessions.com

- **Business Know-How**
  Excellent networking area for MT's. Includes a message board area as well as chats on the subject of Medical Transcription.
  www.businessknowhow.com

- **Health Professions Institute: Current Terms**
  An online list of new medical words and phrases along with definitions.
  Source of SUM medical transcription training program, word books.
  209-551-2112
  www.hpisum.com

- **Lippincott, Williams & Wilkins**
  Source for reference books and MT specialty software.
  800-527-5597
  E-mail: custserve@wwilkins.com

- **Medical Transcription Industry Alliance**
  Provides information about MTIA membership and other helpful medical transcription sites.
  800-543-MTIA
  www.mtia.com

- **Medword: Medical Transcription**
  This site describes the medical transcription profession and provides links to the large amounts of reliable medical information on the Internet.
  www.medword.com

- **MT Daily: The medical transcription networking center**
  This site offers many online resources as well as career information for medical transcriptionists. Very complete source for MT information, excellent message board, MT training sites, national services, etc. This site is available from the MT Forum's first screen.
  www.mtdaily.com

- **MT Desk**
  Informational site with weekly updates to the Alphabetical Index of New Terminology, Weekly Updates of Medical Drugs/Terms, and Medical/Surgical Word Glossary.
  www.mtdesk.com

- **MT Monthly**
  Published since 1993, *MT Monthly* is a 16-page newsletter providing medical transcriptionists with monthly terminology updates, computer help, and articles related to the profession.
  www.mtmonthly.com

- **PMIC**
  Reference books including Medical Phrase Index.
  800-633-7467
  www.pmiconline.com

- **Quail Haven Medical Transcription Links**
  Well-organized links to medical transcription sites on the Internet.
  www.quailhaven.com

- **W.B. Saunders Co.**
  Dorland's reference books.
  6277 Sea Harbor Dr.
  Orlando, FL 32887
  800-545-2522
  www.wbsaunders.com

SPEECH TECHNOLOGY AND MEDICAL TRANSCRIPTION SERVICES

- **Dragon**
  Naturally Speaking speech recognition systems, Medisoft and Medamation electronic medical records software.
  L&H Inc.
  781-203-5000
  www.lhsl.com

- **Dictation Software for Medical and Other Professionals**
  Speech recognition technology providing accurate transcription and HCFA compliant reports.
  219-662-3800
  www.lhsl.com

- **Business Know-How**
  Excellent networking area for MT's. Includes a message board area as well as chats on the subject of Medical Transcription.
  www.businessknowhow.com

- **Expert System Applications, Inc. (ESAI)**
  Offers medical transcription and digital dictation services for doctors, physicians, clinics and hospitals utilizing major transcription vehicles like Lanier, Dictaphone, and DVI.
  440-248-0110
  www.expert-system.com

- **ITS Speech**
  Solutions for the medical and legal communities dictation needs. Site's goal is to provide a completely seamless transition from traditional dictation services to speech recognition and speech to text based technologies.
  202-366-0408
  www.its.dot.gov

- **Lairds Medical Transcription School**
  At home medical transcription training since 1980. Approved by the United States of America Department of Education.
  800-209-9899
  www.lairdsschool.com

- **Medical Data Capture**
  MedSpeak VRE integrates continuous speech recognition and relational database to create real time electronic medical records (EMR) with a user friendly interface for healthcare providers.
  www.md-it.com

- **Medical Dictation and Transcription**
  Specializes in speech recognition software for the medical and legal professions.
  www.pucservice.com

- **Medical Transcription**
  Medical and legal transcription services, digital dictation, 24 hours 7 days a week. Transcriptionists can have their own virtual dictation services, e-mail, 800 numbers, wholesale prices.
  www.medicaltranscription.org

- **MediTalk Medical Dictation and Practice Management Software**
  Medical speech recognition software from Duostar.
  www.duostar.net

- **MediTalk/Quicknotes**
  MediTalk has medical dictation and practice management software, and medical speech recognition software from Duostar. In addition, they offer general speech consulting for small and medium size businesses with a specialty in Quincy Meditalk patient records and Dragon "Naturally Speaking" speech recognition software.
  714-969-7632
  www.voiceautomated.com

- **Medpro Solutions — Speech Recognition Specialists**
  Providing L&H Medical solutions, speech recognition and medical billing software. Authorized Dragon Systems Premier Partner.
  516-679-7765
  www.medprosolutions.net

- **medQ inc**
  Offering Medspeak, PACS, Radworks, RIS, speech dictation, recognition and other software for the medical field.
  214-221-6330
  www.medq.com

- **Network Based Dictation/Transcription Service**
  Provides ability for doctors to use standard PC (with sound card) to send patient information to server.
  www.theprogrammers.com

- **Prophysys, Inc.**
  Medical systems using Dragon Naturally Speaking.
  513-381-2633
  www.prophysys.com

- **RVC Medical Transcription and Dictation Services**
  RVC Services offers speech recognition software for the medical and legal professions.
  www.rvcservice.com

- **Speech Machines**
  A speech-to-data medical transcription application service provider.
  www.speechmachines.com

- **Talk Technology**
  Fully integrated windows-based, speech recognition workflow solutions for medical reporting.
  www.talktechnology.com

- **Wilson Technology**
  Offers complete hardware and software for turnkey speech recognition computer systems for the medical industry.
  www.wilsontech.net

- **Winscribe Digital Dictation**
  WinScribe offers enterprise digital dictation systems with workflow routing of speech to text transcription.
  www.winscribe.com

GEAR FOR LONG DISTANCE TELECOMMUTING

- **Road Warrior — Gear for the Mobile Professional™**
  International modem and power adapters, telecouplers, cellular phone and laptop accessories, PDA accessories, and a good selection of white papers in the support area.
  www.roadwarrior.com

- **Globalstar**
  Satellite-based voice and data communications
  www.globalstar.com

- **KVH Industries, Inc.**
  TracVision (mobile television) and TracPhone (mobile telephony)
  www.kvh.com

- **Nokia**
  Accessories (PC card and connector) to make your Nokia cellular phone modem capable. Search by model number; not all models can interface with a modem. More efficient to phone than use their website.
  www.nokia.com

- **Audiovox Corporation**
  Wide range of personal electronics including modem-ready cellular phones (Audiovox 9000). Search the site for "data accessories."
  www.audiovox.com

- **Modern Living, USA**
Cellular accessories and original equipment. Provides fax and data accessories for brands from Audiovox to Uniden. Helpful articles on modems, chargers, and more.
www.mod-usa.com

LAPTOP/DESKTOP RESOURCES

- **Laptop Travel**
Laptop, palmtop, and cellular accessories, including vehicle desks, security cables and alarms, screen shades, and more.
www.laptoptravel.com

- **iGo (affiliated with Road Warrior)**
Laptop, palmtop, and cellular accessories, including digital line testers, socket multipliers, inverters, emergency power supplies, voice recorders, and more. Ask for a print catalog.
www.igo.com

- **Hello Direct**
Known for headsets, Hello Direct also offers digital line testers, voice recorders, and adapters.
www.hellodirect.com

SENDING/RECEIVING DICTATION/DOCUMENTS

- **MedRemote, Inc.**
Internet-based system for file (voice & data) transfers, includes tracking/management features.
www.medremote.com

- **Spantel, LLC**
Internet-based system for file (voice & data) transfers, includes tracking/management features.
www.spantel.com

- **Vianeta Communications**
  Internet-based system for file (voice & data) transfers, includes tracking/management features.
  www.vianeta.com

- **Hilgraeve, Inc. (product: Hypersend)**
  Low-volume use of this secure internet file (voice & data) transfer system is free. Higher volume available by subscription. Limited tracking features.
  www.hypersend.com

CONNECTION SPOTS

- **Kinko's**
  Internet connectivity and other office support functions from locations nationwide. Call toll-free number and ask to have a national location directory mailed to you.
  www.kinkos.com

- **Office Depot**
  Some locations offer PC stations. Call ahead, not offered in all locations. No Internet access that we know, but fax and printing services available.
  www.officedepot.com

- **Cybercafe.com**
  Database of over 4000 cybercafes worldwide. Phone ahead as cybercafes pop in and out of existence frequently.
  www.cybercafe.com

- **Flying J, Inc.**
  "Roadside hospitality" services, AKA truck stops. Telephones, Internet kiosks, copy centers, fax machines, and more. Use website to find national locations.
  www.flyingj.com

OVERSEAS TRAVEL — STARTING POINTS

- **The Escape Artist**
  Products and information for expatriates.
  www.escapeartist.com

UNITED STATES CHAMBERS OF COMMERCE
(Courtesy of World Chamber of Commerce Directory, 970-663-3231)

- **ALABAMA** (Business Council of Ala.)
  William F. O'Connor, Jr., President
  2N. Jackson; P.O. Box 76
  Montgomery, 36101-0076
  334-834-6000; Fax 334-262-7371
  www.bcatoday.org

- **ALASKA** (Alaska State C of C)
  Pamela La Bolle, President
  217 2nd St., #201
  Juneau, 99801-1267
  907-586-2323; Fax 907-463-5515
  E-mail: asccjuno@ptialaska.net
  www.alaskachamber.com

- **ARIZONA** (Arizona C of C)
  James Apperson, Pres./CEO,
  Public Policy & Legislative Issues Only
  1221 E. Osborn Rd., #100
  Phoenix, 85014-5539
  602-248-9172; Fax 602-265-1262
  E-mail: info@azchamber.com
  www.azchamber.com

- **ARKANSAS** (Arkansas State C of C)
  Ron Russell, Pres./CEO
  410 S. Cross; P.O. Box 3645
  Little Rock, 72203-3645
  501-374-9225; Fax 501-372-2722
  E-mail: rrussell@ascc-aia.org
  E-mail: statechamber-aia.dina.org

- **CALIFORNIA** (California State C of C)
  Allan Zaremberg, President
  1215 K St., #1400; P.O. Box 1736
  Sacramento, 95812-1736
  916-444-6670; Fax 916-444-6685
  E-mail: information@calchamber.com
  www.calchamber.com

- **COLORADO** (Col. Assn. of Comm. & Ind.)
  Chuck Berry, Pres./CEO
  1600 Broadway, #1000
  Denver, 80202
  303-831-7411; Fax 303-860-1439
  E-mail: caci@businesscolorado.com
  www.businesscolorado.com

- **CONNECTICUT** (Conn.Bus. & Ind. Assn.)
  Kenneth O. Decko, President
  350 Church Street
  Hartford, 06103-2022
  860-244-1900; Fax 860-278-8562
  www.cbia.com

- **DELAWARE** (Delaware State C of C)
  Suzanne Moore, President
  1201 N. Orange St., #200; P.O. Box 671
  Wilmington, 19899-0671
  302-655-7221; Fax 302-654-0691
  E-mail: dscc@dscc.com; www.dscc.com

- **DISTRICT OF COLUMBIA**
  (Dist. of Columbia C of C)
  Richard Monteilh, President
  1213 K St. N.W.
  District of Columbia, 20005
  202-347-7201; Fax 202-638-6764
  www.dcchamber.org

- **FLORIDA** (Florida C of C)
  Frank M. Ryll, Jr., President
  136 S. Bronough St.; P.O. Box 11309
  Tallahassee, 32302-3309
  805-425-1200; Fax 805-425-1260
  E-mail: policy@flchamber.com
  www.flchamber.com

- **GEORGIA** (Georgia C of C)
  Lindsay Thomas, President
  235 Peachtree St. N.E., #900
  Atlanta, 30303-1504
  404-223-2264; Fax 404-223-2290

- **HAWAII** (C of C of Hawaii)
  Stanley Hong, President
  1132 Bishop St., #402
  Honolulu, 96813-2830
  808-545-4300; Fax 808-545-4309
  www.cochawaii.com

- **IDAHO** (Idaho Assn. of Chambers of C.)
  Carol Waller, President
  P.O. Box 2368
  Boise, 83701
  E-mail: cwaller@micron.net
  208-472-5221; Fax 208-472-5201

- **ILLINOIS** (Illinois State C of C)
  311 S. Wacker Dr., #1500
  Chicago, 60606-6619
  312-983-7100; Fax 312-983-7101
  E-mail: info@ilchamber.org
  www.ilchamber.org

- **INDIANA** (Indiana C of C)
  Christopher Lamothe, Pres./CEO
  115 W. Washington St., #850S
  Indianapolis, 46204-3407
  317-264-3110; Fax 317-264-6855
  E-mail: clamothe@indianachamber.com
  www.indianachamber.com

- **IOWA** (Iowa Assn. of Bus. & Industry)
  Jim Aipperspach, President
  904 Walnut St., #100
  Des Moines, 50309-3503
  515-242-4700; Fax 515-242-4832
  E-mail: abi@iowaabi.org
  www.iowaabi.org

- **KANSAS** (Kansas C of C & Ind.)
  Ed Bruske, Pres./CEO
  835 S.W. Topeka Blvd.
  Topeka, 66612-1671
  785-357-6321; Fax 785-357-4732
  E-mail: kcci@kansaschamber.orgw
  www.kansaschamber.org

- **KENTUCKY** (Kentucky C of C)
  Ken Oilschlager, President
  464 Chenault Rd.
  P.O. Box 817
  Frankfort, 40602-0817
  502-695-4700; Fax 502-695-6824
  E-mail: kcc@kychamber.com
  www.kychamber.com

- **LOUISIANA** (Louisiana Assn. of
  Business & Industry)
  Daniel Juneau, President
  3113 Valley Creek Dr.
  P.O. Box 80258
  Baton Rouge, 70898-0258
  225-928-5388; Fax 225-929-6054
  www.labi.org

- **MAINE** (Maine State C of C)
  Dana F. Connors, President
  7 University Drive
  Augusta, 04330-9412
  207-623-4568; Fax 207-622-7723
  E-mail: info@mainechamber.org
  www.mainechamber.org

- **MARYLAND** (Maryland C of C)
  Kathleen T. Snyder, Pres./CEO
  60 West St., #100
  Annapolis, 21401-24798
  410-269-0642; Fax 410-269-5247
  E-mail: mcc@mdchamber.org
  www.mdchamber.org

- **MASSACHUSETTS**
  (No State Chamber)

- **MICHIGAN** (Michigan C of C)
  James Barrett, President
  600 S. Walnut St.
  Lansing, 48933-2200
  517-371-2100; Fax 517-371-7224
  E-mail: info@michamber.org
  www.michamber.org

- **MINNESOTA** (Minnesota State C of C)
  David Olson, President
  30 E. 7th St., #1700
  Saint Paul, 55101-4901
  651-292-4650; Fax 651-292-4656
  www.mnchamber.org

- **MISSISSIPPI** (Mississippi Economic
  Council)
  Blake Wilson, President
  666 North St., #104
  P.O. Box 23276
  Jackson, 39225-3276
  601-969-0022; Fax 601-353-0247
  www.mcc.ms

- **MISSOURI** (Missouri C of C)
  Daniel P. McHan, President
  428 E. Capitol Ave.
  P.O. Box 149
  Jefferson City, 65102-0149
  573-634-3511; Fax 573-634-8855
  E-mail: DMchan@Mochamber.org
  www.Mochamber.org

- **MONTANA** (Montana C of C)
  Webb Brown, President
  2030 11th Ave.
  P.O. Box 1730
  Helena, 59624-17301
  406-442-2405; Fax 406-442-2409
  E-mail: info@montanachamber.com
  www.montanachamber.com

- **NEBRASKA** (Nebraska C of C & Ind.)
  Barry L. Kennedy, CAE, President
  P.O. Box 95128
  Lincoln, 68509-5128
  402-474-4422; Fax 402-474-5681
  E-mail: nechamber@nechamber.com
  www.nechamber.com

- **NEVADA** (Nevada State C of C)
  David Howard, Legislative Affairs
  Director
  P.O. Box 3499
  Reno, 89505
  702-686-3030; Fax 702-686-3038

- **NEW HAMPSHIRE** (Business and
  Industry Assn. of New Hampshire)
  John D. Crosier, President
  122 N. Main
  Concord, 03301
  603-224-5388; Fax 603-224-2872
  www.nhbia.org

- **NEW JERSEY** (New Jersey C of C)
  Joan Verplanck, President
  216 W. State Street
  Trenton, 08608-1214
  609-989-7888; Fax 609-989-9696
  www.njchamber.com

- **NEW MEXICO** (Assn. of Commerce
  & Industry of New Mexico)
  John A. Carey, President
  P.O. Box 9706
  Albuquerque, 87119-9706
  505-842-0644; Fax 505-842-0734
  E-mail: aci@nm.net
  www.aci.nm.org

- **NEW YORK** (No State Chapter)

- **NORTH CAROLINA** (North Carolina Citizens for Business & Industry)
  Phillip J. Kirk, Jr., President
  225 Hillsborough St., # 460
  P.O. 2508
  Raleigh, 27602-2508
  919-836-1400; Fax 919-836-1425
  www.nccbi.org

- **NORTH DAKOTA** (Greater North Dakota Assn.)
  Dale O. Anderson, President
  2000 Schafer St.
  P.O. Box 2639
  Bismarck, 58502
  701-222-0929; Fax 701-222-1611
  E-mail: gnda@gnda.com
  www.gnda.com

- **OHIO** (Ohio C of C)
  Andrew E. Doehrel, President
  P.O. Box 15159
  Columbus, 43215-0159
  614-228-4201; Fax 614-228-6403
  www.ohiochamber.com

- **OKLAHOMA** (The State Chamber, Oklahoma's Assn. of Business & Industry)
  Richard P. Rush, CCE, Pres./CEO
  330 N.E. 10th St.
  Oklahoma City, 73104-3200
  405-235-3669; Fax 405-235-3670
  E-mail: drush@okstatechamber.com
  www.okstatechamber.com

- **OREGON** (Associated Oregon Industries)
  Richard Butrick, President
  1149 Court St. N.E.
  Salem, 97301
  503-588-0050; Fax 503-588-0052
  E-mail: aoi@aoi.org
  www.aoi.org

- **PENNSYLVANIA** (Pennsylvania Chamber of Business and Industry)
  Floyd W. Warner, President
  417 Walnut St.
  Harrisburg, 17101-1902
  717-255-3252; Fax 717-255-3298
  E-mail: info@pachamber.org;
  www.pachamber.org

- **PUERTO RICO** (Puerto Rico C of C)
  Edgardo Bigas, Exec. Vice President
  P.O. Box 9024033
  San Juan, 00902-4033
  787-721-6060; Fax 787-723-1891
  E-mail: info@pachamber.org;
  www.pachamber.org

- **RHODE ISLAND** (No State Chapter)

- **SOUTH CAROLINA** (South Carolina State C of C)
  S. Hunter Howard J., Pres./CEO
  1201 Main St., #1810
  Columbia, 29201-3254
  803-799-4601; Fax 803-779-6043
  E-mail: chamber@sccc.org;
  www.scchamber.net

- **SOUTH DAKOTA** (South Dakota Chamber of Commerce & Industry)
  David Owen, President
  P.O. Box 190
  Pierre, 57501-0190
  605-224-6161; Fax 605-224-7198
  E-mail: sdchamber@dtgnet.com

- **TENNESSEE** (Tennessee Assoc. of Bus.)
  Dave Goetz, President
  611 Commerce St., #3030
  Nashville, 37203-3742
  615-256-5141; Fax 615-256-6726
  E-mail: info@tennbiz.org
  www.tennbiz.org

- **TEXAS** (Texas Assn. of Business & Chambers of Commerce)
  Bill Hammond, President
  1209 Nueces
  Austin, 78701
  512-447-6721; Fax 512-477-0836
  E-mail: bhammond@tabcc.org
  www.tabcc.org

- **UTAH** (Utah State C of C)
  Mr. Chris Dallin, Chairman
  P.O. Box 457
  Centerville, 84014-0457
  801-295-6944; Fax 801-298-1114
  www.davischamberof commerce.com

- **VERMONT** (Vermont State C of C)
  Christopher G. Barbieri, President
  P.O. Box 37
  Montpelier, 05601-0037
  802-223-3443; Fax 802-223-4257
  E-mail: info@vtchamber.com;
  www.vtchamber.com

- **VIRGIN ISLANDS** (St. Thomas-St. John C of C)
  Joe S. Aubain, Exec. Director
  6-7 Dronningens Gade
  P.O. Box 324
  00804-0324
  340-776-0100; Fax 340-775-0588
  E-mail: chamber@islands.vi
  www.chamber.vi

- **VIRGINIA** (Virginia C of C)
  Hugh D. Keogh, President
  9 S. Fifth St.
  Richmond, 23219
  804-644-1607; Fax 804-783-6112
  E-mail: chamber@vachamber.com
  www.vachamber.com

- **WASHINGTON**
  (Assn. of Washington Business)
  Don Brunell, President
  1414 S. Cherry; P.O. Box 658
  Olympia, 98507-0658
  360-943-1600; Fax 360-943-5811
  E-mail: donb@awb.org
  www.awb.org

- **WEST VIRGINIA** (West Virginia C of C)
  Stephen Roberts, President
  P.O. Box 2789
  Charleston, 25330-2789
  304-342-1115; Fax 304-342-1130
  E-mail: forjobs@wvchamber.com;
  www.wvchamber.com

- **WISCONSIN**
  (Wisconsin Manufacturers & Commerce)
  James S. Haney, President
  501 E. Washington Ave.
  P.O. Box 352
  Madison, 53701-0352
  608-258-3400; Fax 608-258-3413
  E-mail: wmc@wmc.org
  www.wmc.com

- **WYOMING** (No State Chapter)

OUR FAVORITE REFERENCE BOOKS

To stay on medical transcription's cutting edge, keep your library well stocked with the **latest editions** of top quality references, especially medical specialty reference books. Our favorites are the following titles:

Pharmaceutical Books

- *Quick Look Drug Book,* Lippincott, Williams & Wilkins
- *Saunders Pharmaceutical Word Book,* Drake/Drake, Harcourt Int'l. (W. B. Saunders Co.)
- *Mosby's Nursing Drug Reference*
     You can never have too many drug books!

Medical Books from Harcourt International (W. B. Saunders Co.)

- *Dorland's Gastroenterology Wordbook*
- *Dorland's Illustrated Medical Dictionary*
- *Dorland's Immunology/Endocrinology Wordbook*
- *Dorland's Medical Speller*
- *Dorland's Neurology Wordbook*
- *Dorland's Obstetrics/Gynecology Wordbook*
- *Dorland's Orthopedic Wordbook*
- *Dorland's Radiology Wordbook*
- *The Surgical Word Book*, Tessier, C.
- *A Word Book in Pathology and Laboratory Medicine*, Sloan/Dusseau

Books from Lippincott, Williams and Wilkins (LWW)

- *Stedman's Abbreviations, Acronyms & Symbols*
- *Stedman's Endocrinology Words*
- *Stedman's GI & GU Words*
- *Stedman's Laboratory Test Handbook*
- *Stedman's Medical Dictionary*
- *Stedman's Medical Eponyms*
- *Stedman's OB-GYN & Genetics Words*
- *Stedman's Ophthalmology Words*

- *Stedman's Orthopaedic & Rehab Words*
- *Stedman's Pathology & Lab Medicine Words*
- *Stedman's Surgical and Medical Equipment Words*

Medical Word Books from other publishers

- *Current Medical Terminology*, Pyle, Health Professions Institute
- *The Dictionary of Eye Terminology,* MedBioworld On Line Dictionaries
- *Internal Medicine Words*, Danna, Rayve Productions Inc.

Other Essential References

Some other essential references for the medical transcription library include grammar and punctuation references such as:

- *The Elements of Style*, Strunk/White, MacMillan
- *Errors in English and Ways to Correct Them*, Shaw, Harper and Row
- *The Manual of Medical Transcription*, Sloan/Fordney, W. B. Saunders Co.
- *Medical Transcription Guide — Do's & Don'ts*, Fordney & Diehl, 2nd Edition, March 1999, W. B. Saunders Co.

Also necessary are a good collegiate dictionary, medical dictionary, anatomy book, abbreviations, acronyms and symbols book, and the list goes on. An excellent medical transcription resource list and catalog are available through the American Association for Medical Transcription (AAMT) (see publishers' contact numbers below).

- **AAMT Medical Transcription Resource Library** (latest edition)
  (A comprehensive medical transcription reference list)
- **AAMT Success Catalog**

We have also found the following directory helpful.

- **The Little Blue Book**
  (published by Physician's Telephone Directory)
  302 West Main Street, Suite 206
  Avon, CT 06001-9962
  860-409-7000
  Fax 860-674-8893

PUBLISHERS SPECIALIZING IN HEALTH CARE BOOKS

In addition to the above, other publishing houses specialize in health care books. To obtain a list of available titles, contact the following publishers.

- **American Association for Medical Transcription (AAMT)**
  P.O. Box 576187
  Modesto, CA 95355 2
  209-551-0883
  Fax 209-551-9317
  E-mail: aamt@sna.com

- **F.A. Davis Co.**
  1915 Arch Street
  Philadelphia, PA 19103
  800-523-4049

- **Facts and Comparisons**
  Subs. of Wolters Kluwer U.S. Corp.
  111 West Port Plaza, Ste.423
  St. Louis, MO 63146-3098
  800-223-0554

- **Harcourt International**
  (formerly W. B. Saunders Company)
  Curtis Center,
  Independence Square West
  Philadelphia, PA 19106
  215-238-7800

- **Health Professions Institute**
  P.O. Box 801
  Modesto, CA 95353
  209-551-2112

- **Houghton Mifflin Company**
  Two Park Street & One Beacon St.
  Boston, MA 02107
  800-725-5000

- **J.B. Lippincott**
  227 East Washington Square
  Philadelphia, PA 19106
  800-638-3030 (orders);
  800-441-4526 (office)

- **Lippincott, Williams & Wilkins (LWW)**
  (formerly Williams & Wilkins)
  351 W. Camden Street
  Baltimore, Maryland 21201-2436
  800-638-3030
  Fax 301-223-2400

- **Merriam-Webster, Inc.**
  47 Federal Street
  Springfield, MA 01102
  413-734-3134

- **Physicians' Desk Reference**
  Division of Medical Economics Data
  Five Paragon Drive
  Montvale, NJ 07645
  800-232-7379

- **Rayve Productions Inc.**
  P.O. Box 726
  Windsor, CA 95492
  800-852-4890

- **Rittenhouse**
  P.O. Box 1565
  511 Feheley Street
  King of Prussia, PA 19406
  800-624-7627
     or
  P.O. Box 458
  Sterling Rd.
  S. Lancaster, MA 01561

OTHER RESOURCES FOR HEALTH CARE BOOKS

Other helpful resources for health care reference books include the following:

- **J.A. Majors Books**
  1401 Lakeway Drive
  1220 W. Walnut
  Lewisville, TX 75057
     or
  Compton, CA 90220
  800-633-1851
  310-608-2358

- **L&M Bookstore**
  1716 N. Main Avenue
  San Antonio, TX 78212
  210-222-1323
  Fax: 210-222-1580
  800-285-1323

PRODUCTS & SERVICES

- **Beck Office Furniture**
  800-202-7876

- **C.H.A.R.T.S.**
  (Cassettes, headsets and related
  transcription supplies)
  P. O. Box 3284
  Springfield, MO 65808
  800-994-3210; fax 417-881-1872

- **DAK Systems Consulting**
  Voice Recognition Consultants
  505 Madera Drive
  San Mateo, CA 94403
  650-345-9900

- **DataCal Enterprises, LLC**
  (Resource for WP 5.1)
  531 E. Elliott Road
  Chandler, AZ 85225
  800-223-0123

- **Dictaphone Corporation**
  3191 Broadbridge Avenue
  Stratford, CT 06497-2559
  203-381-7124
  Fax 203-386-8597

- **Dragon Systems** (DragonDictate)
  888-81DRAGON
  Fax: 802-872-3138

- **Eloquently Speaking**
  (Speech Recognition)
  800-245-2133

- **Individual Software**
  (Audio training cassettes)
  4255 Hopyard Road, Suite 2
  Pleasanton, CA 94588-9900
  800-822-3522

- **McMillan and Co.**
  Professional Organizing
  Personal Assets Inventory Workbook
  12021 Wilshire Blvd., Suite 670
  West Los Angeles, CA 90025
  310-391-7392
  Fax 310-478-7049

- **MouseMitt International**
  P.O. Box 67370
  Scotts Valley, CA 95067
  800-489-6488
  E-mail: mousemitt@mousemitt.com

(Products and Services continued)

- **Opus Communications**
  Resources for Health care
  Professionals
  200 Hoods Lane
  Marblehead, MA 01945
  800-650-6787; Fax 781-639-2982

- **Paper Direct**
  800-A-PAPERS
  205 Chubb Avenue
  Lyndhurst, NJ 07071

- **Phillips Speech Processing**
  365 Crossways Park Drive
  Woodbury, NY 11797
  516-921-9310
  Fax: 516-921-9319
  E-mail: 04075.3212@compuserve.com

- **Sylvan Software**
  5144 N. Academy Blvd., Suite 531
  Colorado Springs, Colorado 80918
  800-235-9455

- **Transcription Gear**
  (Transcription Equipment)
  888-834-2392

CATALOGS

- **AAMT**
  Success Catalog
  AAMT, P.O. Box 576187
  Modesto, CA 95357-6187
  209-551-0883

- **Sears**
  800-267-3277
  (Office Essentials for Your Home or
  Business. Discounted office
  equipment and furniture.)

- *Computer Shopper*
  Coastal Associates Publishing
  280 28th Street
  New York, NY 10016
  800-274-6384

Computer Shopper offers information
and merchandise from a variety of
suppliers. Good for general reference,
money-saving tips on mail order supplies, and sources. If an item exists,
it is probably listed here.)

- **Crutchfield Personal Office**
  Crutchfield Corporation
  1 Crutchfield park
  Charlottesville, VA 22906
  800-521-4050

CONTINUING EDUCATION

- **American Association for Medical Transcription (AAMT)**
  P.O. Box 576187
  Modesto, CA 95357

- **American Health Information Management Association**
  (formerly American Medical Record Association)
  919 North Michigan Avenue
  Chicago, Il 60611-1683

- **Guide to Alternative Colleges and Universities**
  Garrett Park Press
  Garrett Park, MD 20766

- **The Weekend Education Source Book**
  Wilbur Cross/Harper & Row
  153 E. 53rd St.
  New York, NY 10022

- **Directory of Accredited Private Home Study Schools**
  National Home Study Council
  1601 18th Street NW
  Washington, D.C. 29009

MAGAZINES AND NEWSPAPER PUBLICATIONS

- *Advance for Health Information Professionals*
  Merion Publications, Inc.
  650 Park Avenue West
  King of Prussia, PA 19406
  215-265-7812

- *Business Week*
  McGraw-Hill Bldg.
  1221 Avenue of the Americas
  New York, NY 10020

- *Business Week Online*
  Through Amazon.com

- *Changing Times*
  Kiplinger Washington Editors, Inc.
  Editors Park, MD 20782

- *For the Record*
  3801 Schuylkill Road
  Spring City, PA 19475
  800-278-4400

- *The Futurist* — World Future Society
  7910 Woodmont Ave., Suite 450
  Bethesda Branch
  Washington, D.C. 20014

- *Home Business Magazine*
  714-968-0331

- *Home Office Computing*
  730 Broadway
  New York, NY 10003

- *Money*
  3435 Wilshire Blvd.
  Los Angeles, CA 90010

- *ZiffDavis Smart Business*
  Through Amazon.com

Bibliography

ABC'S of WordPerfect 5, The. Alameda, CA: Sybex.

Avila, Donna. *Donna's Home-made Surgical Reference*. 20th ed. St. Helena, CA: Homemade Press, 1991.

Baumback, Lawyer, Kelley. *How To Organize and Operate a Small Business*. 5th ed. New York: Prentice-Hall, Inc., 1973.

Blanchard, Kenneth and Robert Lorber. *Putting the One Minute Manager To Work*. New York: William Morrow Co., 1984.

Bohigian, Valerie. *Real Money From Home. How to Start, Manage, and Profit from a Home-Based Service Business*. New American Library, 1985.

Brody, Herb. "The Body In Question," *PC Computing*. March 1989.

Business Plan for Homebased Businesses, The. #MPl5. Washington D.C.: Small Business Administration.

Business Use of Your Home, #587. Washington, D.C.: Internal Revenue Service.

Calem, Robert E. "When Leasing or Renting Makes Sense," *Home Office Computing*. March 1991.

Danna, Minta, MT, *Internal Medicine Words*. Windsor, CA: Rayve Productions Inc., 1997.

Deken, Joseph. *The Electronic Cottage*. New York: William Morrow Co., 1981.

DeLorenzo, Barbara. *Pharmaceutical Terminology*. 2nd Edition. Slack, Inc., 1988.

Dorland's Medical Dictionary, 27th ed. Philadelphia: W. B. Saunders Co., 1988.

Edwards, Paul and Sarah. *Working From Home - Everything You Need to Know About Living and Working Under the Same Roof*. Los Angeles: Jeremy P. Tarcher, Inc., 1985.

Feldman, E. and Beverly Neuer. *Home Based Businesses*. New York: Ballantine Books, 1982.

Fordney, Marilyn and Marcy Diehl. *Medical Transcription Guide*. Philadelphia: W. B. Saunders Co., 1990.

Frohbieter-Mueller. *Your Home Business Can Make Dollars and Sense*. Radnor, PA: Chilton Book Company, 1990.

Glossbrenner, Alfred. *How to Get Free Software*. New York: St. Martin's Press, 1984.

Gregory, Helen I. *Finding and Keeping Customers. A Small Business Handbook*. Sedro Woolley, WA: Pinstripe Publishing.

Guide to Hiring Independent Contractors. Sacramento: California Chamber of Commerce, 1991.

Health Professions Institute, Modesto, CA:
     Cardiology Words/Phrases
     GI Words/Phrases
     Orthopedic Words/Phrases
     Psychiatric Words/Phrases
     Radiology Words/Phrases

Holtz, Herman. *The Complete Work-at-Home Companion*. Rocklin, CA: Prima Publishing & Communications, 1990.

Hooper, W.E. *Bookkeeping for Beginners*. Beekman Publishers, Inc., 1970.

Jorgensen, James and Michael G. Rinaldi. *A Clinician's Dictionary of Bacteria and Fungi*. Indianapolis: Eli Lilly & Co., 1986.

Kamoroff, Bernard. *Small-Time Operator*. Laytonville, CA: Bell Springs Publishing, 1990.

Kotler, Phillip and Paul N. Bloom. *Marketing Professional Services*. New York: Prentice-Hall, Inc., 1984.

Lance, Leonard L., Charles Lacy and Warren Flynn. *2002 Quick Look Drug Book*. Baltimore: Williams & Wilkins, 2002.

Lyons, Albert S. and R. Joseph Petrucelli, II. *Medicine. An Illustrated History*. New York: Abradale Press, 1987.

McCann, Ron. *The Joy of Service*. Service Information Source Publications, 1989.

Merck Manual. 14th ed. Robert Berkow, ed. Rahway, NJ: Merck, Sharp & Dohme, 1982.

Milliron, Robert R. *How to Do Your Own Accounting for a Small Business*. Enterprise Del, 1980.

Poynter, Dan. *Word Processors and Information Processing*. Santa Barbara, CA: Para Publishing, 1982.

Pricing Your Products and Service Profitability, #FM13. Washington, D.C.: Small Business Administration.

Pyle, Vera. *Current Medical Terminology*. 3rd ed., Modesto, CA: Prima Vera Publications, 1990.

Ray, Norm. *Easy Financials for Your Home-based Business*. Windsor, CA: Rayve Productions Inc., 1993.

Ray, Norm. *Smart Tax Write-offs*. Windsor CA: Rayve Productions Inc., 2000.

Shaw, Harry. *Errors in English and Ways to Correct Them*. 3rd ed. New York: Harper & Row, 1986.

Sloane, Sheila B. *The Medical Word Book*. 3rd ed., Philadelphia: W. B. Saunders Co., 1982.

Sloane, Sheila B. and John L. Dusseau. *A Word Book in Pathology and Laboratory Medicine*. Philadelphia: W. B. Saunders Co., 1984.

Sloane, Sheila B. *Medical Abbreviations and Eponyms*. Philadelphia: W. B. Saunders Co., 1985.

Stedman's Medical Dictionary. 27th ed. Baltimore: Williams & Wilkins, 2000.

Taber's Cyclopedic Medical Dictionary. 15th ed. Edited by Thomas L. Clayton. Philadelphia: F.A. Davis Co., 1988.

Tax Guide for Small Businesses #2334. Internal Revenue Service. Washington, D.C.

Taylor, Donna M. and Patricia A. Collins. *For Your Information*. Santa Ana, CA: FYI Book Co., 1991.

Tennenhouse, Dan J. *California Health Care Law*. Danville, CA: Contemporary Forums, 1985.

Tessier, Claudia and Sally C. Pittman. *Style Guide for Medical Transcription*. Modesto, CA: American Association for Medical Transcription, 1985.

Tessier, Claudia. *The Surgical Word Book*. Philadelphia: W. B. Saunders Co., 1981.

Webster's College Dictionary. New York: Random House, Inc., 1991.

Whitmyer, Claude, Salli Rasberry and Michael Phillips, *Running a One-Person Business*. Berkeley, CA: Ten Speed Press, 1994.

Wookridge, Susan and Keith London. *The Computer Survival Handbook: How to Talk Back to Your Computer*. Educator Books, Inc., 1973.

WordPerfect Workbook. Orem, Utah: WordPerfect Corp., 1989.

Glossary (Terms related to medical transcription)

AAMT — American Association for Medical Transcription, a national professional transcription association.

Accountant — A person who organizes, maintains or audits the financial records of a company or individual.

Accredited — Status of health care organizations that meet the standards of national accrediting organizations, such as the Joint Commission on Accreditation of Healthcare Organizations (JCAHO) and the National Committee for Quality Assurance (NCQA).

Accredited Records Technician (ART) — An individual who has completed a course of instruction, passed an examination, and achieved entry-level certification in medical records management from the American Health Information Management Association (AHIMA).

Admission — The formal process of registering a patient for service. In a hospital, admission usually involves an overnight stay. In an ambulatory care facility, length of stay is immaterial.

ALOS — Average Length of Stay.

Adaptor — A device for connecting parts having different sizes.

AHA — American Hospital Association.

AHIMA — American Health Information Management Association.

AMA — American Medical Association; Against Medical Advice.

Ambulatory care — All types of health services provided on an outpatient basis, in contrast to services provided in the home or to persons who are inpatients. Many inpatients may be ambulatory, but the term ambulatory care usually refers to patients who travel to locations other than their home to receive services and then depart the same day.

AMLOS — **A**rithmetic **M**ean **L**ength **o**f **S**tay — Average number of days patients within a given DRG stay in the hospital, also referred to as the average length of stay.

Anatomy — The science of the structure of the animal body and the relation of its parts.

Ancillary Services — Inpatient services other than basic room and board and professional services, and hospital outpatient services other than professional services. They include services such as radiology, drug, laboratory, emergency room and home health care.

ANSI — **A**merican **N**ational **S**tandards **I**nstitute.

ASCII — The code used by all personal computers that use a DOS operating system. Provides a common format for saving and importing into various programs.

Authentication (of an entry in a medical record) — The process of confirming the content of a health care entry by such means as written signature, identifiable entry, biometric identifier, or computer key. In practice, authentication usually involves countersigning a verbal or telephone order or signing the typed copy of a dictated document to confirm that it was accurately transcribed.

Authorship (of an entry in a medical record) — The process of identifying a health care practitioner who has released a health care entry for use by writing, dictation, keyboard, or keyless data entry. In practice, authorship usually involves signing — or using some other method besides signing — to indicate authorship and authenticity of a dictated document.

Backlog — An accumulation of unfinished work.

Backup — A copy of a computer program or file, usually stored separately from the original. A form of insurance in case one of the copies becomes lost.

Billing — A statement of money owed for services rendered.

BIN — **Bin**ary.

Bit — **Bi**nary dig**it**. The smallest unit of digital information, represented electronically as either 1 (on) or 0 (off).

Blackout — A period of failure of all electric power.

Blanks — A place or space where something is missing or lacking.

Bookkeeper — One who keeps account books or systematic records of business transactions.

Brochure — A pamphlet used for promotional purposes.

Brownout — Any curtailment of electric power, especially a voltage reduction to prevent a blackout.

Business card — A small card containing the business name, name of owner/operator, address, and telephone number.

Business license — A governmental certificate of permission to operate a business.

Byte — A unit of digital information (eight consecutive bits). Memory and disk capacity are measured in thousands (K) of bytes. One byte is equivalent to approximately one character of text. If a piece has 2000 characters, it needs 2K (kilobytes) of storage.

Call-in-line — A private telephone line and dictating unit specifically used for call-in dictation.

Canned reports or **normals** — A body of a report that can repeatedly be called out and listened to. Although changes can be made to the original, the body of the report need not be redictated each time it is used.

Capital — The net worth of a business; assets minus liabilities of a business.

Capital gain — Profit from the sale of capital assets.

Capitation — The provider receives a fixed payment per member, per month, for which the provider must provide specific services. Though capitation involves less administrative cost than other payment methods, providers must assume the risk that the fixed payment will cover the costs of patient care needs.

Cardiology — The study of the heart and its functions.

Carpal tunnel syndrome — Entrapment of the median nerve at the wrist, caused by accumulative trauma.

Case management — A process through which a single health care professional has the responsibility of monitoring the location and coordination of a patient's overall care to maximize effectiveness, reduce waste of resources, and reduce patient discomfort.

Case mix — The diagnosis-specific makeup of a hospital's workload, which directly influences the lengths of stay and the intensity, cost, and scope of services provided by the hospital.

Cassette — A compact case enclosing audio tape that runs between two reels. It is recordable or playable by inserting it into a recorder or player.

CC — Comorbid Condition; complication.

CEO — Chief Executive Officer.

CFO — Chief Financial Officer.

Character — In typing, any letter, number or symbol.

Character count — Usually consists of adding the number of characters you physically see on a printed page and dividing the total character count by some factor, usually 65, 55, or 50. Usually, spaces and carriage returns (line breaks) are also counted as characters.

Client — A person who engages the services of a professional.

Clinic — A facility or portion thereof used for diagnosis and treatment of outpatients. Also may be loosely defined to include physicians' offices.

Clip art — Copyright-free art, available in books and on diskettes, that can be used and modified without permission.

Closed-end lease — A contract whereby you rent equipment for a specific period of time, and which allows you to purchase the equipment after the last installment has been paid.

CMI — Case-Mix Index — The sum of all DRG relative weights, divided by the number of Medicare cases.

Cold calling — Marketing technique for procuring new clients. Telephoning potential clients directly or visiting their businesses to solicit work.

COMPRO — Competency Profile. An AAMT description of competencies necessary for a medical transcriptionist.

Concurrent review — Case review conducted while a patient is in treatment, as opposed to **retrospective review**, which occurs after treatment and, therefore, cannot affect treatment.

Continuation — In the insurance context, when a covered person who would otherwise lose insurance coverage due to termination of employment, divorce, etc., is allowed to "continue" his or her coverage under conditions specified in the plan, as opposed to under any law. Health care providers must be aware of "continuation" limits.

Confidential — Communicated in confidence.

Contract — An agreement, especially one enforceable by law.

Copiers — Duplicating machines.

Corporation — An association of individuals, created by law and existing as an entity with powers and liabilities independent of those of its members.

CPR — Computer-based Patient Record.

CPRI — Computer-based Patient Record Index.

CPU — Central Processing Unit.

CQI — Continuing Quality Improvement.

Credentialing — The two-pronged process that involves establishing requirements and evaluating individual qualifications for entry into a particular status, such as medical staff membership. First, credentialing considers and establishes the professional training, experience and other requirements for medical staff membership. Second, credentialing obtains and evaluates evidence of the qualifications of individual applicants. Most frequently, credentialing applies to medical staff membership; however, it also applies to the process hospital personnel departments use to evaluate applicants for other positions.

Curriculum vitae — A brief summary of a person's schooling and specialty training. For a physician, this information is required for board certification.

Daisy wheel — A letter quality impact printer which acts much like a typewriter.

Decipher — To make out the meaning of; to decode.

Delivery — To carry transcription to the recipient.

Department — In a hospital, a major unit of the medical staff, headed by a chair, director or chief, usually devoted to providing clinical service in one specialty area.

Departmental QA (or departmental QA/I) — The quality-related activities that, before 1994, the JCAHO required to be carried out by each major medical staff department. This is no longer a JCAHO requirement.

Depreciating — Lessening of price or value due to wear and tear or obsolescence.

Diagnostic related groups (DRGs) — Classification system developed at Yale University using 383 major diagnostic categories (based on the ICD-9 codes) that assigns patients into case types. Designed to facilitate the utilization review process, DRGs are also used to analyze the patient case mix in hospitals and determine their reimbursement policies.

Dictation — Voice recordings to be transcribed.

Digital — A system in which data are stored and transmitted electronically in 1's and 0's for speed and efficiency.

Direct contracting — Individual or groups of employers contract directly with providers for health care services with no managed care intermediary (i.e. HMO, PPO, EPO) to customize services for employees.

Discharge days — For each patient, the total number of inpatient days between admission and discharge dates. In calculating total inpatient days, the day of admission is included in the count, but not the day of discharge.

Discharge summary — Synopsis of a patient's stay in the hospital.

Disk — The storage medium for programs and files. A "hard" disk is generally not removable; a "floppy" disk is removable.

Disk drive — The computer device that holds a disk, gets information from it, and saves information on it.

DOS — Date of Service.

Dot matrix printer — A printer which creates characters or graphics in dots through the use of a print head that contains varying numbers of pins. An impact printer.

Download — To receive a computer file electronically.

Downloadable font — A set of instructions defining a family of letters (a font) that is stored in a computer and sent (downloaded) to an output device such as a printer.

dpi — dots per inch — The more dpi, the sharper the image (the higher the resolution).

DRG — Diagnosis Related Group — A classification system used to categorize patients according to clinical coherence and expected resource intensity, as indicated by their diagnoses, procedures, age, sex, and disposition. The system was established and is revised annually by the U.S. Health Care Financing Administration.

DSL — Digital Subscriber Line — Technology that enables high-speed transmission of digital data over standard telephone lines.

E-Codes — Supplementary classification of ICD-9-CM, containing external causes of injury and poisoning.

EDI — Electronic Data Interchange.

Editing — The art of preparing and arranging materials for the medical record or for publication.

EIN — Employer Identification Number. Needed for tax purposes.

Electronic books — Books that are read and experienced on a computer, with or without an interactive element.

Electronic mailbox — The address on a computer network where people pick up messages sent by other computer users.

Entrepreneur — A person who organizes, manages and assumes responsibility for a business or other enterprise.

Ergonomics — The study of movement.

Errors and Omissions Policy — An insurance policy, much like malpractice coverage, for the medical transcriptionist.

ES — Electronic Signature.

Ethics — A system of moral standards or values; essential quality; conforming to the standards of a given group or profession.

Facility — Buildings, including the physical plant, equipment and supplies used in providing health services. Major types of health facilities include hospitals and nursing homes.

Fax (Facsimile transmission) — Graphic images or printed matter that are scanned and sent electronically via telephone wires.

Fax machine — A duplicating machine that electronically transmits printed matter or graphic images via telephone wires.

Fee-for-Service (FFS) — A traditional payment system in which the physician or hospital bills the patient or insurer for each visit and service provided.

Fictitious name statement — Required by law for businesses using a name other than that of the business owner.

Floppy disk — A removable diskette, either 3-1/2", 5-1/4", or 8", used to store approximately one megabyte of computer information.

Flier / flyer — A small handbill used in procuring business accounts.

Format — The overall style of a printed document including paper type, size, layout, fonts, margins, and other document requirements.

Freelancer — A self-employed medical transcriptionist.

Freestanding — Not part of a hospital (neither structurally connected to nor organizationally considered part of a hospital); not hospital-based.

Fry — To damage or destroy electronic circuitry with excessive heat or current.

Gastroenterology — The study of the stomach and intestines and their diseases.

Gateway — A device that connects different types of networks and performs protocol translation.

Going rate — The usual and customary fee charged for a particular service in a specific area or locale.

Gross Line — Also known as a "visual line count." Every line on the page that has text counts as a "line" and (usually, but not always) every blank line does not.

Grouper — Software program that assigns DRGs.

Hard copy — The paper version of what's been generated on a computer.

Hard disk — The rigid disk in a computer that stores programs and large amounts of data.

Hardware — The physical components of a computer system, such as a computer, monitor, disk drive, and printer.

HCFA — Health Care Financing Administration. A division of the Department of Health and Human Services that administers Medicare and certain aspects of Medicaid. HCFA is responsible for determining which facilities meet federal quality standards for providing health care to beneficiaries.

HCPCS, HCFA — Health Care Common Procedural Coding System; Health Care Financing Administration.

HCQIA — Health Care Quality Improvement Act.

HCWS — Healthcare workers.

HFMA — Healthcare Financial Management Association.

HIPAA — Health Insurance Portability and Accountability Act.

HIS — Hospital Information System.

HMO — Health Maintenance Organization — A legal entity or organized health care system that provides directly or arranges for a comprehensive range of basic and supplemental health care services to a voluntarily enrolled population in a geographic area on a primarily prepaid and fixed periodic basis. This term is defined by federal law in the Health Maintenance Organization Act of 1973 (Public Law 93-222).

Home Health Services — Home medical services.

Hospice — A facility that cares for terminally ill patients, with more emphasis on meeting the psychosocial needs of patients and families.

Hospital — Generally, an institution with an organized medical staff whose primary function is to provide diagnostic and therapeutic inpatient services for a variety of medical conditions, both surgical and nonsurgical.

ICD-9-CM — International Classification of Diseases — Modification developed in the United States based on the official version of the World Health Organization's International Classification of Diseases, 9th Revision, and designed for classification of morbidity and mortality information for statistical reporting purposes and information retrieval.

Icons — Symbols on a computer screen.

Impact printer — Printers which use either a daisy wheel or print thimble as the typing element. Sometimes called a letter quality printer.

Indemnification — A negotiated contract provision under which one party to the contract agrees to pay any judgments, costs and attorney fees incurred by the other for acts or omissions that are the fault of the first. It is important for providers to insist on "mutual" indemnification provision in any contract with a managed care entity.

Information superhighway — The global information and communications network that includes the Internet and other networks and switching systems such as networks for telephone, cable, and satellite communications.

Inkjet printer — Nonimpact printer that uses ink sprays to produce legible copy.

Interface — Software designed to communicate specific information between the digital dictation system and the department's information system.

Internet — An enormous international interconnected set of computer networks that links government agencies, universities, corporations and individuals.

IRA — **I**ndividual **R**etirement **A**ccount.

IRS — **I**nternal **R**evenue **S**ervice.

JCAHO — **J**oint **C**ommission on **A**ccreditation of **H**ospitals **O**rganization.

The Joint — A commonly used, informal term for the Joint Commission on Accreditation of Healthcare Organizations (JCAHO).

Keyboard — A row or set of keys, as on a piano, typewriter or computer terminal used to enter data into a computer.

Kilobyte (1024 bytes) — Common measure of memory capacity (a double-spaced type-written page used about 1.5K).

LAN — **L**ocal **A**rea **N**etwork.

Laser — A device that produces a very narrow beam of extremely intense light, used in communications and industrial processes.

Laser printer — A high-resolution printer that produces type and graphics of near-typeset quality.

LQ — **L**etter **Q**uality.

Lift-off tape — A tape used with self-correcting typewriters for correcting errors.

Line count — A method used to determine transcription productivity by counting total lines typed, used for billing purposes.

Log sheet — A record of completed transcription.

LTC — Long Term Care — Skilled nursing/intermediate care.

Malpractice — Legal liability against a physician or health care organization resulting from negligent or unprofessional treatment in the practice of a health care profession.

Managed care — A health care plan, such as an HMO-style plan, that attempts to monitor and control the quality, cost effectiveness, and resource utilization of doctors, hospitals, and other health care facilities as they provide service to patients. Also, the organization of various types of health care providers into administrative networks in which they collaborate, refer patients to each other and share funding.

Maximize — Raise to highest degree possible.

Medical staff — The semiautonomous group of physicians, other licensed independent practitioners, and other such health care professionals permitted by state law and a hospital to take responsibility as a group for specified aspects of hospital operation. The medical staff is one of the three key parts of hospital governance. (The other two key parts of hospital governance are the governing board and the hospital administration.)

Medical terminology — The language of medicine.

Megabyte (MB) — Unit of measure of computer memory, equal to 1024 kilobytes or roughly one million bytes.

Mentor — A wise and trusted counselor.

Memory — A computer's information storage site, usually measured in thousands (K) of bytes.

Menu — The lists of options on a computer screen.

Microbiology — The science that deals with the study of microorganisms, including algae, bacteria, fungi, protozoa and viruses.

Microcassette — An audio cassette tape that is smaller than a standard cassette.

Minute of dictation — Every minute dictated is a billing unit.

Modem — A device for transmitting computer data over telephone lines.

Module — A standard or unit for measuring.

Monitor — A computer display screen.

Mouse — A hand-operated pointing device, usually beside the computer keyboard, that enables a computer user to manipulate what is on the screen.

MT — **M**edical **T**ranscriptionist.

Multimedia — Electronic products that use various media (text, graphics, animation, audio) to deliver information. Often these products are also interactive, allowing the user to pick and choose from a variety of information options.
NCQA — **N**ational **C**ommittee on **Q**uality **A**ssurance.

NCR PAPER — Specially treated paper on which an original and two or three copies print simultaneously.

Nerd — A computer fanatic.

Netizens — Internet citizens.

Networking — (1) Technology that connects computers at several different locations and allows communication among them. (2) Communicating with other MTs regarding work practices, standards, and problem solving.

NFIB - **N**ational **F**ederation of **I**ndependent **B**usiness

Nondisclosure statement — In a contract between a medical transcriptionist and her client, the section dealing with confidentiality of the medical record.

Online — A state in which information is accessible electronically, via computers, cable TV or telephone lines.

Open-end lease — A rental agreement allowing the renter the options of purchasing the equipment at a fair market price, renegotiating and extending the lease, or terminating the lease and returning the equipment to the lessor.

Operating system — The program that enables you to run the computer.

Optimize — Make the most of; develop or realize to the utmost extent; obtain the most efficient or optimum use of. DRG optimization helps increase Medicare DRG payments and case-mix index, improve coding quality, reduce PRO risks and improve physician documentation.

Ordinance — An authoritative law or rule, especially one enacted by a municipal body.

OTJ — **O**n-the-**J**ob.

Outpatient — A person who receives medical, dental, or other health-related services in a hospital or other health care institution but who is not lodged there.

Outsourcing (subcontracting) — To transcribe for another person or service.

Page rate — A method used to measure productivity of transcription; used for billing purposes.

Partnerships — Two or more persons associated as principals or contributors of capital in a business.

Patient mix — The different types of patients served in a hospital in terms of such characteristics as age, sex, diagnosis, and residence.

PC — Personal Computer.

PCL — Printer Command Language — The commands for operating printers.

Peer Review — Evaluation of a physician's performance by other physicians, usually within the same geographic area and medical specialty.

Per case — A method of payment in which a provider receives a payment determined by case mix for a particular patient.

Perk — Informal word for "perquisite," a payment, profit or benefit derived from one's employment, in addition to a regular wage or salary. Among other things, independent medical transcriptionists' perks include self-determination and flexible work schedules.

PHI — **P**roteected **H**ealth **I**nformation or **P**rivacy of **H**ealth **I**nformation.

Physical therapy — The study and treatment of the body.

Physiology — The science which treats the functions of the living organism and its parts, and of the physical and chemical factors and processes involved.

Policies and Procedures — Detailed technical directives and guidance that are outlined in documents. Often, policies are statements of purpose or objectives, and procedures are statements of how purposes or objectives will be attained. They usually appear in the same document.

Port — An access path into the digital system for one of the following purposes: Dictate - Transcribe - Listen.

PPO — **P**referred **P**rovider **O**rganization — A health care organization formed by a hospital or physician group to contract with an insurer for health care provided to a defined population. PPOs are not exclusive providers of care to insured groups, but they usually offer lower charges to the insured groups in return for their influence in channeling patients to providers participating in the PPO. (Also see Preferred Provider Organization below.)

Practice Guidelines — Statements, either narrative or pictorial, describing recommended approaches to diagnosis or treatment of specified diseases, injuries, or conditions.

PRD+ — **Pr**oductivity **Plus**, a medical terminology abbreviation program for computers.

Preferred Provider Organization (PPO) — A system designed to be an alternative to HMOs. Health care providers define a population to service at an agreed-upon fee schedule. (Also see PPO above.)

Printer — A machine that receives electronic signals from a computer and responds by printing on paper.

Professional — One who is connected with or engaged in a profession. A person who is an expert.

PRO — **P**eer **R**eview **O**rganization — An organization that reviews appropriateness and quality of care for beneficiaries of the Medicare program.

Profiling — Collection and analysis of an individual practitioner's practice statistics for evaluation purposes.

Program (also, **software, application**) — The coded instructions that enables the computer to perform a desired sequence of operations.

Proofreader — A person employed to detect and mark errors to be corrected.

Programmer — A person adept at developing a systematic plan or set of instructions for the solution of a problem by a computer. One who prepares computer programs or supplies a computer with a program.

Provider — A person or organization that provides health care services (e.g., physician, hospital, home health agency).

Quality — Grade of excellence.

Quality assessment/improvement (QA/I) — The term adopted by the JCAHO in 1993 to describe activities required of hospitals to monitor and maintain quality of patient care.

Quality of care — Evaluation of the performance of medical providers according to the degree to which the process of care increases the probability of outcomes desired by patients.

Quantity — Amount.

Radiology — That branch of the health sciences dealing with radioactive substances and radiant energy, and with the diagnosis and treatment of disease by means of both ionizing and nonionizing radiations.

RAM — **R**andom **A**ccess **M**emory. The amount of computer memory, measured in thousands (K) of bytes. Also, computer memory that stores information temporarily while you are working on it.

Ream — Five hundred sheets of paper.

Registered Record Administrator (RRA) — The recognition awarded by the AHIMA to individuals who possess the required credentials and pass the required examination that demonstrate competence in the management of health information record departments.

Reimbursement — Repayment of money spent; compensation for expenses.

Retrospective review — The determination of medical necessity, coverage, or payment for services that have already been rendered.

RIS — **R**adiology **I**nformation **S**ystem.

Reprint — Reproducing transcribed reports which were previously printed.

Rerecord — The ability to repeat record work onto a cassette central recorder. Some systems need to be monitored as they rerecord.

Risk management — An administrative activity aimed to prevent the loss of hospital resources resulting from actual or alleged accidents, neglect, or incompetence.

Rolodex™ — A file box or wheel for holding business cards, clients' names and telephone numbers. Filed items can be readily added or deleted.

ROM — **R**ead **O**nly **M**emory. Programs or instructions that are permanently stored in a computer.

Router — A device that connects segments of networks that use the same protocols.

RSI - **R**epetitive **S**train **I**njury. Caused from cumulative trauma at the computer.

Save — To store information on disk.

Seminar — An educational course or meeting.

Service — Work performed for another or a group.

SNF — **S**killed **N**ursing **F**acility — A health facility or a distinct part of a hospital that provides skilled nursing care and supportive care to patients whose primary need is for skilled nursing care on an extended basis. It provides 24-hour inpatient care and, as a minimum, includes medical, nursing, dietary and pharmaceutical services, as well as activity programs.

Software — Programs, procedures and data used for the operation of a computer system.

SOHO — Small office, Home office.

Sole proprietor —A one-person business owner.

Standard mileage allowance —Standard set by the IRS to facilitate the determining of car expenses as a tax-deduction.

Standard of care — A legal standard defined as the level of care provided by the majority of physicians in a particular clinical situation.

Subcontract (outsource) — To transcribe for another person or service.

SUM — Home study medical transcription program created by Health Professions Institute.

Surge protector — A portable device containing electrical outlets that protects equipment plugged into it from a surge in current.

Tampering — To make changes in order to falsify.

TAT — Turnaround time. The time between dictation and completion of transcription.

Tax deduction — An item which can be subtracted from income in calculating taxable income.

Tax preparer — One who is in business to complete tax returns for a fee.

Tax shelter — Investing a portion of otherwise taxable income in programs designed to defer taxation of income.

Template — A pre-designed pattern or grid for printed items such as letters, medical reports, invoices, brochures, and newsletters.

Thermal printer — A printer that uses heat to imprint paper.

Toner — Laser printer "ink" made of fine plastic particles.

TQM — Total Quality Management.

Trademark — A word or symbol distinguishing the product of one company from those of competitors, usually registered with the government to assure its exclusive use by its owner.

Transcriber — The machine used to listen to dictation in order to transcribe.

Transcription — The art or process of transcribing.

Transcriptionist — Person who transcribes.

Transcription pool — A group of transcriptionists usually working in a specified area.

Turnaround time — The specified time when completed work is to be delivered; the time between dictation and completion of transcription.

24/7 or 24-7 — Continuously. Short for 24 hours a day, 7 days a week.

UHDDS — **U**niform **H**ospital **D**ischarge **D**ata **S**et — The hospital discharge data set periodically issued by the U.S. Department of Health and Human Services.

Upload — To electronically send a computer file.

Users — An unfortunate reference to those who use computers.

Utilities program — A specialized computer program used to manage information on computer disks.

Utilization Review (UR) — The examination and evaluation of the efficiency and appropriateness of any health care service.

V-Codes — Supplementary classification of ICD-9-CM, containing factors influencing health states and contact with health services.

Video telephony — Telephones that also broadcast video images.

Video card — A printed circuit board that is installed in a computer to drive the monitor display.

Virtual reality — A computer simulation usually experienced through headgear, goggles and sensory gloves that lets the user feel he or she is present in another place.

Virus — In reference to computers, a corrupting influence, a "bug" in the software program which can cause it to malfunction.

WAN — Wide Area Network.

Windows — In some computer programs, sections of the screen (sometimes overlapping) that enable one to work with multiple applications at once.

WordPerfect™ — A computer software program for word processing.

Wordstar™ — A computer software program used in word processing.

Workers' Compensation —An insurance policy for employees injured while performing their job duties.

WYSIWYG (pronounced wizzy-wig) — What you see is what you get — Computer systems in which what you see on the computer screen is as it will appear on the printed (hard) copy.

Zoning — An area divided off or somehow differentiated from adjoining zones. Any specific area or district, as one in a city under certain restrictions, especially with regard to building.

Appendix

- Exhibit A: AAMT Model Job Description: Medical Transcriptionist
  (Reproduced with permission from AAMT.)

- Exhibit B: Budget Worksheet
  You may photocopy this worksheet to use for your budget preparation. You can enlarge it to 150% for an 8½ x 11" page. (Reproduced from the book *Easy Financials for Your Home-based Business*).

- Exhibit C: Sample Contract

- Exhibit D: Sample Contract Addendum — HIPAA Compliance Business Associate Agreement

Exhibit A: AAMT Model Job Description

AMERICAN ASSOCIATION
FOR MEDICAL TRANSCRIPTION

AAMT Model Job Description:

MEDICAL TRANSCRIPTIONIST

The *AAMT Model Job Description* is a practical, useful compilation of the basic job responsibilities of a medical transcriptionist. It is designed to assist human resource managers, department managers, supervisors, and others in recruiting, supervising, and evaluating individuals in medical transcription positions.

The *AAMT Model Job Description* is not intended as a complete list of specific duties and responsibilities. Nor is it intended to limit or modify the right of any supervisor to assign, direct, and control the work of employees under supervision. The use of a particular expression or illustration describing duties shall not be held to exclude other duties not mentioned that are of a similar kind or level of difficulty.

Position Summary: Medical language specialist who interprets and transcribes dictation by physicians and other healthcare professionals regarding patient assessment, workup, therapeutic procedures, clinical course, diagnosis, prognosis, etc., in order to document patient care and facilitate delivery of healthcare services.

Knowledge, skills, and abilities:
1. Minimum education level of associate degree or equivalent in work experience and continuing education.
2. Knowledge of medical terminology, anatomy and physiology, clinical medicine, surgery, diagnostic tests, radiology, pathology, pharmacology, and the various medical specialties as required in areas of responsibility.
3. Knowledge of medical transcription guidelines and practices.
4. Excellent written and oral communication skills, including English usage, grammar, punctuation, and style.
5. Ability to understand diverse accents and dialects and varying dictation styles.
6. Ability to use designated reference materials.
7. Ability to operate designated word processing, dictation, and transcription equipment, and other equipment as specified.
8. Ability to work independently with minimal supervision.
9. Ability to work under pressure with time constraints.
10. Ability to concentrate.
11. Excellent listening skills.
12. Excellent eye, hand, and auditory coordination.
13. Certified medical transcriptionist (CMT) status preferred.

Working conditions:
General office environment. Quiet surroundings. Adequate lighting.

Physical demands:
Primarily sedentary work, with continuous use of earphones, keyboard, foot control, and where applicable, video display terminal.

AAMT gratefully acknowledges Lanier Voice Products, Atlanta, Georgia, for funding the development of the *AAMT Model Job Description: Medical Transcriptionist.*

For additional information, contact AAMT, P.O. Box 576187, Modesto, CA 95357-6187. Telephone 209-551-0883 or 800-982-2182. FAX 209-551-9317.

AAMT Model Job Description (*continued*)

AAMT Model Job Description: Medical Transcriptionist

Job responsibilities:	*Performance standards:*
1. Transcribes medical dictation to provide a permanent record of patient care.	1.1 Applies knowledge of medical terminology, anatomy and physiology, and English language rules to the transcription and proofreading of medical dictation from originators with various accents, dialects, and dictation styles.
	1.2 Recognizes, interprets, and evaluates inconsistencies, discrepancies, and inaccuracies in medical dictation, and appropriately edits, revises, and clarifies them without altering the meaning of the dictation or changing the dictator's style.
	1.3 Clarifies dictation which is unclear or incomplete, seeking assistance as necessary.
	1.4 Flags reports requiring the attention of the supervisor or dictator.
	1.5 Uses reference materials appropriately and efficiently to facilitate the accuracy, clarity, and completeness of reports.
	1.6 Meets quality and productivity standards and deadlines established by employer.
	1.7 Verifies patient information for accuracy and completeness.
	1.8 Formats reports according to established guidelines.
2. Demonstrates an understanding of the medicolegal implications and responsibilities related to the transcription of patient records to protect the patient and the business/institution.	2.1 Understands and complies with policies and procedures related to medicolegal matters, including confidentiality, amendment of medical records, release of information, patients' rights, medical records as legal evidence, informed consent, etc.
	2.2 Meets standards of professional and ethical conduct.
	2.3 Recognizes and reports unusual circumstances and/or information with possible risk factors to appropriate risk management personnel.
	2.4 Recognizes and reports problems, errors, and discrepancies in dictation and patient records to appropriate manager.
	2.5 Consults appropriate personnel regarding dictation which may be regarded as unprofessional, frivolous, insulting, inflammatory, or inappropriate.
3. Operates designated word processing, dictation, and transcription equipment as directed to complete assignments.	3.1 Uses designated equipment effectively, skillfully, and efficiently.
	3.2 Maintains equipment and work area as directed.
	3.3 Assesses condition of equipment and furnishings, and reports need for replacement or repair.
4. Follows policies and procedures to contribute to the efficiency of the medical transcription department.	4.1 Demonstrates an understanding of policies, procedures, and priorities, seeking clarification as needed.
	4.2 Reports to work on time, as scheduled, and is dependable and cooperative.
	4.3 Organizes and prioritizes assigned work, and schedules time to accommodate work demands, turnaround-time requirements, and commitments.
	4.4 Maintains required records, providing reports as scheduled and upon request.
	4.5 Participates in quality assurance programs.
	4.6 Participates in evaluation and selection of equipment and furnishings.
	4.7 Provides administrative/clerical/technical support as needed and as assigned.
5. Expands job-related knowledge and skills to improve performance and adjust to change.	5.1 Participates in inservice and continuing education activities.
	5.2 Provides documentation of inservice and continuing education activities.
	5.3 Reviews trends and developments in medicine, English usage, technology, and transcription practices, and shares knowledge with colleagues.
	5.4 Documents new and revised terminology, definitions, styles, and practices for reference and application.
	5.5 Participates in the evaluation and selection of books, publications, and other reference materials.
6. Uses interpersonal skills effectively to build and maintain cooperative working relationships.	6.1 Works and communicates in a positive and cooperative manner with management and supervisory staff, medical staff, co-workers and other healthcare personnel, and patients and their families when providing information and services, seeking assistance and clarification, and resolving problems.
	6.2 Contributes to team efforts.
	6.3 Carries out assignments responsibly.
	6.4 Participates in a positive and cooperative manner during staff meetings.
	6.5 Handles difficult and sensitive situations tactfully.
	6.6 Responds well to supervision.
	6.7 Shares information with co-workers.
	6.8 Assists with training of new employees as needed.

Exhibit B: Budget Worksheet

Budget   Year

	Jan	Feb	Mar	Apr	May	June	July	Aug	Sept	Oct	Nov	Dec	Total
1 Sales													
2 Cost of sales													
3 Gross profit													
4 Gross margin %													
Operating expenses:													
5 Advertising & promotion													
6 Auto expense													
7 Commissions & fees													
8 Insurance													
9 Legal & accounting fees													
10 Office expense													
11 Rentals & leases													
12 Repairs & maintenance													
13 Supplies													
14 Taxes & licenses													
15 Travel													
16 Meals & entertainment													
17 Salaries expense													
18 Bank service charges													
19 Postage & freight													
20 Telephone													
21 Dues & reference material													
22 Utilities													
23 Independent contractors													
24 Cleaning & maintenance													
25 Conventions & trade shows													
26 Bad debts													
27 Other:													
28 Other:													
29 Other:													
30 Other:													
31 Depreciation													
32 Total operating expense													
33 Operating income													
34 Interest income -- plus													
35 Interest expense -- minus													
36 Net income before income tax													
37 Provision for income taxes													
38 Net income													

From *Easy Financials for Your Home-based Business*, © Norm Ray, CPA

Exhibit C: Sample Contract

This agreement entered into this date, by and between the subcontractor known as: ———————————————— , herein referred to as Subcontractor, whose address is

———————————————————————————————— ,
telephone is ————————— and the Contractor: ————————————————— .

WHEREAS SUBCONTRACTOR desires to contract with CONTRACTOR to perform said work and/or service, and

WHEREAS the parties desire to set forth their contractual and business arrangement(s)

THEREFORE, this agreement constitutes the said contractual and business arrangements, and the parties contract and agree as follows:

THAT THE SUBCONTRACTOR agrees to perform, abide by and follow the stipulations listed in the remainder of this contract.

Equipment

The subcontractor is responsible for providing all equipment and supplies necessary for any work done, other than supplies given by the client (i.e., stationery indigenous to the client). These supplies provided by the Subcontractor include, but are not limited to, office equipment (i.e., typewriter, computer, transcription equipment, etc.), paper, dictionaries and manuals, ribbons, tools, etc. The subcontractor is also responsible for all repairs on her [his] own equipment.

Any supplies that are necessary from the client must be requested well in advance by the Subcontractor and the Subcontractor is responsible for keeping an adequate supply on hand at all times. This supply must be returned to the Contractor should this contract ever cease.

Any equipment or supplies loaned by the Contractor to the Subcontractor must be returned to the Contractor at the termination of this contract, or final payment of any payment due will be withheld until said items are returned.

Pricing and Payment

Each client's pricing is set separately, according to the individual client. Pricing is by each piece and/or line as set forth in the Work Scope.

Payment for services rendered is on a twice monthly basis. The Subcontractor is responsible for issuing a billing to the Contractor on the 1st of each month for the 16th through the 31st of the previous month, and on the 16th of each month for the 1st through the 15th of that same month. Payment to the Subcontractor from the Contractor is due on the 5th of each month for the pay period of the 16th through the 31st, and on the 20th of each month for the pay period of the 1st through the 15th. If the pay date falls on a weekend or holiday, the Contractor reserves the right to pay on the first working day following the weekend or holiday. If the Subcontractor does not turn in invoices by the dates specified, the Contractor is not responsible to pay by any set date and pay may be late.

A separate billing for each client must be given to the Contractor by the Subcontractor. Each billing must be typewritten and include the name of the client, the dates of the billing, the pages and specific dates of work completed and, if applicable, a description of each piece of work completed, and individual pricing, as well as a total. The Subcontractor must be prepared to back up each billing with copies of work completed should the Contractor or client request any information regarding any services rendered.

Contractor will pay for any work containing errors. Subcontractor is responsible to redo all work containing errors without charge to the client or Agency. If the client should request a redo of typing with minor editing changes that were not the fault of the typist or Agency, then the Subcontractor will provide redo at one-half of the original cost.

Contractor is not responsible to pay for redo work in the case of power outages or faulty equipment. It is the responsibility of the Subcontractor to keep equipment in working order and to provide backup emergency services should a technical problem occur.

Communication with Clients

Subcontractor may not communicate with client directly regarding billing or pricing structure or anything other than a question directly applying to the typing or work procedure, such as terminology, spelling, etc. When communicating with client on the above matters, Subcontractor must identify herself [himself] as being from the agency of the Contractor and in no way represent herself [himself] as her [his] own agency or business.

Noncompete Clause

The clients of the Contractor will remain the clients of the Contractor. At no time in the future may the Subcontractor do any work for the clients in any way, contract or draw business or clients or accounts from anybody in any way connected with any of the clients' relatives, friends, contacts or anybody associated with the client in any way. All referrals are the express property of the Contractor.

Work Scope

The Subcontractor is responsible for keeping a complete Work Scope on each client assigned by the Contractor. This Work Scope is to be given to the Contractor upon termination originated either by the Subcontractor or the Contractor. The Work Scope must be typewritten, include the client's name, address, telephone number, names of contact personnel, list of specific terminology used by that client, and any specialized instructions for that client.

The Subcontractor is responsible for keeping one month of work for each client on file for reference for billing purposes, termination or request of the client for any particular piece of work.

The Subcontractor is responsible to either pick up and drop off the work load of the client(s) at the office or the Contractor, at the office of the client directly according to the times specified, or make specific arrangements with the management of the Contractor.

All completed work dropped off at the office of the Contractor or given directly to the client's office by the Subcontractor must be in individual folders supplied by _____ with _____ logo on them, separated according to each client, neatly labeled and with any necessary instructions for the daily driver.

The Subcontractor is responsible for providing services for the assigned client at all times during the duration of this contract. The Subcontractor is responsible for providing her [his] own backup service in case of illness, vacation, emergency or any possible occurrence that would render the Subcontractor unable to perform. The Subcontractor is responsible for providing all payment arrangements to backup personnel and it is the responsibility of the Subcontractor to ensure that the backup personnel comply with all stipulations contained within this contract. The Subcontractor is held directly responsible for anything her [his] backup may or may not do.

The Subcontractor is responsible for providing liability insurance of at least $500,000 if any kind of bookkeeping services are contracted for by the Contractor with the Subcontractor.

The Contractor expects loyalty, enthusiasm and total support verbally, in action, and in deed from the Subcontractor at all times.

Miscellaneous

The logo, name, promotional material, and advertising associated with the Contractor are exclusively the property of the Contractor. Unauthorized usage of any stationery or materials or unauthorized representation of the Agency of the Contractor or the Contractor itself is strictly prohibited. The Subcontractor cannot use any name similar to or resembling in any way, shape or form the name, advertising methods and appearances or practices of the Contractor.

The Subcontractor gives her [his] permission for her [his] name, picture, and information to be included in any advertising for the Contractor at any time during this contract or after this contract is terminated.

Termination of this Contract

The Subcontractor must give no less than a 7-day notice to the Contractor in writing for termination of this contract. Anything less than a 7-day notice will result in a 50% penalty fee payable to the Contractor and subtracted from the final payment due to the Subcontractor.

Before the termination is effective, Subcontractor must return all supplies and/or equipment belonging to or loaned by or borrowed from the Contractor. The Subcontractor is also responsible for supplying the Contractor with a copy of all work done for any client(s) within the previous two-week period, as well as a complete and detailed work scope as specified previously in this contract. Failure to comply with any portion of this termination stipulation or any portion of this contract may result in withholding of final payment.

Violation of any part of this contract can result in immediate termination by the Contractor without notice. All termination terms other than the 7-day notice would then be applicable for the Subcontractor and final check would be held until terms are complied with.

Contractor reserves the right to remove a client from the Subcontractor without any notice and give to another Subcontractor. Subcontractor also agrees that clients can be dropped at any time due to termination from the client.

The Subcontractor hereby agrees to abide by all of the terms and stipulations set forth in pages one through five of this contract and understand each item fully, as signified by signing below.

_____

Subcontractor   Date

_____

Social Security Number of Subcontractor

_____

Contractor   Date

Exhibit D: Sample Contract Addendum
HIPAA Compliance Business Associate Agreement

Section 1. Use of Protected Health Information. Contractor shall not use Protected Health Information (hereinafter "PHI") received from _____ in any manner that would constitute a violation of the Privacy Standards. Contractor shall further ensure that its officers, employees, contractors and agents do not use PHI received from _____ in any manner that would constitute a violation of the Privacy Standards. Contractor may use PHI for Contractor's proper management and administrative services, or to carry out the legal responsibilities of the Contractor.

Section 2. Disclosure of PHI. Contractor, officer, employees, and agents shall not disclose PHI received from_____ in any manner that would constitute a violation of the Privacy Standards. Contractor may disclose PHI in a manner permitted pursuant to this Privacy Addendum, or as required by law. If Contractor discloses PHI to a third party, Contractor must obtain, prior to making any such disclosure: 1) reasonable assurance from such third party that such PHI will be held confidential as provided pursuant to this Addendum, and only disclosed as required by law or for the purposes for which it was disclosed to such third party: and 2) an agreement from such third party to immediately notify Contractor of any breaches of the confidentiality of the PHI, to the extent it has obtained knowledge of such breach.

Section 3. Safeguards Against Misuse of Information. Contractor agrees that it will implement all appropriate safeguards to prevent the use or disclosure of PHI other than pursuant to the terms and conditions of this Addendum.

Section 4. Reporting of Disclosures and Uses of PHI. Contractor shall, within five (5) days of becoming aware of a disclosure or use of PHI in violation of this Addendum by Contractor, its officers, directors, employees, contractors, or agents, or by a third party to which Contractor disclosed PHI pursuant to Section 2 of this Addendum, report any such disclosure or use to _____.

Section 5. Agreements by Third Parties. If an agent, including a subcontractor, will have access to PHI that is received from, or created by, the Contractor on behalf of _____ , Contractor shall enter into an agreement with such an agent, pursuant to which agreement the agent agrees to be bound by the same restrictions, terms, and conditions that apply to Contractor pursuant to this Addendum with respect to such PHI.

Section 6. Access to Information. Within ____ days of a request by_____ for access to PHI about an individual, Contractor shall make available to_____ such PHI, for so long as information is maintained.

481

Section 7. Availability of PHI for Amendment. Within____days of receipt of a request from_____ for the amendment of an individual's PHI or record regarding an individual, Contractor shall provide such information to _____ for amendment and incorporate any such amendments in the PHI as required.

Section 8. Return and Destruction of PHI. At termination of the Agreement, Contractor shall either return or destroy all PHI received from, or created or received by, Contractor on behalf of _____ that Contractor still maintains in any form. Contractor shall further not retain any copies of such information in any form. In the event such return or destruction is not feasible, Contractor shall 1) provide an explanation in writing to_____ as to why such return or destruction is not feasible; 2) continue to extend the protection required under this Agreement; and 3) limit any further uses and disclosures of the PHI to those purposes that make the return or destruction of the information infeasible. This provision shall survive the termination of this Agreement.

Section 9. Termination for Violation. Notwithstanding any other provisions of the Agreement to the contrary, if_____ determines that Contractor has materially breached or violated its obligations under this Agreement and reasonable efforts to cure the breach or to end the violation are unsuccessful,_____ shall have the right, but not the duty, to terminate this Agreement.

Index